Musculoskeletal Ultrasound in Rheumatic Diseases

Md Abu Bakar Siddiq
Editor

Musculoskeletal Ultrasound in Rheumatic Diseases

A Case-based Review

Springer

Editor
Md Abu Bakar Siddiq
Department of Rheumatology
Royal North Shore Hospital, Northern Clinical School,
Faculty of Medicine and Health, The University of Sydney
Sydney, NSW, Australia

ISBN 978-981-96-5297-6 ISBN 978-981-96-5298-3 (eBook)
https://doi.org/10.1007/978-981-96-5298-3

This Springer imprint is published by the registered company Springer Nature Singapore Pte Ltd.
The registered company address is: 152 Beach Road, #21-01/04 Gateway East, Singapore 189721, Singapore

This synthesis is dedicated to my family, particularly my cherished wife, Dr. Israt Jahan, and my lively sons, Master Zibu and Zabi. Their steadfast support and affection have played a crucial role in my endeavors. I also wish to acknowledge all the physiatrists and physiatry students in Bangladesh, along with the patients who have come to me with their concerns, entrusting me with their care. Finally, I hold dear the memory of the 57 beautiful flowers that once flourished, symbolizing hope and optimism across the nation.

Foreword

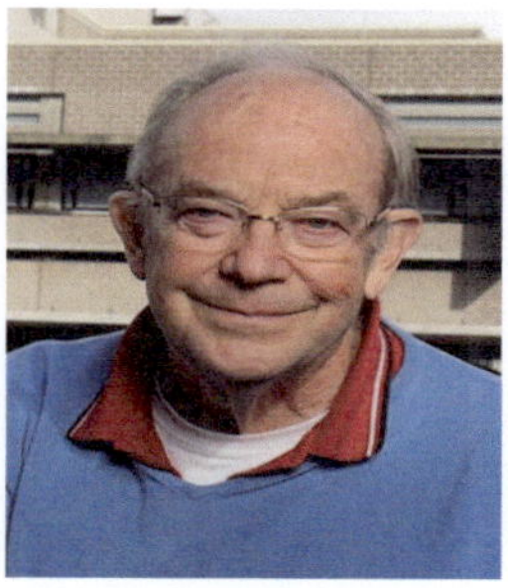

Since the 1970s, the use of ultrasound in rheumatology has become an important asset for clinicians because of its easy accessibility and low cost. New technical developments have made it possible to display in detail muscles, ligaments and tendons, nerves, vessels, and joints and to perform functional assessments of these tissues. Ultrasound currently plays a crucial role in diagnosing and treating patients with rheumatic disorders.

Medical specialists such as radiologists, rheumatologists, physiatrists, and orthopedic surgeons are increasingly applying ultrasound in daily practice, as are health professionals such as physiotherapists, occupational therapists, and foot specialists. For all of them, it is important to stay updated with new advances in the field and to know when to use ultrasound and when further techniques such as MRI are indicated. Clinical cases, such as those presented in this book, will be helpful in educating all who apply ultrasound. Education and continued education regarding new developments and opportunities for ultrasound are highly important. This book will be very helpful for all these aims. This study focuses on the role of ultrasound in rheumatology and presents a series of cases as learning material. It also raises a series of questions related to the reader's knowledge regarding the use of ultrasound in rheumatology.

I am pleased to recommend it not only to all practitioners but also to trainees in the field of rheumatology.

Rheumatologist, Faculty of Behavioral Sciences
Psychology Health, and Technology
University of Twente
Enschede, The Netherlands

Johannes J. Rasker

Preface

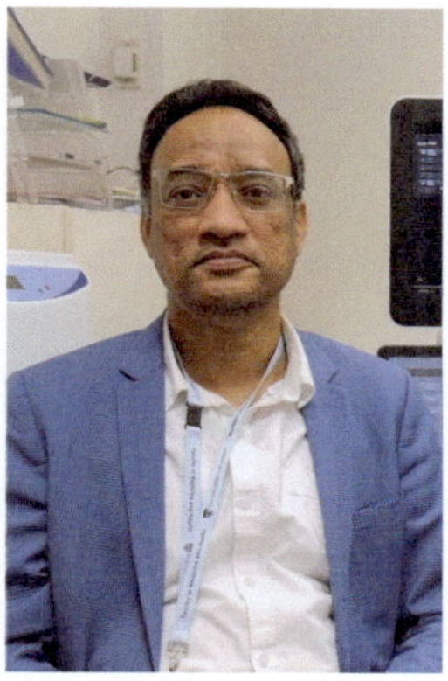

Ultrasound imaging plays a significant role in the diagnosis and monitoring of treatment response in musculoskeletal disorders [1]. Over the years, its use in rheumatic diseases has been increasing, and a growing number of international organizations in the field such as the European Alliance of Associations for Rheumatology (EULAR), the American College of Rheumatology (ACR), and the International League of Associations of Rheumatology (ILAR) have recommended its use [2, 3]. In rheumatology, ultrasound grayscale (B-mode) and Doppler modes are widely used; however, contrast-enhanced ultrasound and superb microvascular imaging could also improve the diagnosis of low-flow tissue pathology and treatment response [4]. Moreover, elastography delineates tissue elastic properties; for example, shear wave elastography can distinguish between arthritis types depending on the elastic properties of the synovial tissue [5]. Outcome measures in rheumatology (OMERACT) first established ultrasound definitions set in 2005 and revised in 2019 [6, 7]; OMERACT ultrasound pathologies associated with rheumatic diseases have been validated and tested for reliability globally [6, 7].

The burden of rheumatic diseases has increased over the last few decades [8]. In Bangladesh, the prevalence of musculoskeletal disorders and related disabilities has also been increasing [9]. This comes with increased diagnostic musculoskeletal ultrasound volume not only within rheumatology but also within physiatry, orthopedics, pain management, and emergency medicine, with the greatest growth in private offices [10]. To mitigate this increased demand, more healthcare professionals with ultrasound expertise are needed. Accurate ultrasound diagnosis of tissue pathology and ultrasound-guided interventions necessitate extensive hands-on experience and valid certifications. As the day progresses, a growing number of bodies and organizations have been involved with certifying physicians in the field, leading to an increase in the number of ultrasound sonographers (physician- and nonphysician-based) worldwide.

X-ray has been the most frequently applied imaging method in rheumatology practice and research over the years; nevertheless, it has poor diagnostic sensitivity in early-stage rheumatic disease; hence, advanced imaging is needed. Magnetic resonance imaging (MRI) and computed tomography (CT) have long been utilized for delineating pathologies involving bones, joints, and intra- and extra-articular soft tissues. However, many patients cannot afford these imaging tools, and in some cases, they are contraindicated as well. For example, in some patients, metallic implants and claustrophobia may hinder MRI, whereas radiation exposure may limit access to CT. Overall, ultrasound (including portable systems) could be a less expensive and suitable alternative in daily practice and research [10]. Further studies on ultrasound validation in rheumatic diseases are still needed.

Before January 2023, I was the only physiatrist in Bangladesh (172 million inhabitants) certified with RMSK (Registered in Musculoskeletal sonography) [11] and POCUS (Musculoskeletal) certifications [11], with Dr. Mohammad Moin Uddin being the second to obtain the RMSK certification. In 2018, the country's first Physiatry Department at Chittagong Medical College launched a musculoskeletal ultrasound (Fujifilm Sonosite M-Turbo) clinic, an innovative initiative spearheaded by the departmental head professor Dr. Md Shawkat Hossain. This significant advancement has motivated numerous other Physiatry departments across the country to adopt similar initiatives. Currently, an increasing number of physicians in Bangladesh are practicing diagnostic musculoskeletal ultrasound and performing ultrasound-guided interventions. To ensure that their practice is both comprehensive and trustworthy, it is crucial to have access to educational materials and continuous medical education (CME), as well as certifications from authentic organizations. I am confident that the environment will continue to improve in the future.

The book *Musculoskeletal Ultrasound in Rheumatic Diseases: A Case-Based Review* includes three sections. *Part I* focuses on the role of ultrasound in general. Six chapters provide a theoretical background of different facets of musculoskeletal ultrasound. Each chapter begins with an abstract that outlines the key subjects to be discussed. Chapter 1 highlights the impact of ultrasound imaging in rheumatology, drawing on recent studies, whereas Chapter 2 discusses ultrasound terminology pertinent to rheumatology, covering aspects such as transducer handling, tissue pathology, intervention landmarks, and advanced imaging methods. Chapter 3 compares ultrasound with other imaging methods. Chapter 4 provides insights into the OMERACT ultrasound outcome measures, detailing their development and updates. Chapter 5 offers comprehensive insights into the artifacts that may arise during musculoskeletal ultrasound practice. Chapter 6 outlines the principles of ultrasound documentation relevant to rheumatology practice and research.

Part II (Chapter 7) presents and discusses a variety of 64 clinical cases. Each clinical case summary has been followed by ultrasound features. We discuss the clinical cases randomly; for example, you may not encounter all cases from a specific region followed by cases from other areas in a systematic order.

Part III (Chapter 8) includes 50 multiple choice questions (MCQs). These MCQs are designed to assess readers' knowledge regarding ultrasound in rheumatology.

It is recommended that readers carefully read the *Parts I* and *II* before attempting the questions in *Part III.*

Additionally, on behalf of the coauthors.

Department of Rheumatology, Royal North Shore Hospital, Northern Clinical School
The University of Sydney Faculty of Medicine and Health
Sydney, NSW, Australia

Md Abu Bakar Siddiq

References

1. Hall MM, Allen GM, Allison S, et al. Recommended musculoskeletal and sports ultrasound terminology: a Delphi-based consensus statement. British J Sports Med 2022; 56:310–319.
2. Kang T, Lanni S, Nam J, Emery P, Wakefield RJ. The evolution of ultrasound in rheumatology. Ther Adv Musculoskelet Dis 2012; 4:399–411.
3. Kane D, Grassi W, Sturrock R, Balint PV. A brief history of musculoskeletal ultrasound: 'From bats and ships to babies and hips'. Rheumatology 2004; 43:931–933.
4. Diao XH, Shen Y, Chen L, et al. Superb microvascular imaging is as sensitive as contrast-enhanced ultrasound for detecting synovial vascularity in rheumatoid arthritis. Quant Imaging Med Surg 2022; 12:2866–2876.
5. Chandel K, Prakash M, Sinha A, Sharma A, Chouhan DK, Sandhu MS. Role of Shear Wave Elastography of Synovium to Differentiate Rheumatoid and Tubercular Arthritis. J Med Ultrasound 2021;30:30–35
6. Wakefield RJ, Balint PV, Szkudlarek M, et al. OMERACT 7 Special Interest Group. Musculoskeletal ultrasound including definitions for ultrasonographic pathology. J Rheumatol 2005; 32:2485–2487.
7. Bruyn GA, Iagnocco A, Naredo E, et al. OMERACT Ultrasound Working Group. OMERACT Definitions for Ultrasonographic Pathologies and Elementary Lesions of Rheumatic Disorders 15 Years On. J Rheumatol 2019; 46:1388–1393.
8. GBD 2021 Osteoarthritis Collaborators. Global, regional, and national burden of osteoarthritis, 1990-2020 and projections to 2050: a systematic analysis for the Global Burden of Disease Study 2021. Lancet Rheumatol 2023; 5:e508–e522.
9. Zahid-Al-Quadir A, Zaman MM, Ahmed S, et al. Prevalence of musculoskeletal conditions and related disabilities in Bangladeshi adults: a cross-sectional national survey. BMC Rheumatol 2020; 4:69.
10. Sharpe RE, Nazarian LN, Parker L, Rao VM, Levin DC. Dramatically increased musculoskeletal ultrasound utilization from 2000 to 2009, especially by podiatrists in private offices. J Am Coll Radiol 2012; 9:141–6.
11. Tins BJ, Butler R. Imaging in rheumatology: reconciling radiology and rheumatology. Insights Imaging 2013; 4:799–810.
12. APCA: Alliance for Physician Certification & Advancement™ (APCA™). Available at: https://www.apca.org/about-apca/. Accessed on August 15, 2024.

Acknowledgments

The process of bringing this book to life was profoundly enriched by the unlimited support of many remarkable individuals, whose involvement was crucial for its successful and timely completion. First, I am thankful to my teacher and primary supervisor, Professor (Dr.) Suzon Al Hasan, a prominent expert in physical medicine and rehabilitation who currently serves at Islami Bank Medical College, Rajshahi, Bangladesh. His steadfast support and invaluable insights have been crucial in shaping my path as a researcher and author in the realm of medical publishing and writing this book. Without his motivation and encouragement, my accomplishments would have remained out of reach. My PhD lead supervisor, Professor (Dr.) David Hunter, Florance and Cope Chair of Rheumatology and Co-Director Sydney Musculoskeletal Health Flagship, University of Sydney, Australia, continually inspires me in my medical research pursuits and provides insightful advice.

Additionally, I am profoundly thankful for the mentorship I received from Professor (Dr.) Amin Uddin A Khan, the former head of the Department at Physical Medicine and Rehabilitation, Chittagong Medical College, Bangladesh, along with Professor (Dr.) Sheikh Ahmed, former professor, Physical Medicine and Rehabilitation, Chattogram Maa-O-Shishu Hospital Medical College, Dr. Md Shawkat Hossain, Professor and Acting Head, Physical Medicine and Rehabilitation, Chittagong Medical College, Professor (Dr.) Abu Taslim, Physical Medicine and Rehabilitation, BGC Trust Medical College, Professor (Dr.) Jahangir Alam Chowdhury, Physical Medicine and Rehabilitation, Chattogram Maa-O-Shishu Hospital Medical College, Associate Professor, (Dr.) M Abdur Rahim, (Dr.) Nitai Prasad Dutta, Physical Medicine and Rehabilitation, Chittagong Medical College, Bangladesh. I sincerely appreciate my friends and colleagues for their love, support, and guidance, which inspired me to embark on the journey of writing this book. My heartfelt appreciation also goes to all my coauthors for their invaluable contributions, particularly to Professor (Dr.) Johannes J. Rasker, who has been a guiding force in my journey since our initial meeting at a rheumatology conference in Dhaka in 2008. In this book, he contributed as a coauthor in three different chapters and helped me find coauthors for the book chapters where appropriate. I appreciate his prompt response to my request for writing the foreword for the book.

I wish to extend my heartfelt gratitude to Dr. Mohammad Moin Uddin, a consultant Physiatrist at Apollo-Imperial Hospital in Chittagong, Bangladesh, for his invaluable contribution of images and clinical data related to 12 distinct clinical cases for Section II. Additionally, I would like to acknowledge Dr. Omer Mala Ahmed from Sulaimanya-Ranya Teaching Hospital in Iraq for providing clinical data on a patient diagnosed with an ulnar nerve epineural cyst through ultrasound.

Contents

Editors and Contributors

About the Editors

Md Abu Bakar Siddiq MBBS, MSc (Rheumatology), FACR, FCPS, RMSK, POCUS (Musculoskeletal), PhD candidate at Department of Rheumatology, Royal North Shore Hospital, Northern Clinical School, University of Sydney Faculty of Medicine and Health, Sydney, New South Wales, Australia; Sydney Musculoskeletal Health, The University of Sydney, Sydney, New South Wales, Australia; Kolling Institute of Medical Research, St Leonards, New South Wales, Australia; School of Health Sports and Professional Practice (Rheumatology), University of South Wales, Pontypridd, United Kingdom; Department of Physical Medicine and Rehabilitation, Brahmanbaria Medical College, Bangladesh

Contributors

George A. W. Bruyn Department of Rheumatology, Reumakliniek Lelystad, Lelystad, The Netherlands

Tergooi MC Hospital, Hilversum, The Netherlands

Syed Atiqul Haq Department of Rheumatology, GreenLife Medical College, Dhaka, Bangladesh

David Hunter Department of Rheumatology, Royal North Shore Hospital, Northern Clinical School, Faculty of Medicine and Health, The University of Sydney, Sydney, NSW, Australia

Sydney Musculoskeletal Health, The University of Sydney, Sydney, NSW, Australia

Win Min Oo Department of Rheumatology, Royal North Shore Hospital, Northern Clinical School, The University of Sydney Faculty of Medicine and Health, Sydney, NSW, Australia

Sydney Musculoskeletal Health, The University of Sydney, Sydney, NSW, Australia

Department of Physical Medicine and Rehabilitation, University of Medicine, Mandalay, Myanmar

Yasser Ragab Department of Radiology, University of Cairo, Cairo, Egypt

Johannes J. Rasker Faculty of Behavioral Sciences, Psychology, Health and Technology, University of Twente, Enschede, The Netherlands

Md Abu Bakar Siddiq Department of Rheumatology, Royal North Shore Hospital, Northern Clinical School, Faculty of Medicine and Health, The University of Sydney, Sydney, NSW, Australia

Sydney Musculoskeletal Health, The University of Sydney, Sydney, NSW, Australia

Kolling Institute of Medical Research, St Leonards, NSW, Australia

School of Health Sports and Professional Practice (Rheumatology), University of South Wales, Pontypridd, United Kingdom

Department of Physical Medicine and Rehabilitation, Brahmanbaria Medical College, Brahmanbaria, Bangladesh

Patricia van der Meijde SonoCare, Apeldoorn, The Netherlands

Part I

Ultrasound in Rheumatology

1 Introduction to Musculoskeletal Ultrasound in Rheumatic Diseases

Md Abu Bakar Siddiq and Patricia van der Meijde

1.1 Background: Musculoskeletal Ultrasound

The definition of musculoskeletal ultrasound (MSUS) is not straightforward, encompassing the diagnosis of pathological changes in various musculoskeletal structures, such as bones, joints, tendons, muscles, bursae, ligaments, cartilage, nerves, fascia, and adjacent soft tissues, as well as guided interventions in rheumatic disorders [1]. In rheumatology practice, B (brightness)-mode ultrasound is utilized, which consists of two primary features: grayscale (GS) pathologies and increased color and power Doppler activity (DA). The frequency-dependent GS technique enables visualization of deep structures by recording ultrasound waves reflecting into body tissues, with GS echoes categorized as isoechoic, hypoechoic, and hyperechoic on the basis of image brightness compared with surrounding structures [2–4]. DA is effective in assessing hyperemia and neovascularity in inflammation, distinguishing between cystic and solid lesions, and can aid in guided biopsy, joint and bursal aspiration, and injection procedures [3]. High-resolution transducers are employed in rheumatic diseases, with lower frequencies (6–9 MHz) used for deeper structures [4], higher frequencies (12–18 MHz) for superficial structures, and 18–24 MHz for smaller structures such as pulleys, tendons, and nerves, depending on the structure being imaged and body habitus [2–4].

M. A. B. Siddiq (✉)
Department of Rheumatology, Royal North Shore Hospital, Northern Clinical School, Faculty of Medicine and Health, The University of Sydney, Sydney, NSW, Australia

Sydney Musculoskeletal Health, The University of Sydney, Sydney, NSW, Australia

Kolling Institute of Medical, Research, St Leonards, NSW, Australia

School of Health Sports and Professional Practice (Rheumatology), University of South Wales, Pontypridd, United Kingdom

Department of Physical Medicine and Rehabilitation, Brahmanbaria Medical College, Brahmanbaria, Bangladesh
e-mail: msid8426@uni.sydney.edu.au

P. van der Meijde
SonoCare, Apeldoorn, The Netherlands

1.2 Ultrasound in Rheumatic Disease: Historical Perspectives

The initial publication on the measurement of acoustic attenuation in normal articular cartilage and periarticular soft tissues via MSUS dates back to 1958 [5]. However, it was not until 1972 that the first B-scan image successfully distinguished between Baker's cyst (BC) and thrombophlebitis [5]. The first demonstration of GS effusion synovitis and synovial hypertrophy (SH)

M. A. B. Siddiq (ed.), *Musculoskeletal Ultrasound in Rheumatic Diseases*,
https://doi.org/10.1007/978-981-96-5298-3_1

in the knee, observed in yttrium-90-treated rheumatoid arthritis (RA), was documented in 1978. In 1988, ultrasound reports highlighted synovitis, tenosynovitis, and bone erosion in the rheumatoid hand [5]. In 1981, the first report presented ultrasound-guided septic shoulder arthritis aspiration in advanced RA [4, 5], followed by the 1988 ultrasound demonstration of rheumatoid nodules and tenosynovitis in RA [4, 5]. Furthermore, in 1989, the description of GS synovial effusion or synovitis in a clinically and radiologically normal hip in RA patients was presented [6, 7]. By 1992, reduced cartilage thickness was measured in both RA and osteoarthritis (OA) patients via ultrasound. However, it was not until 1994 that the first ultrasound power Doppler revealed soft tissue hyperemia in patients with inflammatory arthritis [4]. Toward the end of the year 2000, the potential of ultrasound in diagnosing and monitoring therapeutic responses in rheumatologic conditions piqued the interest of rheumatologists, leading to an increased focus on learning MSUS [5]. Consequently, the formation of the rheumatologist-led EULAR (the European Alliance of Associations for Rheumatology) MSUS working group (WG) in 1998, which organized the first EULAR ultrasound training course in the Netherlands, marked a significant milestone in the field [5].

The initial guidelines for MSUS in rheumatology were established by the EULAR-WG in 2001 [5]. However, owing to a lack of agreement on standard ultrasound pathology definitions and scanning techniques, an international group of rheumatologists formed the ultrasound task force OMERACT (Outcome Measures in Rheumatoid Arthritis Clinical Trial, later renamed Outcome Measures in Rheumatology) to create a consensus set of definitions for ultrasound pathologies in inflammatory joint disease. This effort resulted in the development of the first consensus set of definitions for ultrasound pathologies in inflammatory joint disease in 2005, with subsequent updates in 2019 [8, 9]. The OMERACT ultrasound definitions, which are intended for use in rheumatic diseases, are detailed in Chap. 3.

The inaugural EULAR advanced ultrasound course was introduced in 2006 to cater to the growing number of learners seeking expertise in this field [10]. In 2007, 14th EULAR ultrasound courses were subsequently established, along with educational guidelines outlining the structure of future courses categorized into basic, intermediate, and advanced levels [10]. On the other hand, the progress of MSUS training led by rheumatologists in America was relatively sluggish until 2005, when the Ultrasound Society of North American Rheumatologists (USSONAR) was established to promote training and research in this area [11]. The American College of Rheumatology (ACR) initiated two standalone training conferences in 2010, marking a significant step toward enhancing expertise in MSUS [5]. By 2011, the ACR collaborated with USSONAR to develop a comprehensive training program on MSUS, culminating in a competence exam at the conclusion of the program. In 2012, the ACR subsequently made the decision to implement a distinct certification process specifically tailored for rheumatologists, which was officially launched the following year [4].

1.3 Applications of Ultrasound in Rheumatic Diseases

The use of the ultrasound in the field of rheumatology has been steadily gaining approval from reputable organizations such as the British Society for Rheumatology, ACR, and the EULAR [6]. MSUS enhances the clinical data obtained through physical examinations and proves to be valuable in directing treatment decisions and assessing treatment efficacy. Like magnetic resonance imaging (MRI), ultrasound can detect subclinical synovitis [4, 5].

In 2013, a panel of experts from the EULAR formulated ten recommendations pertaining to the utilization of imaging techniques in the context of RA, with the majority focusing on the diagnosis of joint inflammation, assessment of structural damage, prediction of disease prognosis, and monitoring of disease remission, as outlined in Table 1.1 [2]. When seropositive RA patients were compared with those with seronegative RA, the former group exhibited higher

Table 1.1 Ultrasound in rheumatoid arthritis (RA) [7]

Recommendation 1	When there is diagnostic doubt, conventional radiography, ultrasound, or MRI can be used.
Recommendation 2	The presence of inflammation seen with ultrasound or MRI can be used to predict the progression to clinical RA from the so-called undifferentiated inflammatory arthritis.
Recommendation 3	Ultrasound and MRI are superior to clinical examination in the assessment of joint inflammation; these techniques should be considered for improved detection of inflammation in joints.
Recommendation 4	Conventional radiography of the hands and feet should be the initial imaging technique to detect damage (erosions). However, ultrasound or MRI should be considered for earlier detection of erosions or if radiography is negative.
Recommendation 5	MRI bone edema is a strong independent predictor of subsequent radiographic progression in early RA and should be considered for use as a prognostic indicator. Early joint inflammation detected by MRI or ultrasound as well as joint damage detected by conventional radiography, MRI, or ultrasound can also be considered for the prediction of further joint damage.
Recommendation 6	Inflammation seen on imaging may be more predictive of a therapeutic response than clinical features of disease activity.
Recommendation 7	Since MRI and ultrasound are more effective than clinical examination in detecting inflammation, they may be useful in monitoring disease activity.
Recommendation 8	The periodic use of radiography of the hands and feet should be considered for joint damage monitoring. MRI (and possibly ultrasound), being more sensitive, can also be used to monitor disease progression.
Recommendation 9	If cervical spine is suspected of being involved, it should be periodically evaluated for functional instability by lateral radiograph obtained in the neutral position, maximum flexion, and extension. When the radiograph is positive or specific neurological symptoms and signs are present, MRI should be performed.
Recommendation 10	MRI and ultrasound can detect inflammation that predicts subsequent joint damage, even when clinical remission is present. These methods can be used to assess persistent inflammation.

MRI magnetic resonance imaging, *RA* rheumatoid arthritis

levels of inflammation and joint damage, as detected by ultrasound imaging [12]. Ultrasound has proven to be a valuable tool for visualizing joint inflammation and structural damage not only in RA but also in other rheumatic conditions, such as spondylarthritis (SpA), crystal arthropathies, and connective tissue diseases [2]. The diagnostic significance of ultrasound in identifying large vessel vasculitis has been widely acknowledged, highlighting its crucial role in the assessment and management of various rheumatic conditions [12].

The prevalence and distribution of inflammatory ultrasound biomarkers and structural damage in SpA vary depending on the enthesis distribution [12]. Compared with gout, inflammatory DA is more common in SpA patients, particularly at the Achilles tendon enthesis, whereas structural damage is more prevalent in gout patients [12]. The inclusion of ultrasound tenosynovitis and enthesitis in the Classification Criteria for Psoriatic Arthritis (CASPAR) enhances its diagnostic accuracy for psoriatic arthritis (PsA) [12]. Evidence of subclinical joint inflammation and entheseal involvement has been noted in healthy controls [13] and patients with inflammatory bowel diseases who have not previously experienced inflammatory arthritis [12]. However, there is significant variability in the frequency of these lesions among affected individuals [12].

The correlation between extra-articular structural involvement, such as salivary gland morphology in Sjogren's syndrome (SS), and the clinical and histological features of the disorder has been described in the literature [12]. Studies have shown that ultrasound is a valuable tool for evaluating peripheral neuropathies of rheumatological significance in various conditions, including SS, systemic sclerosis (SSc), RA, PsA, Behcet's syndrome, vasculitis, sarcoidosis, and crystal arthropathies [12]. Researchers have discussed the advantages and limitations of using ultrasound for assessing peripheral neuropathies, particularly in comparison with alternative imaging techniques such as magnetic resonance imaging (MRI), as well as the role of nerve conduction studies in the diagnostic process [12].

1.4 Request for Ultrasound Examination

A written request for an ultrasound examination should include clear clinical details, including signs and symptoms, provisional diagnosis, previous medical history, and clinical diagnosis of known relevant disease and should be made by a licensed healthcare provider; requests should align with legal and local healthcare facility requirements [14].

General Principles An examination request may encompass a comprehensive evaluation of a joint or inspection of a specific anatomical area or structure. For example, a peroneal tenosynovial complex and lateral collateral ligament (LCL) ultrasound examination is requested in patients with a history of lateral ankle sprain with lateral ankle pain and swelling. A thorough joint assessment involves the examination of all intra-articular (IA) components, such as the synovium, bone, cartilage, ligament, and effusion, as well as extra-articular structures, including the bursa, muscle, tendon, ligament, and nerve. Doppler ultrasound can identify hyperemia and active inflammation [14]. Images should be captured perpendicular to the region and along both the short- and long-axes [15]. Dynamic evaluation is utilized to detect structural subluxation, dislocation, and impingement syndrome. Maneuvers such as heel-toe and tilting of the transducer can enhance image quality and prevent anisotropy [15]. Sono-palpation is beneficial for distinguishing between a ganglion cyst and bursal swelling [15].

Indications Indications for musculoskeletal ultrasound are listed below [14]. In Box 1.1, ACR recommendations for common indications are provided [14].

- Pain or dysfunction.
- Soft tissue or bone injury.
- Tendon, ligament, or fascial pathology.
- Arthritis, synovitis, or crystal deposition disease.
- Joint effusion and intra-articular bodies.
- Neurovascular entrapment, injury, neuropathy, mass, or subluxation.
- Evaluation of soft tissue masses, swelling, or fluid collection.
- Detection of foreign bodies in superficial soft tissues.
- Planning and guidance for an invasive procedure.
- Congenital or developmental anomalies.
- Postoperative or postprocedural evaluation.

Box 1.1. A General List of Potential Applications of MSUS in Rheumatic Diseases [4]

Explores	
	Joint synovitis (± Doppler activity)
	Synovial hypertrophy
	Joint effusion
	Bone erosion
	Tenosynovitis (± Doppler activity)
	Enthesitis or other tendon pathology
	Bursitis
	Osteophytes
	Crystalline deposit
	Nerve entrapments (ulnar, median, or tibial nerves)
	Salivary gland pathology in Sjogren's syndrome
Guides and/or assess	
	Treatment response
	Interventional procedure
	Dynamic evaluation of impingement, subluxation, or dislocation

MSUS musculoskeletal ultrasound

– Joint laxity, stiffness, decreased range of motion, or misalignment.

1.5 Joint Specific Examination and Indications

1.5.1 Ultrasound Examination of the Shoulder

Indications Rotator cuff pathologies (partial- or full-thickness tear, calcific tendinitis, tendinosis), biceps tendon pathology (tear, tendinosis, subluxation, and dislocation), subacromial-subdeltoid (SASD) bursal pathologies (hypertrophy/bursitis, impingement), suprascapularis tendon pathologies (tear and impingement), infective and inflammatory synovitis, acromioclavicular joint (ACJ) OA, paralabral cyst, and nerve compression (suprascapular nerve) [16, 17].

Examination Specifications [14]

– All the structures are examined along short and long axes dynamically.
– The long head of the biceps tendon (LHBT) is examined in short and long axes within the bicipital groove and proximally to the IA-glenoid tubercle and distally to the musculotendinous junction. LHBT subluxation-dislocation and subcoracoid impingement can be checked dynamically during shoulder flexion–extension and external–internal rotation. The insertions of the pectoralis major tendon and subscapularis tendon on the humerus can be evaluated at the same time.
– In the oblique plane, the supraspinatus (SST) and infraspinatus (IST) tendons can be scanned. A short-axis view of the LHBT in the rotator interval serves as a landmark for correct orientation to the SST and IST, and more posterior aspects of the IST and teres minor (TM) tendons can be examined by placing the transducer posteriorly at the level of the glenohumeral (GH) joint [14]. Passive internal and external rotation of the patient's arm can facilitate visualization of the IST. The transducer is subsequently adjusted to a transverse orientation and moved slightly distally and inferiorly to examine the trapezoid TM tendon, which is identifiable by its oblique internal echoes that distinguish it from the IST. The teres minor can be further distinguished from the IST because of its wider and more muscular attachment [18].
– Rotator cuff tendinosis is associated with increased thickness and is hypoechoic due to loss of the fibrillar pattern. A transducer that compresses the rotator cuff can detect nonretracted tears. Tendon tear length measured along the long axis and width along the short axis. A partial-thickness tear can be bursal, articular, or intrasubstance. Rotator cuff tears in the SST, IST, and teres minor may follow fatty infiltration and atrophy, should be checked, and compared with those on the contralateral healthy side. The following could be useful tips for differentiating between articular and bursal tears of the rotator cuff [16]: (i) thinning of the tendon; (ii) loss of the typical upper curved shape of the surface of the tendon; (iii) downward displacement or "sagging" of the deltoid muscle; (iv) intrusion of the subacromial-subdeltoid bursa into the space created by the torn tendon; (v) the articular side rim renting tears of supraspinatus, which might show a bull's sign that involves a small, articular surface avulsion adjacent to the tuberosity, which appears as a small, hypoechoic defect with a central hyperechoic line on the articular surface; (vi) intrasubstance or interstitial tear involving volume loss; (vii) cortical irregularity, which is often observed in complete tears; and (viii) in cleavage tears, the tear gap fills with fluid.
– SSAD bursal hypertrophy and effusion should be checked with DA to detect hyperemia, and shoulder abduction with SASD bursal bunching and snapping signifies impingement.
– Posterior scanning can be utilized to assess GH joint effusion. GH effusion is characterized by greater displacement than SH effusion [14]. However, para-labral cysts are frequently misidentified as dilated veins, a

distinction that can be clarified using Doppler imaging [14]. The axillary scan better delineates GH effusion with 60 degrees of internal rotation [19].

- The ACJ should be evaluated for arthritis, infection, or trauma by placing the transducer at the apex of the shoulder over the acromion and distal clavicle obliquely. Sonographic signals help in the diagnosis of ACJ cysts [20].

1.6 Ultrasound Examination of the Elbow

Indications Lateral and medial epicondylitis, inflammatory and infective synovitis, bone erosion, ulnar collateral ligament (UCL) and lateral collateral ligament (LCL) tear, radial nerve compression, cubital tunnel syndrome, pronator teres syndrome, loose body in the joint, olecranon bursitis, snapping tricep syndrome, epitrochlear lymph node, and cellulitis [21, 22].

Examination Specifications [14]

- Both the short and long axes were scanned dynamically.
- The anterior joint recesses are assessed for joint effusion, cartilage thickness, cortical erosion, synovial thickness, and IA bodies.
- Among several alternatives, the distal biceps brachii tendon can be examined dynamically at its attachment to the radial bicipital tuberosity, placing the arm maximally supinated and extended or medially with the elbow flexed and the forearm supinated or laterally using a brachioradialis acoustic window [23]. Isolated bicipito-radial (cubital) bursitis is uncommon and typically occurs alongside a partial tear. The subtendinous bicipito-radial or cubital bursa is situated at the distal insertion of the biceps onto the radial tuberosity, positioned between the biceps attachment and the radius beneath it. Anteriorly, the brachialis muscle, radial and brachial vessels, and median and radial nerves can be scanned [24].
- Laterally, the lateral epicondyle, common extensor tendon origin, origin of the extensor carpi radialis longus and brachioradialis, LCL, and radial nerves (superficial and deep posterior interosseous nerves) can be scanned.
- Medial epicondylitis is less prevalent than its lateral counterpart. Medially, the medial epicondyle, common flexor tendon origin, UCL, and ulnar nerve (UN) in the cubital tunnel are scanned.
- Dynamically, subluxation and dislocation of the UN and adjacent medial head of the triceps muscle with flexion and extension of the elbow can be performed. Dynamic examination could include valgus stress for the UCL and varus stress for LCL integrity.
- The posterior elbow is scanned at 90° flexion for joint effusion, synovial hypertrophy, synovitis, a loose body in the joint cavity, integrity of the triceps brachii tendon, and olecranon bursal pathology.

1.7 Ultrasound Examination of the Wrist and Hand

Indications de Quervains tenosynovitis (dQT), intersection syndrome, nerve sheath tumor, Wartenburg syndrome, scapholunate ligament (SLL) tear, carpal tunnel syndrome (CTS), Guyon's canal syndrome (GCS), ganglion cyst, inflammatory synovitis, extensor carpi ulnaris (ECU), tenosynovitis, etc. [23, 25].

Examination Specifications [14]

- All the structures are scanned on long and short axes and dynamically.
- Volar aspect, flexor digitorum superficialis and profundus tendons, and flexor pollicis longus tendons should lie under the hyperechoic flexor retinaculum (FR) in the carpal tunnel. Dynamic scanning with flexion and extension of the fingers revealed normal tendon motion. The median nerve (MN) lies beneath the FR among these tendons, and bifid or trifid MNs [26] and the accessory muscle belly can be identified incidentally

[23]. The palmaris longus tendon lies superficial to the FR, an important landmark for carpal tunnel intervention.
- On the radial side of the volar wrist, the flexor carpi radialis (FCR) tendon lies superficial to the FR, and the region should be checked for occult ganglion cysts originating from the radiocarpal joint capsule, scaphotrapezial joint, or FCR tendon sheath itself, which should be differentiated from the FCR and the radial artery.
- On the volar ulnar wrist, the triangular fibrocartilage complex (TFCC) should be scanned. The TFCC is deep to the extensor carpi ulnaris (ECU) tendon. The ECU tendon should be viewed in supination and pronation to assess subluxation. In patients with inflammatory arthritis, the ECU tendon should be evaluated for tenosynovitis and rupture. The branches of the UN and ulnar artery are located within the ulnar tunnel (Guyon's canal), which is bordered by the flexor carpi ulnaris (FCU) tendon and pisiform bone on the ulnar aspect of the tunnel [27].
- There are six compartments accommodating nine tendons in the dorsal wrist: compartment 1 (abductor pollicis longus, APL, and excessor pollicis brevis), compartment 2 (extensor carpi radialis longus and extensor carpi radialis brevis), compartment 3 (extensor pollicis longus), compartment 4 (extensor indicis and extensor digitorum), compartment 5 (extensor digiti minimi), and compartment 6 (extensor carpi ulnaris) [28]. The integrity and tendinopathies of the extensor tendons should be checked.
- Moving the transversely positioned transducer distal to Lister's tubercle helps identify the dorsal aspect of the SLL, a potential site for ligament tears and ganglion cysts. dQT with an excessive APL tendon with a positive "lotus root sign" could be incidental [29, 30].
- Volar and dorsal radiocarpal, distal radioulnar, midcarpal, metacarpophalangeal, and interphalangeal joints were examined for effusion synovial hypertrophy, synovial hyperemia, bony erosions, flexor/extensor tendon and pulley integrity, tenosynovitis, and triggering of fingers [23].
- Ultrasound can detect avulsion fractures and Stener's lesions in the thumb [31].

1.8 Ultrasound Examination of the Hip

Indications Hip synovitis, effusion, loose body, septic arthritis, inflammatory arthritis, osteoarthritis, labral tear, hip snapping, muscle tear around the hip, tendinitis (gluteal medius), trochanteric bursitis, pudendal neuropathy, piriformis syndrome. The prosthetic hip is assessed for joint effusion, extra-articular fluid collection, iliopsoas bursitis, or soft tissue masses and/or necrosis (adverse local tissue reaction), and guided fluid aspiration from the joint to exclude infection can be requested. Further examination of the greater trochanter and periarticular soft tissues, including the iliopsoas, gluteus medius, or gluteus minimus muscle, is needed for fluid collection, tendinosis, or tendon tear [32, 33]. Sometimes, gluteal tendon tears and bursitis can be easily missed on the side because of compression of the iliotibial tract, and dynamic ultrasound scanning in the supine position could prevent this pitfall [34].

Examination Specifications [14]

- All the structures are scanned along both the short and long axes dynamically.
- In the supine position with external rotation of the lower extremity, oblique, sagittal long-axis scanning of the femoral head and neck is performed for synovial effusion or synovitis.
- Anterior "hip snapping hip" was revealed dynamically on hip flexion and external rotation for iliopsoas tendon snapping at the acetabular eminence.
- In the lateral decubitus position with the symptomatic side up, the greater trochanter, greater trochanteric bursae, gluteus medius, gluteus maximus, gluteus minimus, iliotibial band, and tensor fasciae latae are scanned. Sono-palpation of the greater tro-

chanter is performed for trochanteric bursitis. An iliotibial band or gluteus maximus muscle snap over the greater trochanter is assessed via dynamic flexion–extension of the hip.

- Medially, the flexed hip in the frog-leg position (external rotation with 45° knee flexion) better visualizes the iliopsoas tendon, adductor muscles, pubic bone and symphysis pubis, and distal rectus abdominis.
- Posteriorly, the extended hip with the knee is scanned along long and short axes for the glutei, hamstring tendons, and sciatic nerve (SN). The glutei are imaged obliquely from their origins to the greater trochanter (gluteus medius and minimus) and linea aspera (gluteus maximus, GM). The SN is scanned at the greater sciatic foramen, deep to the GM; it can be followed distally, midway between the ischial tuberosity and the greater trochanter, superficial to the quadratus femoris muscle.
- The piriformis muscle runs obliquely from the anterior surface of the sacrum to the medial surface of the superior facet of the greater tuberosity of the femur [35]. A transducer placed obliquely over the long axis could be scanned between the greater sciatic notch and greater tuberosity, and 90° rotations of the probe are needed for axial scanning [36].

1.9 Ultrasound Examination of the Knee

Indications Inflammatory arthritis, septic arthritis, osteoarthritis, gout, pseudogout, loose body in the joint, pigmented villionodular synovitis, lipoma arborescence, bursitis, (suprapatellar, prepatellar, and infrapatellar), BC, pesanserine bursitis, meniscal pathology, Osgood Schlatter disease, etc. [37].

Examination Specifications [14, 15]

- All the structures are scanned along short and long axes dynamically.
- The patient was supine with partial knee flexion (20–30°); the quadriceps and patellar tendinopathy, the suprapatellar recess for effusion, the distal femoral trochlear cartilage for cartilage thickness, and the prepatellar and infrapatellar bursae for effusion and bursal thickening were scanned and evaluated with copious gel and minimal transducer compression.
- The medial collateral ligament, pes anserine tendons and bursa, and medial patellar retinaculum are scanned medially. The anterior horn and body of the medial meniscus are scanned accurately with valgus stress.
- Later, the patient remained supine with the ipsilateral leg internally rotated. The popliteus tendon, biceps femoris tendon, patellar retinacula, fibular collateral ligament, lateral meniscus (LM), and iliotibial band are scanned. LM pathology could be checked for varus stress. The common peroneal nerve exits the posterior knee area and can be better scanned at the fibular neck.
- Posterior knee scans are performed while patients are lying prone, and the semimembranosus muscle, medial and lateral gastrocnemius muscles, tendons, and bursa are examined. The BC popliteal region arises from the joint cavity between the medial head of the gastrocnemius and semimembranosus tendon. Dilated BC may lodge with impacted or free loose bodies and may sometimes be confused with popliteal vein thrombophlebitis; however, compressible, superficial BC is distinctive from deeper veins with increased DA. Poorly compressible ganglion cysts deep to the gasctronemius muscle and close to the joint line are sometimes confused with BC. The integrity of the posterior horn of the meniscus could be checked posteriorly. The tibial insertion of the posterior cruciate

ligament may be identifiable in a sagittal oblique plane in this position [37].

1.10 Ultrasound Examination of the Ankle and Foot

Indications Septic arthritis, inflammatory arthritis, gout, osteoarthritis, hemophilic arthropathy, lateral and medial collateral ligament tear, peroneal tenosynovitis, peroneal tendon split, Morton's neuroma, tarsal tunnel syndrome, retrocalcaneal bursitis, Achilles tendinopathy, plantar fasciitis, and extensor tenosynovitis [38].

Examination Specifications [14]

- All the structures are scanned on long and short axes dynamically.
- Anteriorly, the tibialis anterior, extensor hallucis longus, extensor digitorum longus, and peroneus tertius tendons are scanned for integrity and tendinopathies (tendinosis and tenosynovitis). The anterior joint recess is scanned for effusion, synovial hypertrophy, synovitis, a loose body, increased cartilage thickness, and bone erosion.
- The tibialis posterior, flexor digitorum longus (FDL), and flexor hallucis longus (FHL) tendons are scanned medially (anterior to posterior). The tibial nerve identifies between the FDL tendon anteriorly and the FHL tendon posteriorly and can be followed proximally to assess the medial and lateral plantar nerves. The deltoid ligament is scanned longitudinally from its attachment at the medial malleolus to the navicular, talus, and calcaneus.
- The peroneus longus (PL) and brevis (PB) tendons are identified proximal to the lateral malleolus. At the cuboid groove, the PL turns medially along the plantar aspect of the foot and inserts at the base of the first metatarsal (MTB) and medial cuneiform bones. The PB tendon inserts at the base of the fifth MTB.
- Subluxation of the PL and PB is checked dynamically on the dorsiflexion of the ankle and eversion of the subtalar joint. The anterior inferior tibiofibular ligament, anterior talofibular ligament, and calcaneofibular ligament are examined dynamically for integrity in the background of lateral ankle sprain.
- In the prone position, feet extending over the end of the table with a rolled towel placed under the ankles posterior and inferior heel are scanned for Achilles tendon integrity, Haglund deformity, tendinopathy, retro-calcaneal and retro-Achilles bursal effusion, and plantar fascial pathology.
- In the foot, the metatarsophalangeal joints and proximal interphalangeal joints are evaluated on the plantar and dorsal sides for effusion, synovial hypertrophy, synovial hyperemia, and bony erosions. The transducer is placed on the long and short axes of the plantar aspect of the first interdigital space, and the examiner applies digital pressure dorsally. In Morton's neuroma, manual compression of the forefoot with plantar imaging transverse to the metatarsals (Mulder's maneuver) displaces a neuroma in a plantar direction along with a palpable click. The intermetatarsal bursa lies on the dorsal aspect of the interdigital nerve and should be differentiated from Morton's neuroma [39].

1.11 Specifications of a Peripheral Nerve Examination

A nerve is composed of fascicular hypoechoic longitudinal neuronal fascicles interspersed with hyperechoic interfascicular connective tissue and perineurium, which is best visualized in the short-axis plane [40]. Nerves exhibit less mobility than adjacent tendons during dynamic examination. When a nerve passes through fibro-osseous tunnels, it appears more hypoechoic; entrapment neuropathies typically occur within these tunnels, such as the cubital and ulnar tunnels for the ulnar nerve, the carpal tunnel for the median nerve, the fibular neck for the common peroneal nerve, and the tarsal tunnel for the tibial nerve

[40]. Ulnar nerve subluxation can occur within the cubital tunnel region. Static subluxation or dislocation of a nerve can be identified via ultrasound, but an intermittently subluxating or dislocating nerve requires dynamic examination [40]. In some cases, adjacent tendons (dQT may correlate with Wartenberg's syndrome) [29], soft tissues (paral cysts compress the suprascapular nerve at the suprascapular notch), bony spurs (the medial epicondyle of the humerus may impinge the UN at the cubital tunnel), or accessory muscles (the carpal tunnel may cause carpal tunnel syndrome) may contribute to compressive neuropathies [26, 41]. The sonographic appearance of peripheral nerve sheath tumors can vary, although they mostly share the common features of being hypoechoic and homogeneous, with posterior acoustic enhancement and peripheral nerve continuity [14, 40].

1.12 Specifications of a Soft Tissue Mass

Soft tissue masses may exhibit poor compressibility, as observed in ganglion cysts, or good compressibility, as observed in bursal swelling [14, 41]. A cystic mass that is compressible and shows increased DA indicates bursal inflammation, whereas a ganglion cyst appears avascular and inert during power Doppler scanning [14, 41]. Dynamic evaluation is essential for assessing the relationship between soft tissue and adjacent structures. The deep investing fascia plays a crucial role in differentiating between superficial and deep soft tissue masses [14, 41].

1.13 Specifications of MSUS-Guided Interventions

Ultrasound-guided intervention for rheumatic disease represents an optimal method for treatment [42]. The intervention process should encompass a comprehensive review of previous images, obtaining informed consent from the patient, and following aseptic procedures [43]. Ultrasound guidance allows direct visualization of the needle, enabling precise monitoring of its trajectory and accurate placement at the target area [42]. Additionally, Doppler ultrasound aids in delineating hyperemia and increased vascularity, which are indicative of inflammation and infection [2, 4]. If any skin area along the target pathway is hyperemic, an alternative procedure should be considered to prevent the spread of infection (Box 1.2). It is essential to select the shortest pathway to the region of interest, taking into account the absence of adjacent neurovascular structures and optimizing needle visualization [42]. Furthermore, slight "to and fro" movement of the needle can enhance its visualization [42]. The implementation of a virtual convex bundle enhances visualization through the cross-beam effect, even when a left or right in-plane approach is employed, resulting in only a slight reduction in the frame rate. Alternatively, the use of needle guidance software, which combines beam steering and needle enhancement, may lead to a more significant decrease in the frame rate.

While the in-plane technique is preferred, the out-of-plane technique can also be utilized. Doppler ultrasound is particularly beneficial when performing a biopsy of a partially necrotic

Box 1.2 Preparations to Conduct Interventions with Direct Imaging Guidance in Infection [43]

Prevention of spread of infection during ultrasound-guided interventions
Disinfection of the hands (L) or handwashing and disinfection (H)
Gloves (L), alternatively sterile gloves (H).
Sterile preparation of equipment (L, H).
Disinfection of the injection site (L, H).
For US-guided interventions Maintenance of at least 0.5 cm between the probe/gel[a] and the needle (L) or. Extensive disinfection of the probe and use of antiseptic instead of gel (L). Sterile vinyl foil cover for the ultrasound probe and sterile gel (H).
Face masks† and cap (H).
Sterilized wraps with opening to expose the applicable site only (H).

[a]The use of sterile gel for ultrasound-guided interventions is recommended by some national authorities. †Obligatory for patients and healthcare providers in several countries during the COVID-19 pandemic. L, low risk of infection; H, high risk of infection

Table 1.2 Overview of imaging-guided interventions for musculoskeletal diseases [42]

Intervention	Comparator	Results for intervention
IA injections in sacroiliitis and ACJ arthritis	Periarticular	Superior for short-term and long-term pain
Shoulder joint injections in adhesive capsulitis	SASD bursa	Superior for short-term and long-term pain. Mixed results for efficacy
Subscapularis muscle injection in scapular pain	Scapulothoracic bursa	No difference in safety and efficacy
Medial access for knee injections in OA	Midlateral/superolateral access	No difference in safety and accuracy
Ultrasound in-plane injection in knee OA	Ultrasound out-of-plane	No difference in accuracy, adverse events, or procedural time
Bone biopsy in suspected osteomyelitis	Paravertebral soft tissue	No difference in tissue acquisition
Intratendon sheath injection in trigger fingers	Extra tendon sheath	No difference in safety and efficacy
Intraepineurium injections in CTS	Extraepineurium	Superior for symptom severity and efficacy
Ulnar access for injection in CTS	Midline/radial access	Inferior for long-term pain reduction compared with radial access
Injection above the median nerve in CT	Injection under the median nerve	No difference in safety and efficacy

ACJ, acromioclavicular joint, *CTS* carpal tunnel syndrome, *IA* intra-articular, *OA* osteoarthritis, *SASD* subacromial/subdeltoid

Box 1.3 EULAR Ultrasound-Guided Interventions in Musculoskeletal Diseases [42]

Overarching principles

A. The imaging technique should be optimized according to the procedure and the anatomical site taking into account potential side effects, radiation exposure, availability, expertise, and costs.

B. Imaging-guided interventional procedures should be conducted under adequate aseptic conditions.

C. Complex imaging-guided interventional procedures should be conducted with adequate assistance by technical personnel.

Specific points to consider

1. Imaging should be preferred over palpation to guide targeted* interventional procedures at peripheral joints and periarticular structures in patients with RMDs.
2. Ultrasound should be used as the first imaging modality for interventional procedures at peripheral joints. Fluoroscopy may be used as an alternative.
3. Imaging should be preferred over palpation to guide targeted* injections at structures encompassing peripheral nerves. Ultrasound should be the preferred imaging modality.
4. Imaging should be used to guide targeted* injections at the spine.
5. Imaging should be preferred over palpation for targeted* injections of the sacroiliac joint(s).
6. Healthcare professionals performing imaging-guided interventional procedures must have adequate skills in the respective imaging technique and the interventional procedure.

[a]Targeted interventions are defined as procedures requiring a high level of precision to reach a specific anatomical area such as injection of small ganglia, cysts, or tenosynovitis, including aspiration of small amounts of fluid or synovial biopsy; †Levels of evidence were downgraded (from level 2 to level 3) because of bias related to randomization, outcome assessment (trials and nonrandomized studies), the population of interest (cross-sectional studies), and inadequate adjustment of potential confounders; *EULAR* European Alliance of Associations for Rheumatology, *RMDs* rheumatic diseases

mass, as it helps identify areas of vascularity with adequate viable histologic specimens [2, 4, 14]. The EULAR points to consider for image-guided interventions in rheumatic and musculoskeletal diseases are summarized in Box 1.3 [42], while Table 1.2 provides an overview of image-guided interventions in rheumatic diseases [42].

1.14 Specifications for Ultrasound Examination for the Detection of Foreign Bodies

Foreign objects usually appear brighter on ultrasound than nearby soft tissues do and can produce an acoustic shadow (in the case of wood) or a comet tail artifact (in the case of glass or metal) [12]. If foreign bodies are not removed, they can lead to the development of a hypoechoic soft tissue inflammatory reaction, granulation tissue, or abscess [12, 44]. Ultrasound is an effective tool for locating foreign bodies, with superficial bodies being best visualized via a high-frequency linear-array transducer and ample gel, whereas deeper foreign bodies require a lower-frequency transducer [44]. Increased DA indicates surrounding hyperemia and inflammation [12, 44].

To summarize, within the field of musculoskeletal disorders, there is a growing utilization of ultrasound. This technology is valuable for the detection of soft tissue lesions, covering a range of structures such as muscles, tendons, ligaments, bursa, nerves, and synovial tissue. Additionally, it is effective in the identification of intra-articular pathologies, such as joint effusion and the existence of intra-articular bodies. Through the use of ultrasound guidance, healthcare providers can guarantee precise needle placement during joint and soft tissue injections, ultimately improving clinical effectiveness.

Conflict of Interest MAB is supported by a Faculty of Medicine and Health Executive Dean Stipend scholarship, University of Sydney, Australia, for his PhD course.

References

1. Hall MM, Allen GM, Allison S, et al. Recommended musculoskeletal and sports ultrasound terminology: a Delphi-based consensus statement. British J Sports Med. 2022;56:310–9.
2. Newman JS, Adler RS. Power Doppler sonography: applications in musculoskeletal imaging. Semin Musculoskelet Radiol. 1998;2:231–40.
3. van den Berg R, Ohrndorf S, Kortekaas MC, et al. What is the value of musculoskeletal ultrasound in patients presenting with arthralgia to predict inflammatory arthritis development? A systematic literature review. Arthritis Res Ther. 2018;20:228.
4. Cannella AC, Kissin EY, Torralba KD, Higgs JB, Kaeley GS. Evolution of musculoskeletal ultrasound in the United States: implementation and practice in rheumatology. Arthritis Care Res (Hoboken). 2014;66:7–13.
5. Kang T, Lanni S, Nam J, Emery P, Wakefield RJ. The evolution of ultrasound in rheumatology. Ther Adv Musculoskelet Dis. 2012;4:399–411.
6. Kane D, Grassi W, Sturrock R, Balint PV. A brief history of musculoskeletal ultrasound: 'from bats and ships to babies and hips'. Rheumatology. 2004;43:931–3.
7. Płaza M, Nowakowska-Płaza A, Pracoń G, Sudoł-Szopińska I. Role of ultrasonography in the diagnosis of rheumatic diseases in light of ACR/EULAR guidelines. J Ultrason. 2016;16:55–64.
8. Wakefield RJ, Balint PV, Szkudlarek M, OMERACT 7 Special Interest Group, et al. Musculoskeletal ultrasound including definitions for ultrasonographic pathology. J Rheumatol. 2005;32:2485–7.
9. Bruyn GA, Iagnocco A, Naredo E, OMERACT Ultrasound Working Group, et al. OMERACT definitions for ultrasonographic pathologies and elementary lesions of rheumatic disorders 15 years on. J Rheumatol. 2019;46:1388–93.
10. Naredo E, Bijlsma J, Conaghan P, et al. Recommendations for the content and conduct of European league against rheumatism (EULAR) musculoskeletal ultrasound courses. Ann Rheum Dis. 2008;67:1017–22.
11. Samuels J, Abramson S, Kaeley G. The use of musculoskeletal ultrasound by rheumatologists in the United States. Bull NYU Hosp Jt Dis. 2010;68:292–8.
12. Di Matteo A, Dejaco C. Editorial: ultrasound in rheumatology-A polyhedric imaging tool. Front Med (Lausanne). 2023;10:1150111.
13. Elnady B, El Shaarawy NK, Dawoud NM, et al. Subclinical synovitis and enthesitis in psoriasis patients and controls by ultrasonography in Saudi Arabia; incidence of psoriatic arthritis during two years. Clin Rheumatol. 2019;38:1627–35.
14. The AIUM. Practice parameter for the performance of the musculoskeletal ultrasound examination. J Ultrasound Med. 2023;42:E23–35.
15. Siddiq AB, Rahim MA. Knee pain examined under musculoskeletal ultrasonography: experience from a community-based rheumatology practice – a cross-sectional study. J Open Rheumatol. 2023; https://doi.org/10.2174/18743129-v17-230223-2022-10.
16. Singh JP. Shoulder ultrasound: what you need to know. Indian J Radiol Imaging. 2012;22:284–92.
17. Jiang L, He J, Chen CPC, et al. The ultrasonographic features of shoulder pain patients in a tertiary hospital in South China. Biomed Res Int. 2020;2020:3024793.
18. Holling A. Sonography of the rotator cuff: an overview. JDMS. 2001;17:144–50.
19. Schmidt W, Schicke B, Krause A. Which ultrasound scan is the best to detect glenohumeral joint effusions? Ultraschall Med. 2008;29(Suppl 5):250–5.
20. Gilani SA, Mehboob R, Bacha R, Gilani A, Manzoor I. Sonographic presentation of the geyser sign. Case Rep Med. 2019;2019:5623530.
21. Konin GP, Nazarian LN, Walz DM. US of the Elbow: indications, technique, normal anatomy, and pathologic conditions. Radiographics. 2013;33:E125–47.
22. Konarski W, Poboży T, Kotela A, Hordowicz M, Poboży K. Ultrasound in the differential diagnosis of medial Epicondylalgia and medial elbow pain – imaging findings and narrative literature review. Healthcare. 2022;10:1529.
23. Dębek A, Czyrny Z, Nowicki P. Sonography of pathological changes in the hand. J Ultrason. 2014;14:74–88.
24. Konin G, Nazarian LN, Walz DM. US of the elbow: indications, technique, normal anatomy, and pathologic conditions. Radiographics. 2013;33:E125–47.
25. Plotkin B, Sampath SC, Sampath SC, Motamedi K. MR imaging and US of the wrist tendons. Radiographics. 2016;36:1688–700.
26. Siddiq MAB, Hossain Parash MT. Incidental trifid median nerve unveiled in a lactating mother. Cureus. 2019;11:e5809.
27. Olchowy C, Soliński D, Łasecki M, Dąbrowski P, Urban S, Zaleska-Dorobisz U. Wrist ultrasound examination – scanning technique and ultrasound anatomy. Part 2: ventral wrist. J Ultrason. 2017;17:123–8.
28. Olchowy C, Łasecki M, Zaleska-Dorobisz U. Wrist ultrasound examination – scanning technique and ultrasound anatomy. Part 1: dorsal wrist. J Ultrason. 2015;15:172–88.
29. Siddiq MAB. de Quervain's tenosynovitis with accessory abductor pollicis Longus Tendon and

'Wartenberg's syndrome' – a case report. Curr Rheumatol Rev. 2023;19:230–4.
30. Singh JP, Kumar S, Kathiria AV, Harjai R, Jawed A, Gupta V. Thumb ultrasound: technique and pathologies. Indian J Radiol Imaging. 2016;26:386–96.
31. Mattox R, Welk AB, Battaglia PJ, Scali F, Nunez M, Kettner NW. Sonographic diagnosis of an acute Stener lesion: a case report. J Ultrasound. 2015;19:149–52.
32. Clausen S, Kjær S, Fredberg U, Terslev L, Hartvigsen J, Arnbak B. Ultrasound imaging in patients with hip pain and suspected hip osteoarthritis: an inter-rater and intra-rater reliability study. BMJ Open. 2020;10:e038643.
33. Probyn L, Flores D, Rowbotham E, Cresswell M, Atinga A. High-resolution ultrasound in the evaluation of the adult hip. J Ultrason. 2023;23:e223–38.
34. Manske RC, Wolfe C, Page P, Voight ML, Bardowski E. The utilization of diagnostic musculoskeletal ultrasound in the evaluation of gluteus medius tendon pathology: a perspective for rehabilitation providers. Int J Sports Phys Ther. 2024;19:642–5.
35. Siddiq MA, Hossain MS, Uddin MM, et al. Piriformis syndrome: a case series of 31 Bangladeshi people with literature review. Eur J Orthop Surg Traumatol. 2017;27:193–203.
36. Zhang W, Luo F, Sun H, Ding H. Ultrasound appears to be a reliable technique for the diagnosis of piriformis syndrome. Muscle Nerve. 2019;59:411–6.
37. Razek AA, Fouda NS, Elmetwaley N, Elbogdady E. Sonography of the knee joint. J Ultrasound. 2009;12:53–60.
38. Artul S, Habib G. Ultrasound findings of the painful ankle and foot. J Clin Imaging Sci. 2014;4:25.
39. Klontzas ME, Koltsakis E, Kakkos GA, Karantanas AH. Ultrasound-guided treatment of Morton's neuroma. J Ultrason. 2021;21:e134–8.
40. Lawande AD, Warrier SS, Joshi MS. Role of ultrasound in evaluation of peripheral nerves. Indian J Radiol Imaging. 2014;24:254–8.
41. Griffith JF. Practical approach to ultrasound of soft tissue tumors and the added value of MRI: how I do it. J Ultrason. 2023;23:e299–312.
42. Dejaco C, Machado PM, Carubbi F, et al. EULAR points to consider for the use of imaging to guide interventional procedures in patients with rheumatic and musculoskeletal diseases (RMDs). Ann Rheum Dis. 2022;81:760–7.
43. AIUM practice parameter for documentation of an ultrasound examination. J Ultrasound Med. 2020;39:E1–E4.
44. Tantray MD, Rather A, Manaan Q, Andleeb I, Mohammad M, Gull Y. Role of ultrasound in detection of radiolucent foreign bodies in extremities. Strategies Trauma Limb Reconstr. 2018;13:81–5.

2 Ultrasound Definitions in Rheumatology Practice

Md Abu Bakar Siddiq and Win Min Oo

2.1 Introduction

Optimal ultrasound image acquisition relies heavily on proficiently handling the transducer and executing precise movements [1]. The four fundamental movements commonly employed during ultrasound scanning are slide, rock, tilt (fan), and rotation [1]. While OMERACT provides ultrasound definitions, it has limitations, as it does not cover pathologies associated with muscle, ligament, or meniscal pathology or pathological changes due to infection [1]. This chapter expands on ultrasound pathology definitions in accordance with European Alliance of Associations for Rheumatology (EULAR) guidelines, incorporating a more comprehensive array of information [1, 2]. Ultrasound-guided definitions also encompass injection techniques, needle movement, and procedural aspects [1]. The evolution of ultrasound technology has led to substantial progress in its utility within clinical practice and research settings [2]. Innovations such as contrast-enhanced power Doppler (CEPD) and superb microvascular imaging (SMI) have played pivotal roles in enhancing the sensitivity of detecting low-flow vascularity [2, 3]. Moreover, elastography has proven to be effective in diagnosing alterations in tissue properties within inflamed synovial tissue. These advancements collectively aid in the diagnosis of diseases and monitoring of treatment responses [2]. In this chapter, terminologies related to advanced imaging have also been demonstrated.

M. A. B. Siddiq (✉)
Department of Rheumatology, Royal North Shore Hospital, Northern Clinical School, Faculty of Medicine and Health, The University of Sydney, Sydney, NSW, Australia

Sydney Musculoskeletal Health, The University of Sydney, Sydney, NSW, Australia

Kolling Institute of Medical Research, St Leonards, NSW, Australia

School of Health Sports and Professional Practice (Rheumatology), University of South Wales, Pontypridd, United Kingdom

Department of Physical Medicine and Rehabilitation, Brahmanbaria Medical College, Brahmanbaria, Bangladesh
e-mail: msid8426@uni.syndey.edu.au

W. M. Oo
Department of Rheumatology, Royal North Shore Hospital, Northern Clinical School, Faculty of Medicine and Health, The University of Sydney, Sydney, NSW, Australia

Sydney Musculoskeletal Health, The University of Sydney, Sydney, NSW, Australia

Department of Physical Medicine and Rehabilitation, University of Medicine, Mandalay, Myanmar

M. A. B. Siddiq (ed.), *Musculoskeletal Ultrasound in Rheumatic Diseases*,
https://doi.org/10.1007/978-981-96-5298-3_2

2.2 Definitions of Ultrasound Terminologies

A. **Transducer Manipulation Terminologies** [1].
   Slide: The transducer is moved across the body surface in any direction to capture images.
   Heel–toe: the transducer is moved along a fixed point in the long axis, changing the angle of insonation away from 90° to the skin surface while maintaining contact with the skin. This technique eliminates anisotropy.
   Tilt: The transducer is moved along a fixed point in the short axis, changing the angle of insonation away from 90° to the skin surface while maintaining contact with the skin. This technique eliminates anisotropy.
   Compression: The sonographer or sonologist applies force on the transducer toward the patient's body to compress the tissues to differentiate synovial effusion from synovial hypertrophy.
   Rotation: The transducer is rotated in either a clockwise or counterclockwise direction along a fixed center axis.
   Pivot: The transducer is pivoted in either a clockwise or counterclockwise direction along a fixed axis at the end of the transducer.
   Stand-off: The transducer is not in direct contact with the skin surface but is placed on a layer of acoustic coupling gel or other acoustic medium, with an angle of insonation at 90° to the skin surface.
   Oblique stand-off: The transducer is not in direct contact with the skin surface but is placed on a layer of acoustic coupling gel or other acoustic medium, with the angle of insonation away from 90° to the skin surface.
   Sono-palpation: Force is applied on the transducer toward the patient's body to elicit symptom provocation, such as pain.
B. **Ultrasound Definitions of Tissue Pathologies** [1].
   (i) **Tendon**
   Tendinopathy: Distressing ailments of the tendon or tendon sheath, encompassing tendinosis, tendinitis, and tendon tear.
   Tendinosis: The tendon appears abnormally hypoechoic without disruption of the tendon fibers, potentially showing an enlargement in the diameter of the tendon, with or without Doppler imaging flow.
   Tendinitis: An abnormally hypoechoic tendon may sometimes be observed, along with potential increased flow on Doppler imaging.
   Calcific tendinopathy: Calcific deposits in tendons; for example, calcium hydroxyapatite appears as a well-defined, globular, and hyperechoic focus within the tendon, with the possibility of variable shadowing. Small punctate or linear calcifications within the tendon may also be caused by calcium pyrophosphate dihydrate deposition disease or degenerative calcification.
   Tenosynovitis: An inflammation of the synovial sheath enveloping a tendon. It is characterized by the expansion of the tendon sheath caused by the presence of fluid with variable echogenicity. This fluid accumulation can occur with or without synovial hypertrophy, and Doppler imaging may reveal an increase in blood flow in certain cases.
   Stenosing tenosynovitis: Hypoechoic thickening of the pulley or retinaculum accompanied by potential hyperemia with or without additional tendinosis and tenosynovitis.
   Paratenonitis: Focal or diffuse abnormal hypoechogenicity surrounding the tendon, with potential increased flow observed on Doppler imaging.
   Tear: Disruption of tendon fibers, which can be classified as either partial thickness (interstitial, intrasubstance, bursal, or articular) or full thickness (focal or complete). In cases where a tubular tendon is involved, a longitudinal split tear may also be described. The extent of hypoechoic or anechoic tendon fiber disruption is delineated by the categories listed in the definition. Longitudinal tears exhibit a hypoechoic or anechoic abnor-

mality that is aligned parallel to the long axis of the tendon.

Avulsion: Tearing of a tendon at its point of attachment to a bone or a fracture occurring at the site where a tendon is attached.

(ii) **Muscle**

Strain: Characterize muscle injuries; however, because of its ambiguous definition, its application varies inconsistently across different cases.

Tear: Heightened echogenicity in intact muscle tissue or as partial or complete disruption of muscle or musculo-tendinous structures, potentially accompanied by hemorrhage of varying echogenicity. Doppler imaging may reveal increased flow in the affected area.

Contusion: Injured muscle with disrupted muscle fibers can create an area with mixed echogenicity, which appears hyperechoic in acute cases and anechoic in chronic cases. Additionally, the presence of a hematoma can cause a mass effect, and Doppler imaging may reveal an increase in blood flow.

Myositis ossificans: Initially, appearing hyperechoic, it progresses to form a hypoechoic mass-like region within the muscle, with hyperechoic foci evolving into an echogenic outer rim that may exhibit acoustic shadowing. Doppler imaging may reveal an increase in blood flow.

Myositis: Elevated muscle echogenicity with potential alterations in muscle architecture, increased muscle size during acute episodes, and variable heightened flow on Doppler imaging.

Pyomyositis: Presence of a muscle abscess, which is a circumscribed heterogeneous fluid collection exhibiting a range of echogenicity from anechoic to hyperechoic. Additionally, it is increased through transmission, and increased peripheral flow is often observed on Doppler imaging.

Fatty infiltration: Accumulation of fat within muscle tissue due to various factors, such as disuse, dysfunction, injury, or denervation. When muscle size is also reduced, the term atrophy is used to describe the condition. This may present as diffuse increased muscle echogenicity along with a potential decrease in muscle size in cases of atrophy.

(iii) **Ligament**

Sprain: Sprains are often used interchangeably to describe various types of ligament injuries.

Tear: Damage to ligament fibers, which can range from partial to complete disruption of the ligament. The extent of disruption can be observed through stress imaging, with variations in echogenicity and ligament thickness. Doppler imaging may reveal increased flow in cases of tear.

Avulsion: Ligament is torn at its attachment to the bone or when a fracture occurs at the ligament attachment site.

(iv) **Synovium and Bursa**

Effusion: Anechoic and compressible accumulation; however, they may have different echogenicity levels depending on their composition.

Synovial hypertrophy and synovitis: Thick, hypoechoic, and poorly compressible synovium (synovial hypertrophy) with increased Doppler signal (synovitis).

Synovial proliferation: Thickening of the synovium due to noninflammatory causes, such as pigmented villonodular synovitis, lipoma arborescens, and synovial chondromatosis, which may often be mineralized. Like in synovial hypertrophy, the echogenicity of the thickened synovium is variable, and it appears as noncompressible or minimally compressible synovial thickening or mass-like structures. The flow on Doppler imaging can also vary.

Bursitis: Inflammation of a bursa. The presentation of bursitis can vary depending on the underlying pathology, which can include effusion, synovial hypertrophy, synovial proliferation, and synovitis.

Doppler imaging may reveal increased flow in cases of bursitis.

Hyperemia: An elevation in blood flow, which can be attributed to the development of new blood vessels (neovascularity) in conditions such as tendinosis and tumors or to the expansion of blood vessels (vasodilation) due to inflammation in instances such as inflammatory synovitis or infection.

(v) **Nerve**

Neuropathy: Neuropathy is a comprehensive term that encompasses various nerve conditions. The nature of these conditions varies depending on the specific pathological process involved.

Compressive neuropathy: Nerve dysfunction resulting from nerve entrapment or extrinsic impingement. This condition is identified by the hypoechoic appearance of the nerve, which is caused by epineural edema. Additionally, there may be fascicular enlargement, typically proximal to the compression site, and sometimes distal as well.

Transection: Partial or complete discontinuity of a nerve caused by the disruption of some or all its fascicles. In cases of transection, there is a discontinuity of the nerve fascicles, which may lead to retraction of the nerve. At the retracted end, there may be focal or mass-like thickening, which is known as a neuroma.

Neuroma: Focal enlargement of an injured nerve or fascicle, often associated with nerve or fascicular retraction. It is characterized by hypoechoic focal nerve or fascicle enlargement at the site of injury.

Neuritis: Neuritis is the inflammation of a nerve, which can be observed in inflammatory, infectious, or autoimmune conditions. Neuritis is identified by an abnormally hypoechoic nerve and may present increased flow on Doppler imaging.

(vi) **Fascia**

Fasciopathy: Various fascial conditions, with the presentation varying depending on the specific pathological process involved.

Fasciosis: A chronic condition that is histologically characterized by degeneration, collagen necrosis, angiofibrotic hyperplasia, chondroid metaplasia, and fibrosis. On ultrasound, hypoechoic thickening of the fascia, calcification, and increased flow on Doppler imaging are possible features.

Fasciitis: Inflammation of the fascia, presenting with hypoechoic thickening of the fascia and possibly increased flow on Doppler imaging.

Tear: A tear in the fascia involves injury to the fascial fibers, which can range from partial to complete disruption. Tears may exhibit variable echogenicity and thickness, along with possible hemorrhages of variable echogenicity. Complete disruption may result in loss of tension, and increased flow on Doppler imaging is also a potential finding.

(vii) **Bone**

Osteophytes: Bony outgrowths located at the edge of a synovial joint that are often observed in patients with osteoarthritis. This bony excrescence is typically hyperechoic and found at the periphery of a synovial articulation.

Enthesophytes: Bony growth is situated at the attachment site of a tendon, ligament, or fascia and is commonly associated with overuse, tension, previous injury, or adjacent tendinosis. This hyperechoic bony excrescence can be well defined or ill defined, potentially showing erosions and increased flow on Doppler imaging.

Erosion: Cortical discontinuity found in a subsynovial or enthesis location, often because of inflammation caused by infection or inflammatory arthritis. This loss of continuity in the hyperechoic cortical bone surface may be accompanied by synovial hypertrophy. Additionally, Doppler imaging may reveal an increase in flow in the affected area.

Subluxation: Partial displacement of a structure from its usual anatomical position, particularly evident during dynamic movements. It is crucial to avoid using the nonstandard terms "sublux" and "subluxed" and instead utilize "subluxate" and "subluxation" in accordance with accepted English language conventions.

Dislocation: Complete displacement of a structure from its regular anatomical position, which is particularly noticeable during dynamic maneuvers.

C. **Definitions of Ultrasound-Guided Procedural Landmarks**

Consensus statements on ultrasound-guided procedural landmarks have been developed by the American Institute of Ultrasound in Medicine (AIUM) and the American Medical Society for Sports Medicine (AMSSM) via the Delphi method. These statements provide a standardized framework for healthcare experts, ensuring accurate identification of landmarks during ultrasound-guided interventions. These are presented in Table 2.1 [1].

Table 2.1 Ultrasound terms for guided intervention

Term	Definition
Needle/device terminology	
In-plane	Needle/device aligned with the long axis of the transducer
Out-of-plane	Needle/device aligned perpendicular to the long axis of the transducer
Jiggling	Rapid, low-amplitude movement of the needle/device in the plane of insertion to facilitate needle visualization
Rotation	Rotating the needle will result in the bevel alternately facing up and down, thus enabling identification of the needle tip
Stylet movement	Small movements of a stylet in and out of the tip of the needle to improve needle tip visualization; the stylet should not be modified to allow it to advance beyond the needle tip when using this technique for visualization
Procedure technique descriptions	
Aponeurotomy	Cutting an aponeurosis, either completely or incompletely, using a needle, scalpel, or other device
Aspiration	The act of removing fluid, calcification or other crystalline material, blood, pus, or other substance from the body typically using a needle and syringe, catheter, or another device
Barbotage	Repeated injection and aspiration of fluid to break up and remove calcification, usually within a tendon
Brisement	The injection of fluid into the space between a tendon and its paratenon or sheath; brisement has also been used to refer to injection of saline or other fluid into a joint to break down adhesions (e.g., in treatment of adhesive capsulitis)
Debridement	The removal of necrotic, degenerative, or infected tissue from a region or given tissue of the body
Dry needling	A procedure, generally used as part of manual physical therapy, where a small gauge needle is inserted into a muscle or other soft tissue structure to treat myofascial pain
Fasciotomy	Cutting fascia, either completely or incompletely, using a needle, scalpel, or other device
Fenestration	The act of repetitive puncture of a soft tissue structure with a needle or other device
Fragmentation	The use of a needle or other device to break up calcified and/or bony tissue
Hydrodissection	Technique by which saline or other sterile fluid is injected to separate tissues or tissue planes from each other
Injection	The act of delivering a fluid or other substance into the body, typically using a needle and syringe, catheter, or another device

(continued)

Table 2.1 (continued)

Term	Definition
Lavage	Washing out using saline or other sterile solution; irrigation is an acceptable alternate term
Neurolysis	There are distinct definitions of neurolysis. An appropriate modifier is recommended to clearly describe the procedure performed
Chemical neurolysis	The application of chemical agents to a nerve in order to cause temporary or permanent degeneration of targeted nerve fibers
Hydroneurolysis	The injection of saline or other sterile fluid to free nerves from surrounding tissue/adhesion; the term "nerve hydrodissection" is an acceptable alternate term
Surgical neurolysis	The surgical freeing of nerves from surrounding tissue/adhesion
Physical neurolysis	The application of physical energy (e.g., heat or cold) to a nerve in order to cause temporary or permanent degeneration of the targeted nerve fibers
Plantar fasciotomy	Cutting the plantar fascia, either completely or incompletely, using a needle, scalpel, or other device
Tendon scraping	The process of abrading the surface of a tendon or paratenon with a needle, scalpel, or other device, with the goal of separating the tendon from neovessels, neonerves, and/or adjacent soft tissues
Tenotomy	Cutting tendon tissue, either completely or incompletely, using a needle, scalpel, or other device
Trigger finger release	Cutting the pulley and associated tendon sheath responsible for the stenosis using a needle, scalpel, or other device
Terms to avoid	
Minimally invasive, ultra minimally invasive, and microinvasive	These are relative and imprecise terms without formal definitions. Therefore, their use is not recommended. The exact procedure should be described including technique and tool(s) used
Needling	This is an inconsistent term that has been used to describe a range of procedures from dry needling of myofascial trigger points to tenotomy or fasciotomy procedures. The use of a more precise term is recommended. "Needling" should only be used in conjunction with "dry needling" as previously defined
Peppering	This term has been used to describe a type of fenestration procedure (often involving a tendon) alone or in conjunction with an injection. The use of more precise terms such as "tenotomy," "fasciotomy," or "fenestration" is recommended
Percutaneous	This term refers to a procedure performed through the skin. Due to lack of specificity associated with this term, its use in isolation is not recommended. Rather, the exact procedural technique should be described including tool(s) used and approach

2.3 Definitions Related to Advanced Ultrasound Imaging

Superb Microvascular Imaging (SMI) Imaging techniques play crucial roles in the diagnosis, monitoring, and prognosis of rheumatic diseases. For example, magnetic resonance imaging (MRI) has been useful in the early diagnosis of axial spondyloarthritis, whereas positron-emission tomography (PECT) is helpful in the diagnosis of large vessel vasculitis, and dual-energy computed tomography (DECT) is effective in detecting crystal deposition in patients with crystal arthropathy [2]. In addition, ultrasound has also made significant contributions to the field of rheumatology and is now considered an extension of clinical examination [2].

Ultrasound further helps in monitoring inflammatory arthritis treatment [2]. In rheumatoid arthritis (RA), ultrasound PD can identify subclinical inflammatory activity in patients in clinical remission [2]. This finding holds prognostic value, as it can help predict disease flares and structural damage [2]. However, conventional PD may not always detect low-flow synovial vascularity, necessitating the use of new techniques such as SMI [3]. Compared with PD, SMI offers greater resolution, greater sensitivity for slow-flow vessels, and fewer motion artifacts and could be a valuable tool in cases where PD fails [2, 3]. SMI has shown promise in detecting superficial thrombophlebitis in Behcet's disease [4].

In patients with knee OA, the SMI and PD are significantly correlated with knee injury and osteoarthritis outcome scores, radiographic features, MRI effusion-synovitis, and Hoffa's synovitis scores [3]. However, SMI appears to detect low-grade inflammation in OA disease better than PD and is significantly correlated with symptoms, radiographic features, and MRI synovitis [5]. In a recent meta-analysis, the SMI was proven to be useful for characterizing low-flow vascularity, and increasing evidence indicates that the SMI is a noninvasive and low-cost tool for prognostic assessment, especially in patients with inflammatory arthritis. Preliminary findings also suggest potential interest in evaluating the effect of treatment [6]. The added clinical value of SMI over PD is still not clear [5].

Contrast-Enhanced Ultrasound Contrast-enhanced ultrasound (CEUS) involves the administration of intravenous contrast agents consisting of microbubbles/nanobubbles of gas and is useful for accurate detection of microcirculation, synovial thickness, and tissue selection in ultrasound-guided synovial biopsy [7, 8]. Another experimental study reported greater synovial hypervascularity and hyperplasia with CEUS than with unenhanced ultrasound [9]. CEUS also enables the evaluation of enhancement kinetics to increase the detection of disease activity [9]. The diagnostic performance of SMI was recently compared with that of CEUS in rheumatoid arthritis (RA) for both clinically active patients and patients in remission [10]. The study revealed that the detection rate of synovial vascularity was greater with CEUS than with SMI, with no significant difference between the two modalities. Furthermore, in patients with RA in clinical remission, CEUS results in a higher synovial vascularity rate than does SMI, with no significant difference between the two modalities [10]. The vascularity scores of SMI and CEUS are positively associated with elevated serum biomarkers in patients with active RA but not in those with clinical remission [10]. Further studies are needed for large-scale application in day-to-day clinical practice [8].

Elastography In the realm of ultrasound technology, elastography has become a valuable tool for quantitatively studying the mechanical and microenvironmental properties of tissue [11]. This method is commonly categorized into two types: strain elastography (SE) and shear wave elastography (SWE) [11]. SE focuses on changes in tissue texture when exposed to an external force, offering a semiquantitative analysis of tissue resistance based on a reference tissue [11]. In contrast, the SWE provides a quantitative evaluation by detecting fluctuations in internal shear wave velocities [11]. SE heavily relies on user input, whereas SWE is not influenced by user factors [11].

SWE is currently being extensively researched to assess the qualitative and quantitative elastic properties of muscles, tendons, nerves, ligaments, and different types of tumors [12]. One of the significant applications of SWE is its ability to distinguish between RA and tuberculous arthritis by analyzing the elastic properties of the synovium [12]. In an initial pilot study conducted in Latin America, the mean SWE and elastic modulus in the synovium of RA patients were significantly lower than those in the control group [13]. The risk of liver fibrosis in RA patients treated with methotrexate (MTX) has been revealed via ultrasound elastography (acoustic radiation force impulse, ARFI) [14], but no evidence of an increased occurrence of liver fibrosis among RA patients receiving MTX treatment has been reported [14].

Notably, ultrasound ARFI is more sensitive than grayscale ultrasound and is valuable in the diagnosis of Sjögren's syndrome (SS) as well as in screening for skin involvement in systemic sclerosis (SSc) and psoriasis [15]. SWE is strongly correlated with disease activity and offers greater reliability than the modified

Rodnan skin score (mRSS), thereby serving as a valuable tool in the diagnosis of SSc [16]. In the case of SS, there is a positive correlation between SWE and minor salivary gland biopsy (MSGB) findings, particularly in areas with increased lymphoid infiltration. This correlation highlights the ability of SWE to accurately reflect the histopathological chronicity of MSGB in SS patients [17].

Muscle stiffness, as determined by SWE, does not appear to be linked to muscle weakness in individuals with RA [18]. In the context of idiopathic inflammatory myopathy (IIM), ultrasound has proven to be a valuable diagnostic screening tool, particularly in cases where inclusion body myositis or necrotizing autoimmune myopathy is suspected [19]. In healthy controls, age was inversely correlated with shear wave speed (SWS), and PD individuals aged 50 years or older presented lower SWS than did those below the age of 50 [20].Like high-frequency ultrasound, SWE has the potential to serve as an imaging biomarker for the diagnosis of IIM by detecting abnormal muscle thinning, enhanced muscle echo intensity, and reduced muscle shear wave velocity [20].

Elastography is a valuable technique for diagnosing and managing soft tissue rheumatism [11, 22, 23]. For example, SWE has been shown to accurately identify latent trigger points in myofascial pain syndrome [11]. Both SE and SWE are equally effective in diagnosing lateral epicondylitis (LE) [21]. SWE is particularly useful for monitoring the therapeutic response in LE [22]. While a limited number of studies have investigated quantitative elastography in patients with Achilles tendinopathy, none have demonstrated the diagnostic superiority of elastography in patients with Achilles tendon pathologies in clinical practice [23]. Further validation studies are necessary to evaluate the discrimination, reliability, and feasibility of elastography in various rheumatic conditions.

In summary, there has been a growing trend in the application of ultrasound for diagnosing rheumatic ailments. Elastography aids in assessing tissue elasticity, whereas compared with power Doppler, contrast-enhanced and superb microvascular imaging techniques improve the detection of tissue vascularity in inflammatory rheumatic disorders.

Conflict of Interest MAB is supported by a Faculty of Medicine and Health Executive Dean Stipend scholarship, University of Sydney, Australia for his PhD course.

References

1. Hall MM, Allen GM, Allison S, et al. Recommended musculoskeletal and sports ultrasound terminology: a Delphi-based consensus statement. Br J Sports Med. 2022;56:310–9.
2. Almeida DE, Costa E, Cerqueira M. Advances in ultrasound imaging in rheumatology – what do they mean and what challenges do they pose? The example of microvascular imaging. J Ultrasound Med. 2022;41:785–7.
3. Yu X, Li Z, Ren M, Xi J, Wu J, Ji Y. Superb microvascular imaging (SMI) for evaluating hand joint lesions in patients with rheumatoid arthritis in clinical remission. Rheumatol Int. 2018;38:1885–90.
4. Kayadibi Y, Ozguler Y, Melikoglu M, et al. OP0169 vessel wall inflammation detected with superb microvascular imaging in Behcet syndrome. Ann Rheum Dis. 2023;82:112–3.
5. Oo WM, Linklater JM, Bennell KL, et al. Superb microvascular imaging in low-grade inflammation of knee osteoarthritis compared with power Doppler: clinical, radiographic and MRI relationship. Ultrasound Med Biol. 2020;46:566–74.
6. Seskute G, Jasionyte G, Rugiene R, Butrimiene I. The use of superb microvascular imaging in evaluating rheumatic diseases: a systematic review. Medicina (Kaunas). 2023;11(59):1641.
7. Czarniecki M, Campos A, McKay L, et al. Contrast-enhanced ultrasound. Radiopaedia.org. Accessed 13 Jul 2024. https://doi.org/10.53347/rID-27413.
8. Gong Y, Huang Y, Su Y, He J, Chen S. Value of contrast-enhanced ultrasonography in evaluating rheumatoid arthritis: preliminary research based on an animal model. Med Sci Monit. 2021;27:e931327.
9. Liu H, Huang C, Chen S, et al. Value of contrast-enhanced ultrasound for detection of synovial vascularity in experimental rheumatoid arthritis: an exploratory study. J Int Med Res. 2019;47:5740–51.
10. Diao XH, Yan Shen Y, Chen L, et al. Superb microvascular imaging is as sensitive as contrast-enhanced ultrasound for detecting synovial vascularity in rheumatoid arthritis. Quant Imaging Med Surg. 2022;12:2866–76.

11. Ertekin E, Kasar ZS, Turkdogan FT. Is early diagnosis of myofascial pain syndrome possible with the detection of latent trigger points by shear wave elastography? Pol J Radiol. 2021;86:e425–31.
12. Chandel K, Prakash M, Sinha A, Sharma A, Chouhan DK, Sandhu MS. Role of shear wave Elastography of synovium to differentiate rheumatoid and tubercular arthritis. J Med Ultrasound. 2021;30:30–5.
13. Sedano O, Sedano J. AB1547 shear-wave elastographic ultrasound of second metacarpophalangeal in synovium of rheumatoid arthritis. Ann Rheum Dis. 2023;82:2007.
14. Feuchtenberger M, Kraus L, Nigg A, et al. Methotrexate does not increase the risk of liver fibrosis in patients with rheumatoid arthritis: assessment by ultrasound elastography (ARFI-MetRA study). Rheumatol Int. 2021;41:1079–87.
15. Martins-Rocha T, Azzolin I, Serban T, Massazza G, Iagnocco A. New applications of sonoelastography in rheumatology: where are we now? Rheumatology. 2019;58:765–9.
16. Cai R, Lin Z, Xu D, Sun Y, Cui L, Mu R. The value of shear wave elastography in diagnosis and assessment of systemic sclerosis. Rheumatol Adv Pract. 2023;7:rkad075.
17. Park Y, Oh M, Lee YS, et al. Salivary ultrasonography and histopathologic evaluation of secondary Sjögren's syndrome in rheumatoid arthritis patients. Sci Rep. 2023;13:11339.
18. Alfuraih AM, Tan AL, O'connor P, et al. FRI0631 muscle stiffness and weakness in rheumatoid arthritis – a shear wave elastography study. Ann Rheum Dis. 2019;78:1013.
19. Paramalingam S, Needham M, Raymond W, et al. Muscle shear wave elastography, conventional B mode and power Doppler ultrasonography in healthy adults and patients with autoimmune inflammatory myopathies: a pilot cross-sectional study. BMC Musculoskelet Disord. 2021;22:537.
20. Li M, Guo R, Tang X, Huang S, Qiu L. Quantitative assessment of muscle properties in polymyositis and dermatomyositis using high-frequency ultrasound and shear wave elastography. Quant Imaging Med Surg. 2023;13:428–40.
21. Hong S, Hahn S, Yi J, Park EJ, Bang JY. Comparing the clinical application of strain elastography and shear wave elastography for the evaluation of lateral epicondylitis. J Clin Ultrasound. 2023;51:123–30.
22. Elsayed M, Hafez MRM, Ibrahim MAH. Ultrasound with shear wave elastography in diagnosis and follow-up of common extensor tendinopathy in cases with lateral epicondylitis: a cross-sectional analytic study. Egypt J Radiol Nucl Med. 2022;53:236.
23. Mifsud T, Gatt A, Micallef-Stafrace K, Chockalingam N, Padhiar N. Elastography in the assessment of the Achilles tendon: a systematic review of measurement properties. J Foot Ankle Res. 2023;16:23.

Diagnostic Imaging Tools in Rheumatology Practice, with a Focus on Comparison with Ultrasound

3

Md Abu Bakar Siddiq, Syed Atiqul Haq, David Hunter, Yasser Ragab, and Johannes J. Rasker

3.1 Introduction

Conventional radiography (CR) is commonly utilized in rheumatic disease diagnosis [1–5]. Radiology features, including reduced joint space width, osteophytes, subchondral sclerosis and cysts, cortical erosions, cortical breach, juxta-articular osteopenia, soft tissue swelling, and joint dislocation or subluxation, help in the diagnosis of musculoskeletal disorders [1, 2]. However, X-rays cannot depict active synovial inflammation in arthritis, necessitating the use of more advanced imaging modalities [6, 7], such as magnetic resonance imaging (MRI), computed tomography (CT)/dual-energy computed tomography (DECT), ultrasound, and arthroscopy [8–10].

Grayscale ultrasound combined with the power Doppler technique improves the visualization of low-flow vascularity in synovial inflammation [6, 7]; nevertheless, it cannot replace the role of MRI in such a context [6, 7]. Contrast-enhanced (CE) MRI (CE-MRI), DECT, and ultrasound superb microvascular imaging (SMI) further detect low-

M. A. B. Siddiq (✉)
Department of Rheumatology, Royal North Shore Hospital, Northern Clinical School, Faculty of Medicine and Health, The University of Sydney, Sydney, NSW, Australia

Sydney Musculoskeletal Health, The University of Sydney, Sydney, NSW, Australia

Kolling Institute of Medical Research, St Leonards, NSW, Australia

School of Health Sports and Professional Practice (Rheumatology), University of South Wales, Pontypridd, United Kingdom

Department of Physical Medicine and Rehabilitation, Brahmanbaria Medical College, Brahmanbaria, Bangladesh
e-mail: msid8426@uni.sydney.edu.au

S. A. Haq
Department of Rheumatology, GreenLife Medical College, Dhaka, Bangladesh

D. Hunter
Department of Rheumatology, Royal North Shore Hospital, Northern Clinical School, Faculty of Medicine and Health, The University of Sydney, Sydney, NSW, Australia

Sydney Musculoskeletal Health, The University of Sydney, Sydney, NSW, Australia

Y. Ragab
Department of Radiology, University of Cairo, Cairo, Egypt

J. J. Rasker
Faculty of Behavioral Sciences, Psychology, Health and Technology, University of Twente, Enschede, The Netherlands

M. A. B. Siddiq (ed.), *Musculoskeletal Ultrasound in Rheumatic Diseases*,
https://doi.org/10.1007/978-981-96-5298-3_3

flow vascularity in inflamed synovium [6–8, 11, 12]. MRI and ultrasound further help monitor treatment efficacy in patients with arthritis [13].

MRI and DECT are effective modalities for assessing cortical erosions and subchondral bone marrow lesions (BMLs), as well as for monitoring the full extent of intra-articular (IA) ligaments, areas where ultrasound has limited applicability [6, 7, 11]. In contrast to conventional arthroscopy, the IA ultrasound technique offers quantitative assessments of cartilage integrity and thickness [14]. Delayed gadolinium-enhanced MRI of cartilage and T2 mapping could serve as valuable alternative diagnostic methods for differentiating between healthy and compromised cartilage [15]. This chapter emphasizes the role of CR, MRI, CT, and arthroscope compared with ultrasound in the field of rheumatology.

3.2 Radiology

X-rays are widely used in rheumatology practice and research [1, 2]. In clinical settings, the focus is on describing specific features, whereas in research, various radiological scores are used to document joint space width, joint ankylosis, bone erosion, sclerotic changes, osteophyte formation, and fractures, which aid in diagnosing disease and measuring disease progression [1].

In *osteoarthritis (OA)*, characteristic features include radiographic joint space narrowing, marginal osteophytes, subchondral cysts, sclerosis, and deformities [2]. OA may be associated with pseudogout (calcium pyrophosphate dihydrate, CPPD) and CR can reveal increased radio-opacity within the articular cartilage, with fibrocartilage (e.g., meniscus and triangular fibrocartilage complex of the wrist) being observed in approximately 40% of cases, with a higher prevalence as age advances [3].

Pseudogout can sometimes be mistaken for gout, which is characterized by radiographic soft tissue swelling, bone erosion with sclerotic changes, and overhanging bony edges (Fig. 3.1) [4]. In preclinical research, dark-field radiography has shown promise in detecting crystals in gout, although its effectiveness in clinical research has yet to be fully established [5].

The role of CR in the diagnosis of autoimmune arthritis is significant [6, 7]. In the case of *rheumatoid arthritis (RA)*, X-ray imaging reveals features such as juxta-articular osteopenia, erosive changes, diminished joint space, and deformities [6]. Conversely, *psoriatic arthritis* (PsA) is characterized by distinct manifestations, including dactylitis, joint ankylosis, bone erosion, periosteal reactions, and the presence of an ivory phalanx (increased radiodensity due to periosteal and endosteal bone formation) [7]. Enthesitis around the joints of the fingers and toes but also the knees are found not only in PsA patients [16–18] but also in psoriasis patients without overt PsA [19]. These may be visualized with CR but rather with MRI and ultrasound. In advanced PsA, severe erosive changes, including pencil-in-cup deformities and telescoping fingers associated with arthritis mutilans [7, 16], can also be found in RA patients, especially after long-term corticosteroid treatment [20]. In the vertebral column, CR may reveal chunky bridging osteophytes (additional layer on the anterior longitudinal ligament) in diffuse idiopathic skeletal hyperostosis, whereas ankylosing spondylitis (AS) typically presents with thinner, marginal, and symmetrical syndesmophytes, indicative of ossification at the enthesis of the anterior longitudinal ligament and the annulus fibrosus [7, 21].

Enthesitis is the diagnostic hallmark of spondyloarthritis (SpA) [22]. Within the context of SpA, heel discomfort resulting from conditions such as plantar fasciitis and Achilles tendinitis may lead to radiological evidence of bone erosion in the calcaneus, a distinguishing feature between SpA and mechanical heel pain [22]. Enthesitis may manifest at both the lateral and medial aspects of the elbow, complicating the differentiation from mechanical to lateral and medial epicondylitis, respectively, thus necessitating advanced imaging techniques for accurate diagnosis [22].

Noninflammatory focal soft tissue rheumatism can impact various other anatomical regions, including the trigger finger, tendinopathy, plantar fasciitis, ligament tear, subacromial subdeltoid bursitis, de Quervain's tenosynovitis, frozen shoulder syndrome, myofascial pain syndrome, carpal tunnel syndrome, and radial neuritis [23, 24], where conventional X-ray is inadequate, thereby requiring more sophisticated imaging modalities (Fig. 3.1) for diagnosis and treatment monitoring. For example, in shoulder adhesive capsulitis, ultrasound-guided anterior hydrodilatation is more effective than the posterior approach [25].

Osteoporosis (OP) is diagnosed based on bone mineral density, and X-ray can reveal osteopenia [24]. In the presence of risk factors, radiological osteopenia and reduced vertebral body height provide diagnostic clues for OP [26]. Increased radiological bone density with osteosclerosis is observed in PsA, Paget's disease, fluorosis, metastasis, systemic sclerosis, osteopoikilosis, etc. [20]. CR cannot be used to make an early diagnosis but rather results in structural changes at the advanced disease stage [27]. Sometimes, other techniques, such as MRI, are needed for differentiation. An inexpensive method to measure osteoporosis is calcaneal quantitative ultrasound, which is often applied in developing countries; this method can be recommended as a prescreening method for osteoporosis to reduce the number of dual-energy X-ray absorptiometry measurements [28].

If a patient is suspected of having early RA, examination via X-ray of the hands and feet shows rather poor sensitivity to define radiological erosion typical for RA, especially in seronegative patients with normal acute-phase reactant levels [6, 29]. As early RA manifestations are nonosseous in nature, ultrasound and MRI have been shown to be superior to radiographs and CT [30]. Identifying radiological changes in AS takes years and is not useful in early cases [31].

The ability of ultrasound and clinical investigations, as well as CR, to detect *rheumatoid synovitis* has been explored [32]. In early synovitis, grayscale ultrasound has been shown to be more efficient than clinical methods [32]. A systematic review of the literature highlighted the diagnostic superiority of MRI, PET, and ultra-

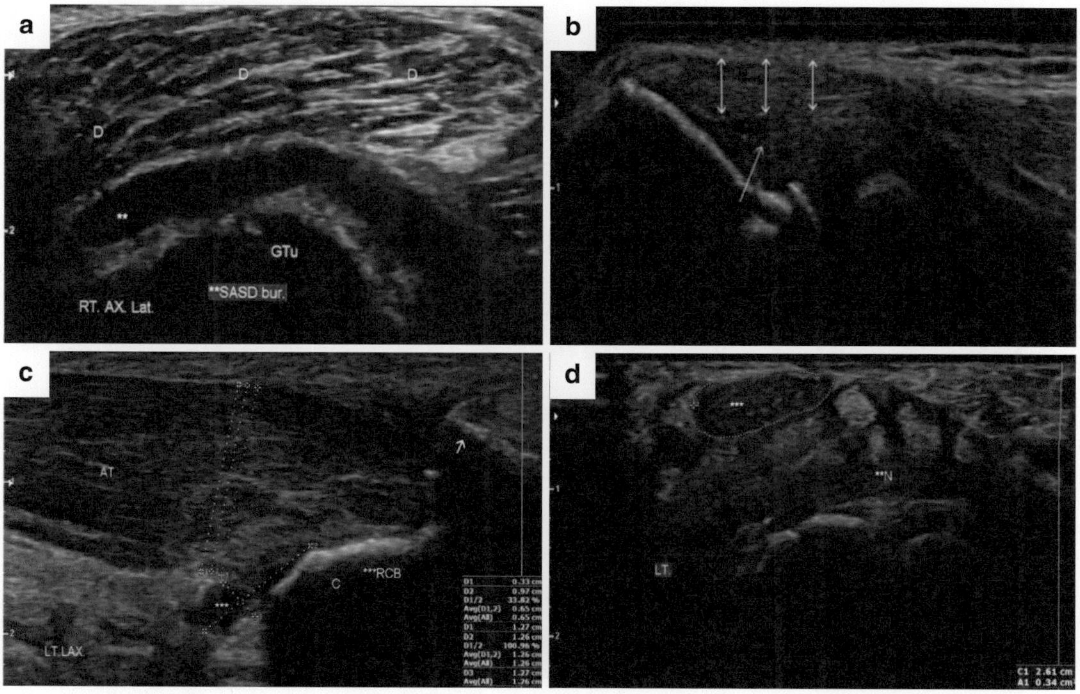

Fig. 3.1 Grayscale ultrasound scan in soft tissue rheumatism. (**a**) Short axis scan of the lateral shoulder reveals SASD bursal wall thickening with anechoic and compressible collection. (**b**) Long axis scan of the lateral elbow shows hypoechoic and thick common extensor tendon (double arrows), RCL tear (white arrow), and distal humeral cortical defect. (**c**) Longitudinal scan of the posterior heel depicts Achilles tendon thick and hypoechoic with loss of fibrillar pattern and anechoic compressible collection in the RCB (asterisks). (**d**) Short axis scan of the volar wrist unveils an increased cross-sectional area of the hypoechoic median nerve at the carpal tunnel (asterisks). *AX* axial, *AT* Achilles tendon, *C* calcaneus, *D* deltoid, *GTu* greater tuberosity, *LAX* long axis, *LT* left, *RCB* retrocalcaneal bursa, SASD subacromial subdeltoid

sound over X-rays in subacromial-subdeltoid bursitis in polymyalgia rheumatica (PMR) [33]. However, study heterogeneity, blinding, and potential bias have impacted the interpretation of these findings [33].

The prevalence of inflammatory and structural changes is high in hereditary *hemochromatosis arthropathy (HHA)* [34]. Overall, ultrasound synovitis and osteophytes are comparable between HHA and hand OA (HOA); however, the extent of cartilage deterioration is significantly greater in HHA than in HOA [34]. Inflammation and cartilage damage scores are most elevated in HHA metacarpophalangeal joints, whereas the scores for osteophytes and grayscale synovitis appear greater in the proximal and distal interphalangeal joints in the HOA group [34].

Ultrasound has proven to be a valuable tool for providing additional diagnostic information in suspected *gout or pseudogout,* especially when traditional laboratory tests and X-ray results are inconclusive (Fig. 3.2) [4]. The EULAR recom-

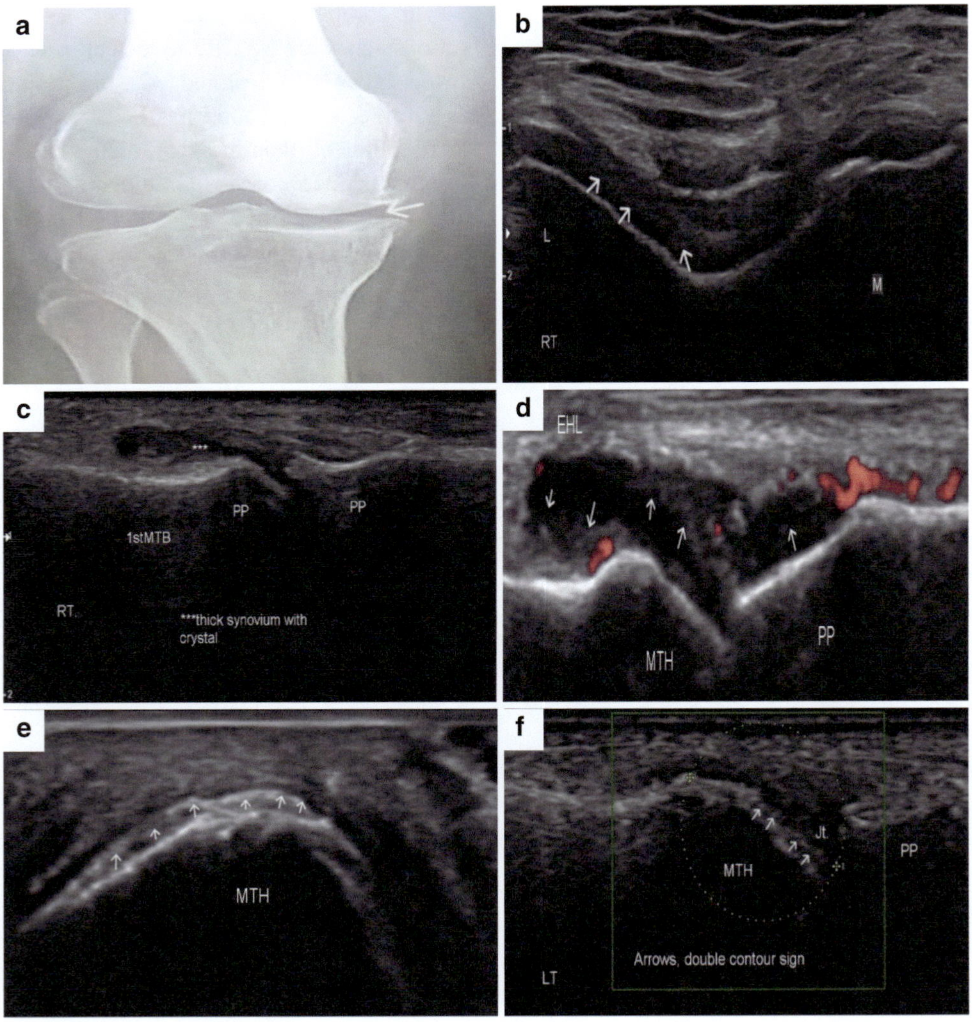

Fig. 3.2 X-ray and grayscale ultrasound scan in pseudogout and gout. (**a**) X-ray antero-posterior knee reveals radioopacity in the medial meniscus (arrow). (**b**) Suprapatellar transverse scan unveiling echogenic femoral condylar cartilage due to CPPD deposition (arrows) in knee OA. (**c**, **d**) Longitudinal ultrasound scans of the anterior first metatarsophalangeal (MTP) joint explore thick and hypoechoic synovial hypertrophy (asterisks) with increased Doppler activity (red spots) in gout (**d**) (**e**, **f**) Short and longitudinal axes scans, respectively show Double contour sign (arrows) over the MTH in clinically diagnosed gout. *EHL* extensor hallucis longus, *LT* left, *MTB* metatarsal bone, *MTH* metatarsal head, *PP* proximal phalanx, *RT* right

mends the use of ultrasound or DECT to evaluate CPPD crystals [10]. Ultrasound and DECT play crucial roles in monitoring crystal accumulation and assessing inflammation [4]. When ultrasound or DECT is unavailable, CR can be utilized to evaluate structural damage associated with gout [10]. Although not used in gout diagnosis routinely, MRI can identify soft tissue inflammation as well as cortical erosion and intraosseous urate crystal deposits [35, 36].

3.3 Computed Tomography

Compared with ultrasound and MRI, standard CT cannot provide detailed differentiation of soft tissues to detect synovitis, enthesitis, or bone marrow edema (BME) [37, 38]. However, the introduction of DECT into clinical rheumatology practice has explored a new avenue for CT imaging [39]. DECT has better sensitivity and specificity than ultrasound in gout diagnosis [31, 40]. Identification of sodium urate crystals in aspirated fluid is the diagnostic gold standard in gout; however, the inclusion of noninvasive DECT improves the diagnostic accuracy of gout classification criteria [10, 40–43], which is useful especially in cases where joint fluid studies are not feasible [10, 40, 41]. Updated criteria demonstrated that both DECT and ultrasound can predict gout flares and monitor treatment efficacy, with ultrasound being the preferred choice for assessing inflammation [10].

Ultrasound has been increasingly used in diagnosing and monitoring treatment efficacy in RA and PsA patients [44]. *Single-photon emission computed tomography* (SPECT/CT) imaging with ^{99m}Tc-glucosamine has high sensitivity for detecting RA synovitis and correlates well with ultrasound scores [44]; 99mTc-glucosamine may effectively evaluate RA activity in the absence of PET/CT cameras for 18F-FDG PET/CT imaging [44]. Currently, ultrasound is preferred in inflammatory rheumatic diseases (Fig. 3.3), with MRI being considered the gold standard. DECT could serve as a valuable complement to both ultrasound and MRI for this purpose [38].

High-resolution peripheral quantitative CT (HR-pQCT) can detect early bone abnormalities (bone density and microstructure), advanced structural changes, anabolic and catabolic bone alterations, joint space width, and treatment efficacy [45]. HR-pQCT further identifies treatment effects depending on changes in erosion volume (repair of erosion or progression of erosion) over time [45]. HR-pQCT appears beneficial where subtle changes are expected in subclinical inflammation [45].

Early identification of *large vessel vasculitis (LVV)* via 2-[18F] FDG-PET/CT in suspected patients can detect vascular activity before visible changes in angiography and LVV progression, aiding in treatment evaluation, relapse recognition, and early vascular complication pinpointing [46]. PET/CT and ultrasound appear to have similar diagnostic accuracies in GCA temporal artery assessment, with PET/CT having lower sensitivity for the parietal branch than ultrasound and histology [47].

Ultrasound is useful in identifying inflammatory synovitis, meniscal extrusion, and cartilage thickness changes in OA [48] (Fig. 3.4); however, ultrasound cannot penetrate cartilage and reach the SCB area, and CT and MRI are useful in these cases [49]. DECT can be used to assess BMD and BME effectively once it is visible only via MRI [48]. Compared with traditional CT, weight-bearing CT enhances the understanding of OA pathophysiology, and photon-counting CT offers higher spatial resolution images with reduced radiation exposure [49].

The semiquantitative weight-bearing CT osteoarthritis knee score (COAKS) is a reliable scoring system for knee OA with strong interobserver agreement for radiographic features [50]. COAKS surpasses conventional MRI and CR in disease severity monitoring in clinical trials [50], and further studies to compare COAKS scoring with CE-MRI delayed uptake images could be performed. The role of SPECT in the decision-making process of OAs is not fully clear [51]. However, *computed tomography arthrography* (CBCT-A) is more reliable than digital radiography for OA diagnosis, with more detailed bone microarchitecture analysis [52]. CT-based summation images (combining CT slices forming 2D images and X-ray images) can be used to detect radiographic hip OA [53].

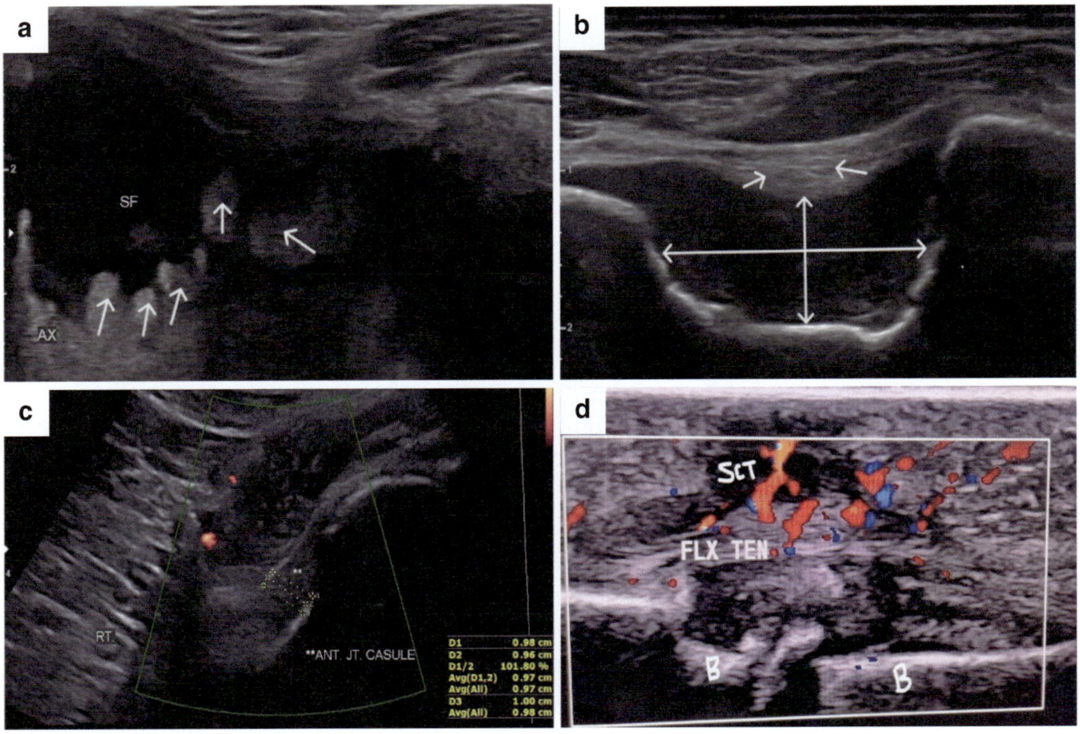

Fig. 3.3 Ultrasound in inflammatory arthritis. (**a**) Short axis grayscale image of anterior knee reveals villous (arrows) synovium in undifferentiated inflammatory synovitis. (**b**) Short axis grayscale scan of the posterior flexed elbow explores synovial hypertrophy (double arrows) in rheumatoid arthritis. (**c**) Anterior oblique longitudinal scan of hip depicts thick and hypoechoic synovial hypertrophy (asterisks) in ankylosing spondylitis. (**d**) Longitudinal scan of the volar aspect of the finger unveils flexor tenosynovitis (Doppler spots around the FLX TEN) in psoriatic dactylitis. *AX* axial, *B* bone, *FLX TEN* flexor tendon, *SCT* subcutaneous tissue, *SF* synovial fluid

^{18}F-FDG-PET/CT enables the quantitative evaluation of *idiopathic inflammatory myositis* (IIM), therefore helping to determine muscle biopsy sites; diagnosing disease, disease activity, and severity; and screening for malignancy and interstitial lung disease in polymyositis (PM) and dermatomyositis (DM) patients [54]. ^{18}F-FDG-PET/CT has good sensitivity for detecting myositis, and tracer uptake values have been shown to be significantly correlated with muscle strength, serum creatinine kinase (CK) levels, and even histopathological severity [55]. The mean CK value appears to be greater in patients with abnormal uptake in PET/CT imaging in IIM; further longitudinal studies should confirm the associations between PET/CT and EMG, MRI, and CK [55]. ^{18}F-FDG PET/CT can discriminate between IIM and nonmuscular diseases and can correlate with serum CK values [57, 58]. Ultrasound has shown high sensitivity in detecting muscle pathology in IIM, but the discrimination of pathology domains and the utility of different ultrasound domains are still contentious [58]. Ultrasound is feasible for identifying a suitable muscle for biopsy, detecting muscle involved in amyopathic DM and active myositis under treatment, and differentiating steroid myopathy from persistent active myositis [58]. In addition to ultrasound, PET-CT plays an important role in the diagnosis of drug-induced myositis, such as sunitinib, a multikinase inhibitor used to treat metastatic renal cell carcinoma [59]. MRI and ultrasound both have value in diagnosing and monitoring treatment efficacy in patients with pyomyositis [60].

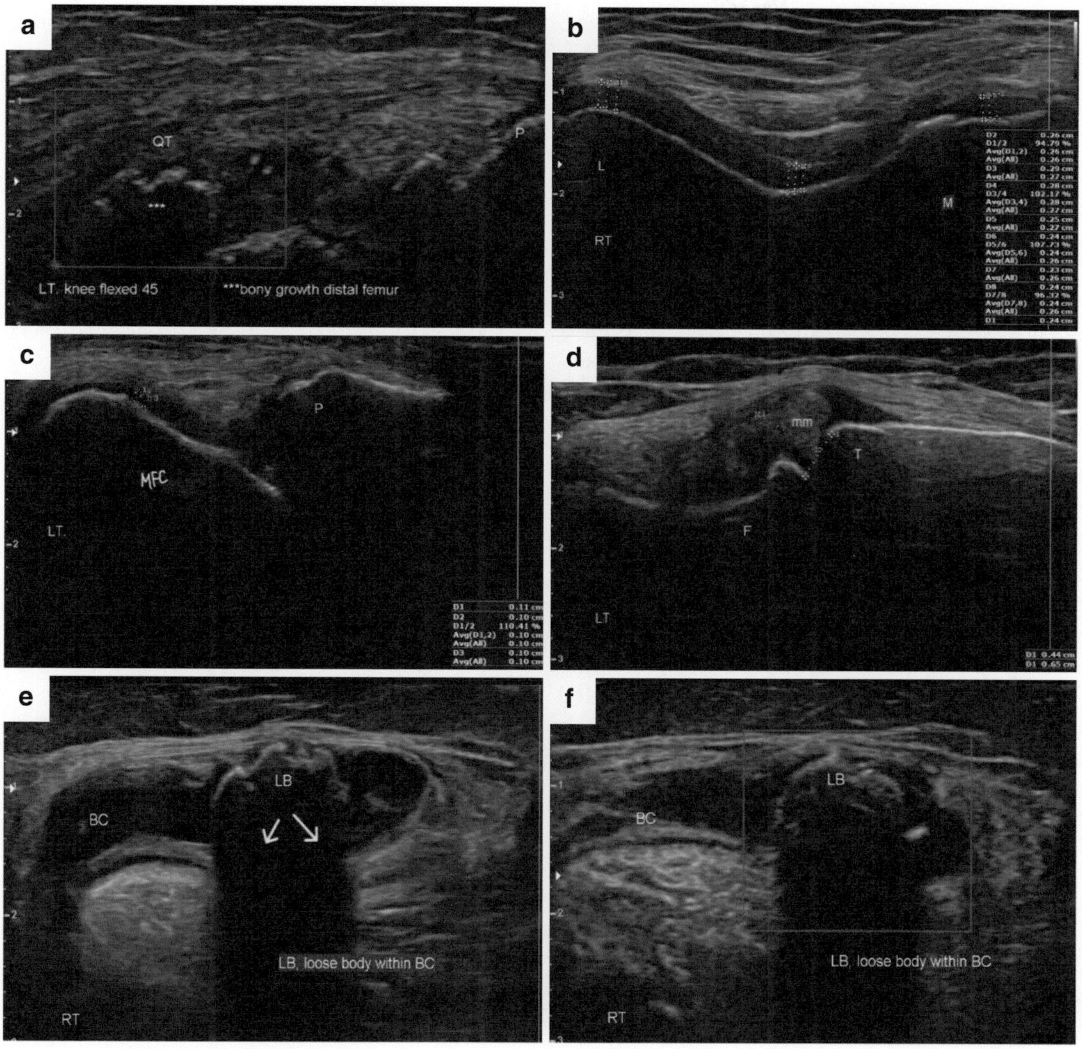

Fig. 3.4 Ultrasound in knee osteoarthritis. (**a**) Longitudinal scan of the anterior semi-flexed knee explores impacted loose body in the anterior joint recess with increased Doppler signal (asterisks). (**b**) Transverse grayscale scan revealing reduced sharpness and thickness of the femoral condylar cartilage, more on the MFC. (**c**) Long axis scan of the flexed knee reveals reduced MFC cartilage thickness. (**d**) Longitudinal scan of the medial knee unveils severe medial meniscal extrusion. (**e**, **f**). Short axis scans of the posterior knee depict beak-shaped BC with LB and increased Doppler activity in the cyst wall. *BC* Baker's cyst, *F* femur, *L* lateral, *LB* loose body, *LT* left, *M* medial, *MFC* medial femoral condyle, *P* patella, *QT* quadriceps tendon, *RT* right, *T* tibia

3.4 Magnetic Resonance Imaging (MRI)

MRI plays a crucial role in the early detection of rheumatic diseases, disease progression, and monitoring of treatment responses during long-term follow-up [61]. MRI can predict cartilage and bone destruction before they are visible via X-ray [61]. High contrast and spatial resolution MRI make it possible to assess the bone marrow, periarticular soft tissues, and articular cartilage thoroughly [61]. CE-MRI and diffusion-weighted imaging provide additional assessments of active synovitis [61]. MRI can detect enthesitis, sacro-iliac joint inflammation, and vertebral body involvement in the axial SpA [61].

MRI and ultrasound imaging modalities have similar levels of diagnostic sensitivity, specificity, and accuracy in diagnosing RA [62]. Compared with CE-MRI, ultrasound shows comparable sensitivity and accuracy in detecting subclinical synovitis and tenosynovitis in RA [63]. MRI and ultrasound findings of inflammatory synovitis are linked to progressive cortical erosions, subclinical inflammation status, and treatment response [63–66]. Nevertheless, the routine use of MRI and ultrasound may have limited benefits in the regular monitoring of early RA [64, 65]. The features of enthesitis on ultrasound include the absence of a normal fibrillar pattern, thickening with a hypoechoic appearance, increased vascularity of tendons, ligaments, and joint capsules at their insertion points on bone, and the presence of bone erosions [66]. Compared with X-ray and MRI, ultrasound has been recognized as a superior imaging modality for identifying enthesitis [66]; nevertheless, CE-MRI could better demonstrate tendon and ligament changes, considering BME and erosions in the context of enthesitis [67].

Ultrasound imaging plays a crucial role in the assessment of *skin and soft tissue infections*, such as abscesses and cellulitis [68, 69] (Fig. 3.5). Ultrasound enhances the accuracy of cellulitis diagnosis and helps its management [69–71]. In cellulitis, ultrasound imaging reveals thickening of the subcutaneous tissue with a loss of the typical hyperechoic epidermis/dermis layer at the surface of the image [69]. Anechoic to hypoechoic fluid can be observed separating the subcutaneous tissue and fat layers, resulting in the sonoappearance of a cobblestone [69].

Diffusion-weighted MR imaging, dynamic CE-MRI, and radiomics analyses can be used to accurately diagnose musculoskeletal infections and measure treatment responses [72]. MRI can overcome the diagnostic confusion between transient synovitis and septic arthritis; for the latter, characteristic changes in the femoral head with BMLs have been noted [73]. To exclude coexisting osteomyelitis, MRI could perform best [74]. Ultrasound-guided aspiration from joints, bursae, and abscesses followed by an analysis of specimens helps to establish a definitive diagnosis [68–71, 75]. After initial radiographs, ultrasound is often used as the next imaging method for soft tissue infections because of its cost-effectiveness, accessibility, portability, and ability to provide real-time guidance for fluid aspiration [76]. However, advanced cross-sectional imaging methods such as MRI and CT have greatly improved radiological assessment in cases where ultrasound use may be limited [74]. Furthermore, CT and MRI allow for a thorough examination of the disease's extent, including the assessment of joint spaces, tendons, and changes in bone that suggest bone involvement [76].

MRI findings indicative of OA can be observed in the asymptomatic knees of healthy young and older adults over the age of 40 [77]. These characteristics include structural abnormalities such as cartilage deterioration, osteophytes, and BMLs, particularly in middle-aged women with nonradiographic knee OA [78]. Additionally, MRI synovitis has been found to contribute significantly to knee pain in early knee OA [78]. Compared with late-stage OA, early knee OA with clinical symptoms and physical examination findings may exhibit the highest sensitivity for detecting medium- to large-scale effusion-synovitis on MRI [78]. Identifying knees at risk of effusion-synovitis in early OA could be achieved through patient-reported symptoms or at least one positive examination finding and one symptom for the purpose of screening or enriching study samples [79]. However, these methods are not suitable for clinical diagnostic use because their diagnostic performance is insufficient [79].

In *juvenile Sjogren syndrome* (JSS), MRI-sialography and fat-suppressed T2-weighted imaging can detect numerous high-intensity spots in the parotid glands (PGs), which tend to decrease with age in the JSS group [80]. Unlike adult SS patients, individuals with JSS rarely exhibit fat areas on MRI or hyperechoic bands on ultrasound in the PGs and submandibular glands [80]. The presence of hyperechoic bands on ultrasound, fat areas on MRI, and reduced salivary flow appear to be linked in JSS [80]. Imaging findings in JSS patients revealed punctate sialectasis, whereas those in adult SS patients displayed fatty degeneration [80]. These distinct imaging

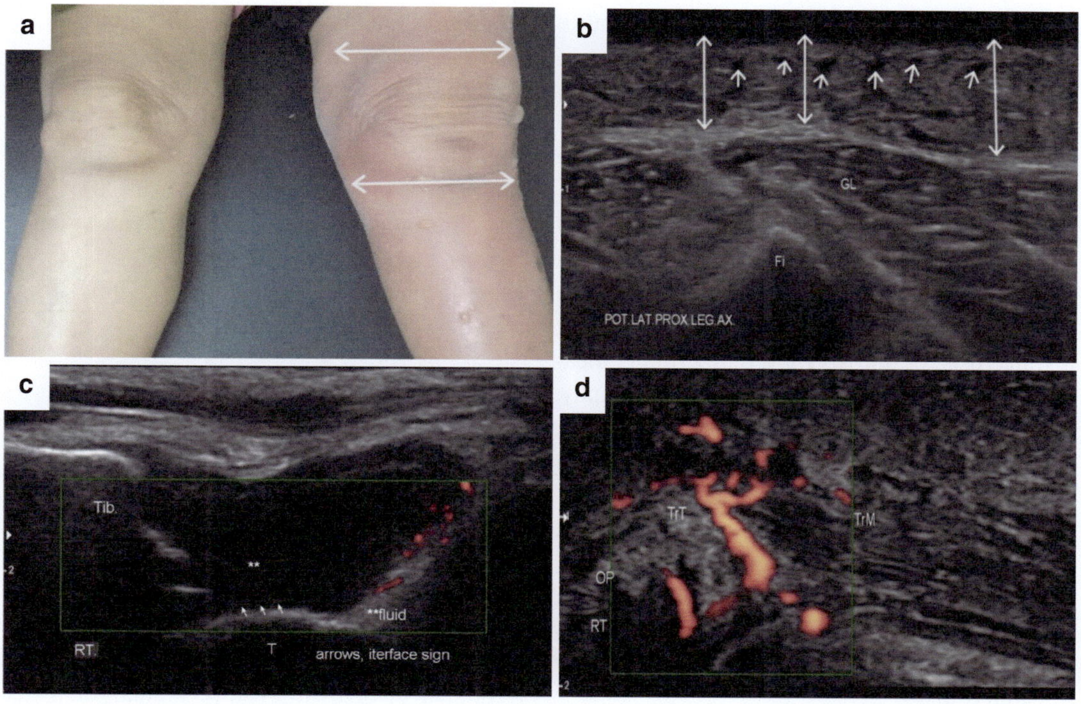

Fig. 3.5 Ultrasound in joint and soft tissue infection. (**a**) Extension of vesicular skin lesions in the left anterior knee and thigh (double arrows). (**b**) Long axis scan of the postero-lateral knee and leg reveals thick and hypoechoic subcutaneous tissue with a cobblestone appearance (double arrows) and hypoechoic-anechoic compressible collection between the fat lobules (single arrows). (**c**) Longitudinal scan of the anterior ankle revealing compressible collection in the talo-crural joint (asterisks) with an increased Doppler signal in synovium. (**d**) Longitudinal scan of the posterior elbow unveils thick and hypoechoic TrM and TrT with increased Doppler activity. *GL* lateral gastrocnemius, *OP* olecranon process, *RT* right, *Tib* tibia, *TrM* tricep's muscle, *TrT* tricep's tendon

findings suggest differences in the stage of glandular lesions between JSS patients and adult SS patients [80]. Both MRI and ultrasound imaging can serve as valuable tools for evaluating the severity of glandular lesions in follow-up examinations in patients with SS [80].

The rheumatoid arthritis MRI score (RAMRIS) and the psoriatic arthritis MRI score (PsAMRIS) are commonly used in clinical trials, and new systems are being developed in ultrasound studies [81]. Considering the potential for a gouty arthritis MRI score (GAMRIS) to measure tophus volume, reducing chronic synovitis and slowing bone erosion progression posttreatment could be beneficial [81]. An alternative strategy might involve creating an ultrasound or CT score for gout, considering each imaging modality's strengths and weaknesses [81]. Compared with CT, MRI can detect all components but may have lower resolution and reproducibility for tophus measurement, whereas ultrasound can reveal most components except for bone edema and some deep tissue tophi, with fair reproducibility for tophus measurement but greater operator dependence [81].

The diagnostic utility of ultrasound in detecting *myositis* is still in its early stages [82]. A recent preliminary investigation indicated that MRI is more effective than ultrasound in identifying muscle irregularities indicative of IIM during the initial diagnosis [83]. Although semiquantitative and qualitative ultrasound methods are able to detect abnormalities in most patients, they assess fewer muscles than MRI does and show changes over a treatment period [83]. The distinct MRI patterns observed in skeletal muscles could be used as markers for distinguishing individuals with DM from those with myositis-specific and myositis-associated autoantibodies [84]. Significant differences in terms of muscle echogenicity of the flexor digitorum profundus and the gastrocnemius muscles have been revealed between IBM patients and healthy controls [84]; further study is needed.

The vastus lateralis muscle in the ultrasound images showed increased echogenicity, which has been linked to fatty infiltration or atrophy on MRI scans, rather than muscle inflammation, myonecrosis, or fibrosis [86]. Furthermore, measurements of shear wave speed elastography, ultrasound-fascial thickness, and muscle bulk were not effective in distinguishing between pathologies seen on MRI and muscle biopsies [58]. PD signals also display a weak correlation with MRI edema, inflammation, or fatty infiltration according to biopsy results [61]. The role of MRI and ultrasound in predicting RA in undifferentiated arthritis patients requires further research [86].

3.5 Arthrography

Prior to the advent of MRI and CT technologies, arthrography served as a valuable method for visualizing joint abnormalities [87]. It may still be incidentally useful to see where leakage, for example, from a Baker's cyst (BC), is going or to see how contrast leaks from an osteoarthritic knee joint into t lymph vessels [87]. Furthermore, arthrograms have demonstrated superior efficacy over ultrasound in detecting BC, particularly smaller cysts that may elude ultrasound detection. Conversely, ultrasound can identify cysts that do not exhibit filling during arthrography [88]. Additionally, arthrography is capable of confirming the existence of a ruptured cyst, whereas ultrasound is adept at highlighting changes in soft tissue and reductions in the distal margins of cysts [88].

Compared with traditional MRI or ultrasound, MR arthrography has been shown to possess enhanced sensitivity and specificity, as indicated by its superior performance in terms of the receiver operating characteristic curve, with ultrasound and MRI ranking lower in effectiveness [88, 89]. In studies focusing on MR arthrography of the glenohumeral joint, a comparison between ultrasound and fluoroscopic guidance has revealed that ultrasound guided injections into the rotator cuff interval yield results comparable to those achieved with fluoroscopic guidance [90]. Given that ultrasound does not expose patients to ionizing radiation, it is regarded as a more advantageous technique for such procedures [90].

3.6 Arthroscopy

Arthroscopic procedures are commonly employed in the field of rheumatology to allow for direct observation of the joint space, enabling a detailed assessment of the synovial tissue, collection of samples for histopathological and microbiological analysis, and the option for therapeutic lavage [91, 92]. This minimally invasive technique involves the use of a small-diameter arthroscope under local anesthesia, which is well received by patients because of its safety profile and low incidence of complications, which are similar to those documented in the orthopedic literature [91, 92]. In the initial prospective questioning arthroscopic debridement study conducted by rheumatologists, the utilization of biological compounds led to a decrease in the necessity for arthroscopic interventions in patients with OA [93]. Certain OA characteristics, such as calcinosis, warrant additional exploration through arthroscopic means [93]. The emergence of advanced "needle scopes" equipped with superior optics presents a promising avenue for upcoming researchers in the field [93].

IA ultrasound and ultrasound, in combination with arthroscopy, can be used to assess articular surface characteristics in OA [14] and improve the diagnostic accuracy for rheumatic diseases [94]. A strong correlation has been demonstrated between urate deposits on cartilage by arthroscopy and the ultrasound-double contour sign [95]. A positive correlation has been revealed between the ultrasound cartilage damage score and Noyes' arthroscopic grading for knee OA; however, a negative ultrasound finding cannot completely exclude this possibility [96].

In adult septic arthritis patients, arthroscopy-guided joint aspiration fluid studies help correct diagnosis and treatment, resulting in low perioperative morbidity, normal hip function restoration, and minimal risk of infection spread [97]. In pediatric septic arthritis, arthroscopic irrigation minimizes repeat surgical irrigations and allows earlier knee ranging and weight-bearing than open irrigation does, without significant differences in knee injury and osteoarthritis outcome score, Lysholm score, range-of-motion, leg length, gait, or radiologic findings between groups at follow-up [98].

The arthroscopic removal and excision of calcifications in the rotator cuff, aided by ultrasound, could improve overall shoulder pain, activity, and range of motion [99]. Arthroscopy and the intra-operative ultra-guided needle technique can be used to accurately pinpoint small calcific deposits [100]. The therapeutic efficacy of ultra-guided puncture and aspiration is not statistically less effective than that of the arthroscopic technique in resolving shoulder calcifying tendonitis [101].

Faster joint effusion decreased in the group treated with arthroscopic lavage than in the non-operated group, as assessed by ultrasound [102].

In summary, medical imaging significantly contributes to rheumatic disease diagnosis. Starting with conventional radiology, computed tomography, magnetic resonance imaging (MRI), and ultrasound help diagnose disease, monitor disease activity, and monitor treatment efficacy. Since radiology cannot label active synovitis and low vascular flow in inflamed synovium, SMI, CE-PD, and CE-MRI could be effective for this purpose. MRI and PET imaging can explore subchondral bone lesions, as observed in infective arthritis, OA, and inflammatory arthritis.

Conflict of Interest MAB is supported by a Faculty of Medicine and Health Executive Dean Stipend scholarship, University of Sydney, Australia, for his PhD course.

References

1. Ezzati F, Pezeshk P. Radiographic findings of inflammatory arthritis and mimics in the hands. Diagnostics. 2022;12:2134.
2. Al Nakshabandi N, Joharji E, El-Haddad H. Radiology in rheumatology. In: Almoallim H, Cheikh M, editors. Skills in rheumatology. Singapore: Springer; 2021. https://doi.org/10.1007/978-981-15-8323-0_5.
3. Miksanek J, Rosenthal AK. Imaging of calcium pyrophosphate deposition disease. Curr Rheumatol Rep. 2015;17:20.
4. Rettenbacher T, Ennemoser S, Weirich H, et al. Diagnostic imaging of gout: comparison of high-resolution US versus conventional X-ray. Eur Radiol. 2008;18:621–30.
5. Scholz J, Roiser N, Braig EM, et al. X-ray dark-field radiography for in situ gout diagnosis by means of an ex vivo animal study. Sci Rep. 2021;11:19021.
6. Kgoebane K, Ally MMTM, Duim-Beytell MC, Suleman FE. The role of imaging in rheumatoid arthritis. SA J Radiol. 2018;22:1316.
7. Crespo-Rodríguez AM, Sanz Sanz J, Freites D, Rosales Z, Abasolo L, Arrazola J. Role of diagnostic imaging in psoriatic arthritis: how, when, and why. Insights Imaging. 2021;12:121.
8. Ulas ST, Ziegeler K, Richter ST, et al. Virtual monochromatic images from dual-energy computed tomography do not improve the detection of synovitis in hand arthritis. Diagnostics (Basel). 2022;12:1891.
9. Kaeley GS, Bakewell C, Deodhar A. The importance of ultrasound in identifying and differentiating patients with early inflammatory arthritis: a narrative review. Arthritis Res Ther. 2020;22:1.
10. Mandl P, D'Agostino MA, Navarro-Compán V, et al. 2023 EULAR recommendations on imaging in diagnosis and management of crystal-induced arthropathies in clinical practice. Ann Rheum Dis. 2024;83:752–9.
11. Jans L, De Kock I, Herregods N, et al. Dual-energy CT: a new imaging modality for bone marrow Oedema in rheumatoid arthritis. Ann Rheum Dis. 2018;77:958–60.
12. Seskute G, Jasionyte G, Rugiene R, Butrimiene I. The use of superb microvascular imaging in evaluating rheumatic diseases: a systematic review. Medicina (Kaunas). 2023;59:1641.
13. Silvagni E, Callegher SZ, Mauric E, et al. Musculoskeletal ultrasound for treating rheumatoid arthritis to target – a systematic literature review. Rheumatology. 2022;61:4590–602.
14. Kaleva E, Virén T, Saarakkala S, et al. Arthroscopic ultrasound assessment of articular cartilage in the human knee joint: a potential diagnostic method. Cartilage. 2011;2:246–53.
15. Rehnitz C, Klaan B, Burkholder I, von Stillfried F, Kauczor HU, Weber MA. Delayed gadolinium-enhanced MRI of cartilage (dGEMRIC) and T_2 mapping at 3T MRI of the wrist: Feasibility and clinical application. J Magn Reson Imaging. 2017;45:381–9.
16. Bakewell C, Aydin SZ, Ranganath VK, Eder L, Kaeley GS. Imaging techniques: options for the

diagnosis and monitoring of treatment of enthesitis in psoriatic arthritis. J Rheumatol. 2020;47:973–82.
17. Elnady B, El Shaarawy NK, Dawoud NM, et al. Subclinical synovitis and Enthesitis in psoriasis patients and controls by ultrasonography in Saudi Arabia incidence psoriatic arthritis during two years. Clin Rheumatol. 2019;38:1627–35.
18. Tan AL, Fukuba E, Halliday NA, Tanner SF, Emery P, McGonagle D. High-resolution MRI assessment of dactylitis in psoriatic arthritis shows flexor tendon pulley and sheath-related enthesitis. Ann Rheum Dis. 2015;74:185–9.
19. Emad Y, Ragab Y, Gheita T, et al. Knee enthesitis and synovitis on magnetic resonance imaging in patients with psoriasis without arthritic symptoms. J Rheumatol. 2012;39:1979–86.
20. Rasker JJ, Cosh JA. Radiological study of cervical spine and hands in patients with rheumatoid arthritis of 15 years duration; an assessment of the effect of corticosteroid treatment. Ann Rheum Dis. 1978;37:529–35.
21. Mader R, Baraliakos X, Eshed I, et al. Imaging of diffuse idiopathic skeletal hyperostosis (DISH). RMD Open. 2020;6:e001151.
22. Sudoł-Szopińska I, Kwiatkowska B, Prochorec-Sobieszek M, Pracoń G, Walentowska-Janowicz M, Maśliński W. Enthesopathies and enthesitis. Part 2: imaging studies. J Ultrason. 2015;15:196–207.
23. Henry TW, Tulipan JE, Beredjiklian PK, Matzon JL, Lutsky KF. Are plain X-Rays necessary in the diagnosis of De Quervain's tenosynovitis? J Wrist Surg. 2021;10:48–52.
24. Roberts S, Dearne R, Keen S, Littlewood C, Taylor S, Deacon P. Routine X-rays for suspected frozen shoulder offer little over diagnosis based on history and clinical examination alone. Musculoskelet Care. 2019;17:288–92.
25. Elnady B, Rageh EM, Hussein MS, et al. In shoulder adhesive capsulitis, ultrasound guided anterior hydrodilatation in rotator interval is more effective than posterior approach: a randomized controlled study. Clin Rheumatol. 2020;39:3805–14. https://doi.org/10.1007/s10067-020-05131-2.
26. Wani IM, Arora S. Osteoporosis diagnosis in knee X-rays by transfer learning based on convolution neural network. Multimed Tools Appl. 2023;82:14193–217.
27. Tins BJ, Butler R. Imaging in rheumatology: reconciling radiology and rheumatology. Insights Imaging. 2013;4:799–810.
28. Li C, Sun J, Yu L. Diagnostic value of calcaneal quantitative ultrasound in the evaluation of osteoporosis in middle-aged and elderly patients. Medicine (Baltimore). 2022;101:e28325.
29. Ulijn E, den Broeder N, Ten Cate D, et al. Limited diagnostic and prognostic value of routine radiographs in newly presenting arthritis suspected of rheumatoid arthritis: a retrospective study. Arthritis Care Res (Hoboken). 2024;76:497.
30. Campos A. Rheumatoid arthritis (musculoskeletal manifestations). https://radiopaedia.org/articles/rheumatoid-arthritis-musculoskeletal-manifestations-2#:~:text=Radiographic%20features,up%20of%20rheumatoid%20arthritis%202. Accessed 1 Aug 2024.
31. Maksymowych WP. The role of imaging in the diagnosis and management of axial spondyloarthritis. Nat Rev Rheumatol. 2019;15:657–72.
32. Zhang YH, Li K, Xiao J, Zhang HD, Zhang XY. Comparison of ultrasound, radiography, and clinical investigations in the diagnosis of early rheumatoid synovitis in patients with nonspecific musculoskeletal symptoms: a multicenter cross-sectional study. Med Sci Monit. 2018;24:4372–8.
33. Mackie SL, Koduri G, Hill CL, et al. Accuracy of musculoskeletal imaging for the diagnosis of polymyalgia rheumatica: systematic review. RMD Open. 2015;1:e000100.
34. Dejaco C, Stadlmayr A, Duftner C, et al. Ultrasound verified inflammation and structural damage in patients with hereditary haemochromatosis-related arthropathy. Arthritis Res Ther. 2017;19(1):243. https://doi.org/10.1186/s13075-017-1448-0.
35. Girish G, Glazebrook KN, Jacobson JA. Advanced imaging in gout. AJR Am J Roentgenol. 2013;201:515–25.
36. Emad Y, Ragab Y, El-Naggar A, et al. Gadolinium-enhanced MRI features of acute gouty arthritis on top of chronic gouty involvement in different joints. Clin Rheumatol. 2015;34:1939–47.
37. Wang X, Oo WM, Linklater JM. What is the role of imaging in the clinical diagnosis of osteoarthritis and disease management? Rheumatology. 2018;57(Suppl 4):iv51–60.
38. Jeka S. Dual-energy computed tomography – possible applications in the diagnosis of rheumatic diseases. Innov Clin Therapy. 2023;9:182–3.
39. Hsu CCT, Kwan GN, Singh D, et al. Principles and clinical application of dual-energy computed tomography in the evaluation of cerebrovascular disease. J Clin Imaging Sci. 2016;6:27.
40. Singh JA, Budzik JF, Becce F, et al. Dual-energy computed tomography vs ultrasound, alone or combined, for the diagnosis of gout: a prospective study of accuracy. Rheumatology (Oxford). 2021;60:4861–7.
41. Sotniczuk M, Nowakowska-Płaza A, Wroński J, et al. The clinical utility of dual-energy computed tomography in the diagnosis of gout-a cross-sectional study. J Clin Med. 2022;11:10.3390/jcm11175249.
42. Khanduri S, Singh V, Pathak V, et al. Comparison between dual-energy computed tomography and ultrasound in the diagnosis of gout. Indian J Musculoskelet Radiol. 2024;6:10–7.
43. Gao X, Gao H, Zhang L, Zhang L. Comparison of diagnostic efficacy of dual-energy CT and ultrasound in gouty arthritis. Int J Rheum Dis. 2023;26:1697–703.

44. Evbuomwan O, Engelbrecht G, Driver C, et al. Head-to-head comparison of ultrasound and ^{99m}Tc-glucosamine SPECT/CT imaging of patients with rheumatoid arthritis: a single center prospective study. Egypt J Radiol Nucl Med. 2023;54:223.
45. Klose-Jensen R, Tse JJ, Keller KK, et al. High-resolution peripheral quantitative computed tomography for bone evaluation in inflammatory rheumatic disease. Front Med (Lausanne). 2020;7:337.
46. Nassarmadji K, Vanjak A, Bourdin V, et al. 18-Fluorodeoxyglucose positron emission tomography/computed tomography for large vessel vasculitis in clinical practice. Front Med (Lausanne). 2023;10:1103752.
47. Rottenburger C, Mensch N, Imfeld S, et al. 18F-FDG PET/CT compared with ultrasound and biopsy for detection of vasculitis of the temporal artery branches. Swiss Med Wkly. 2021;151:w20512.
48. Oo WM, Linklater JM, Bennell KL, et al. Are OMERACT knee osteoarthritis ultrasound scores associated with pain severity, other symptoms, and radiographic and magnetic resonance imaging findings? J Rheumatol. 2021;48:270–8.
49. Fukuda T, Yonenaga T, Miyasaka T, et al. CT in osteoarthritis: its clinical role and recent advances. Skeletal Radiol. 2023;52:2199–210.
50. Turmezei TD, Jeon JH, Akkaya Z, Segal NA. Computed tomography osteoarthritis knee score (COAKS) construction, reproducibility and potential for structural phenotyping. Osteoarthr Imaging. 2023;3(suppl1):100116.
51. Zarringam D, Saris DBF, Bekkers JEJ. The value of SPECT/CT for knee osteoarthritis: a systematic review. Cartilage. 2021;12:431–7.
52. Hamard M, Sans Merce M, Gorican K, Poletti PA, Neroladaki A, Boudabbous S. The role of cone-beam computed tomography CT extremity arthrography in the preoperative assessment of osteoarthritis. Tomography. 2023;9:2134–47.
53. Gebre RK, Hirvasniemi J, van der Heijden RA, et al. Detecting hip osteoarthritis on clinical CT: a deep learning application based on 2-D summation images derived from CT. Osteoporos Int. 2022;33:355–65.
54. Tanaka S, Ikeda K, Uchiyama K, et al. [^{18}F]FDG uptake in proximal muscles assessed by PET/CT reflects both global and local muscular inflammation and provides useful information in the management of patients with polymyositis/dermatomyositis. Rheumatology. 2013;52:1271–8.
55. Selva-O'Callaghan A, Gil-Vila A, Simó-Perdigó M, et al. PET scan: nuclear medicine imaging in myositis. Curr Rheumatol Rep. 2019;21:64.
56. Yildiz H, Lepere C, Zorzi G, Gheysens O, Roodhans F, Pothen L. [^{18}F]FDG-PET/CT in idiopathic inflammatory myopathies: retrospective data from a belgian cohort. Diagnostics. 2023;13:2316.
57. Arai-Okuda H, Norikane T, Yamamoto Y, et al. ^{18}F-FDG PET/CT in patients with polymyositis/dermatomyositis: correlation with serum muscle enzymes. Eur J Hybrid Imaging. 2020;4:14.
58. Paramalingam S, Needham M, Harris S, et al. Muscle B mode ultrasound and shear-wave elastography in idiopathic inflammatory myopathies (SWIM): criterion validation against MRI and muscle biopsy findings in an incident patient cohort. BMC Rheumatol. 2022;6:47.
59. Ritesh RS, Nilendu P, Sneha S, Archi A, Ameya P, Venkatesh R. Sunitinib-induced myositis detected on 18F-FDG PET/CT. Clin Nucl Med. 2022;47:e311–2.
60. Siddiq MAB, Rasker JJ. Piriformis pyomyositis, a cause of piriformis syndrome – a systematic search and review. Clin Rheumatol. 2019;38:1811–21. https://doi.org/10.1007/s10067-019-04552.
61. Weaver JS, Omar I, Mar W, Kauser AS, Mlady GW, Taljanovic M. Magnetic resonance imaging of rheumatological diseases. Pol J Radiol. 2022;87:e93–e112.
62. Jain A, Malhotra A, Chandak S, et al. Comparison of high-resolution ultrasonography with magnetic resonance imaging in rheumatoid arthritis. J Diag Med Sonogr. 2023;39:105–14.
63. Bao Z, Zhao Y, Chen S, et al. Ultrasound versus contrast-enhanced magnetic resonance imaging for subclinical synovitis and tenosynovitis: a diagnostic performance study. Clinics (Sao Paulo). 2020;75:e1500.
64. Sundin U, Sundlisater NP, Aga A, et al. Value of MRI and ultrasound for prediction of therapeutic response and erosive progression in patients with early rheumatoid arthritis managed by an aggressive treat-to-target strategy. RMD Open. 2021;7:e001525.
65. Sundin U, Aga AB, Skare Ø, et al. Conventional versus ultrasound treat to target: no difference in magnetic resonance imaging inflammation or joint damage over 2 years in early rheumatoid arthritis. Rheumatology (Oxford). 2020;59:2550–5.
66. Draghi F, Ferrozzi G, Ballerini D, Bortolotto C. Psoriatic arthritis: ultrasound peculiarities with particular emphasis on enthesitis. J Clin Ultrasound. 2022;50:556–60.
67. Mathew AJ, Østergaard M. Magnetic resonance imaging of enthesitis in spondyloarthritis, including psoriatic arthritis-status and recent advances. Front Med (Lausanne). 2020;7:296. https://doi.org/10.3389/fmed.2020.00296.
68. Perez J, Sorensen S, Rosselli M. Utilisation of musculoskeletal ultrasonography for the evaluation of septic arthritis in a patient presenting to the emergency department with fever during the era of COVID-19. BMJ Case Rep CP. 2021;14:e242370.
69. O'Rourke K, Kibbee N, Stubbs A. Ultrasound for the evaluation of skin and soft tissue infections. Mo Med. 2015;112:202–5.
70. Blanco P, Menéndez MF, Figueroa L, et al. Ultrasound-aided diagnosis of septic arthritis of the elbow in the emergency department. J Ultrasound. 2022;25: L:315–8.
71. Jiang K, Zhang W, Fu G, et al. Ultrasound-guided percutaneous drainage of iliopsoas abscess with sep-

ticemia in an adolescent: a case report and literature review. Front Surg. 2022;9:871292.
72. Spinnato P, Patel DB, Di Carlo M, et al. Imaging of musculoskeletal soft-tissue infections in clinical practice: a comprehensive updated review. Microorganisms. 2022;10:2329.
73. Adam M, Ibrahim B, Khidir R, Elmahdi E, Ahmed S, Ahmed A. Usefulness of MRI findings in differentiating between septic arthritis and transient synovitis of hip joint in children: a systematic review and meta-analysis. Eur J Radiol Open. 2022;9:100439.
74. Lim W, Barras CD, Zadow S. Radiologic mimics of osteomyelitis and septic arthritis: a pictorial essay. Radiol Res Pract. 2021;2021:9912257.
75. Siddiq MAB, Jahan I, Rasker JJ. piriformis syndrome: epidemiology, clinical features, diagnosis, and treatment. In: Iyer KM, editor. Piriformis syndrome. Cham: Springer; 2023. https://doi.org/10.1007/978-3-031-40736-.
76. Altmayer S, Verma N, Dicks EA, Oliveira A. Imaging musculoskeletal soft tissue infections. Semin Ultrasound CT MR. 2020;41:85–98.
77. Culvenor AG, Øiestad BE, Hart HF, et al. Prevalence of knee osteoarthritis features on magnetic resonance imaging in asymptomatic uninjured adults: a systematic review and meta-analysis. Br J Sports Med. 2019;53:1268–78.
78. Ota S, Sasaki E, Sasaki S, et al. Relationship between abnormalities detected by magnetic resonance imaging and knee symptoms in early knee osteoarthritis. Sci Rep. 2021;11:15179.
79. Berlinberg A, Ashbeck EL, Roemer FW, et al. Diagnostic performance of knee physical exam and participant-reported symptoms for MRI-detected effusion-synovitis among participants with early or late stage knee osteoarthritis: data from the Osteoarthritis Initiative. Osteoarthr Cart. 2019;27:80–9.
80. Takagi Y, Sasaki M, Eida S, et al. Comparison of salivary gland MRI and ultrasonography findings among patients with Sjögren's syndrome over a wide age range. Rheumatology (Oxford). 2022;61:1986–96.
81. McQueen FM, Doyle A, Dalbeth N. Imaging in gout–what can we learn from MRI, CT, DECT and US? Arthritis Res Ther. 2011;13:246.
82. Albayda J, van Alfen N. Diagnostic value of muscle ultrasound for myopathies and myositis. Curr Rheumatol Rep. 2020;22:82.
83. Walter AW, Lim J, Raaphorst J, et al. Ultrasound and MR muscle imaging in new onset idiopathic inflammatory myopathies at diagnosis and after treatment: a comparative pilot study. Rheumatology (Oxford). 2022;62:300–9.
84. Ukichi T, Yoshida K, Matsushima S, et al. MRI of skeletal muscles in patients with idiopathic inflammatory myopathies: characteristic findings and diagnostic performance in dermatomyositis. RMD Open. 2019;5:e000850.
85. Abdelnaby R, Mohamed KA, Elgenidy, et al. Muscle sonography in inclusion body myositis: a systematic review and meta-analysis of 944 measurements. Cells. 2022;11:600.
86. de Pablo P, Dinnes J, Berhane S, et al. Systematic review of imaging tests to predict the development of rheumatoid arthritis in people with unclassified arthritis. Semin Arthritis Rheum. 2022;52:151919.
87. Dixon ASTJ, Rasker JJ. Synoviography. In: Clinics in rheumatic Dis, 1: diagnosis and assessment, vol. 2. W.B. Saunders; 1976. p. 129–49.
88. Gompels BM, Darlington LG. Grey scale ultrasonography and arthrography in evaluation of popliteal cysts. Clin Radiol. 1979;30:539–45.
89. de Jesus JO, Parker L, Frangos AJ, Nazarian LN. Accuracy of MRI, MR arthrography, and ultrasound in the diagnosis of rotator cuff tears: a meta-analysis. AJR Am J Roentgenol. 2009;192:1701–7.
90. Ng AW, Hung EH, Griffith JF, Tong CS, Cho CC. Comparison of ultrasound versus fluoroscopic guided rotator cuff interval approach for MR arthrography. Clin Imaging. 2013;37:548–53.
91. Chaturvedi V, Thabah MM, Ravindran V, Kiely PDW. Medical arthroscopy: a tool for diagnosis and research in rheumatology. Int J Rheum Dis. 2017;20:145–53.
92. Goëb V, Walsh CA, Reece RJ, Emery P, Ponchel F. Potential role of arthroscopy in the management of inflammatory arthritis. Clin Exp Rheumatol. 2012;30:429–35.
93. Ike RW, Arnold WJ, Kalunian KC. Arthroscopy in rheumatology: where have we been? Where might we go? Rheumatology (Oxford). 2021;60:518–28.
94. Paresce E, De Lucia O, Bruschi E, Giacomelli L, Epis OM. Use of ultrasound-assisted arthroscopy in rheumatology: an experience in 11 patients with different rheumatic diseases. Expert Opin Med Diagn. 2013;7:309–12.
95. Xie Y, Li L, Luo R, et al. Diagnostic efficacy of joint ultrasonography, dual-energy computed tomography and minimally invasive arthroscopy on knee gouty arthritis, a comparative study. Br J Radiol. 2021;94:20200493.
96. Saarakkala S, Waris P, Waris V, et al. Diagnostic performance of knee ultrasonography for detecting degenerative changes of articular cartilage. Osteoarthr Cartil. 2012;20:376–81.
97. Schröder JH, Perka DKC, Martin H. Arthroscopic treatment for primary septic arthritis of the hip in adults. Adv Orthop. 2016;2016:8713037.
98. Brenton J, Mark L, Eric H, David D. Arthroscopic versus open treatment for acute septic arthritis of the knee in children. Pediatr Infect Dis J. 2018;37:413–8.

99. Rizvi SMT, Qiu D, Lam P, Hackett L, Walton J, Murrell GAC. Ultrasound guided arthroscopic removal of calcific tendonitis: a minimum of 2-year followup. J Clin Med. 2023;12:3114.
100. Martinel V, Fermandois-Maltes P. Arthroscopic ultrasound-guided needling: an effective technique for the treatment of calcific rotator cuff tendinopathy. Arthrosc Tech. 2021;10:e2021–6.
101. Sarasquete RJ, Domínguez GLG, Lobo OC. Ultrasound-guided aspiration puncture vs arthroscopy of the shoulder rotator cuff calcic tendinopathy resolution. Acta Med Austriaca. 2021;19:180–5.
102. Wintzell G, Hovelius L, Wikblad L, et al. Arthroscopic lavage speeds reduction in effusion in the glenohumeral joint after primary anterior shoulder dislocation: a controlled randomized ultrasound study. Knee Surg. 2000;8:56–60.

4 Ultrasound Outcome Measures Tool in Rheumatology (OMERACT)

Md Abu Bakar Siddiq, George A. W. Bruyn, and Johannes J. Rasker

4.1 Background

In recent years, the International League of Associations for Rheumatology (ILAR) has placed significant emphasis on advancing outcome measures within the field of rheumatic diseases, such as rheumatoid arthritis (RA), osteoarthritis (OA), spondyloarthropathy (SpA), systemic lupus erythematosus (SLE), and osteoporosis [1]. This effort has been primarily spearheaded by OMERACT (Outcome Measures for Rheumatoid Arthritis Clinical Trials) [1]. Examples of uniform outcome measures in rheumatology include the OMERACT-OARSI (Outcome Measures in Rheumatology-Osteoarthritis Research Society International) [2], the OMERACT-*systemic lupus erythematosus* (SLE) core outcome sets [3], the Western Ontario and McMasters University Osteoarthritis (WOMAC) index, the Knee Injury and Osteoarthritis Outcome Score (KOOS), and the Patient Reported Outcomes Measurement Information System (PROMIS) physical function scale [4]. To make outcome measures uniform and be able to compare and combine data in statistical analysis, it is necessary to standardize outcome measures in rheumatology worldwide [5]. OMERACT is a worldwide informally organized network that aims to improve outcome measurement in rheumatology [5], to identify pertinent health outcome domains, and to support reliable, practical health outcome measures/scales in rheumatic disorders [5]. The OMERACT meeting is chaired by an executive committee and organizes consensus conferences every 2 years [5]. The first conference was held in 1992 in Maastricht, Netherlands (Fig. 4.1), and building a consensus on some contentious issues in RA clinical trials was one of the three main objectives [5]:

M. A. B. Siddiq (✉)
Department of Rheumatology, Royal North Shore Hospital, Northern Clinical School, Faculty of Medicine and Health, The University of Sydney, Sydney, NSW, Australia

Sydney Musculoskeletal Health, The University of Sydney, Sydney, NSW, Australia

Kolling Institute of Medical Research, St Leonards, NSW, Australia

School of Health Sports and Professional Practice (Rheumatology), University of South Wales, Pontypridd, United Kingdom

Department of Physical Medicine and Rehabilitation, Brahmanbaria Medical College, Brahmanbaria, Bangladesh
e-mail: msid8426@uni.sydney.edu.au

G. A. W. Bruyn
Department of Rheumatology, Reumakliniek Lelystad, Lelystad, The Netherlands

Tergooi MC Hospital, Hilversum, Netherlands

J. J. Rasker
Faculty of Behavioral Science, Psychology, Health and Technology, University of Twente, Enschede, The Netherlands

M. A. B. Siddiq (ed.), *Musculoskeletal Ultrasound in Rheumatic Diseases*,
https://doi.org/10.1007/978-981-96-5298-3_4

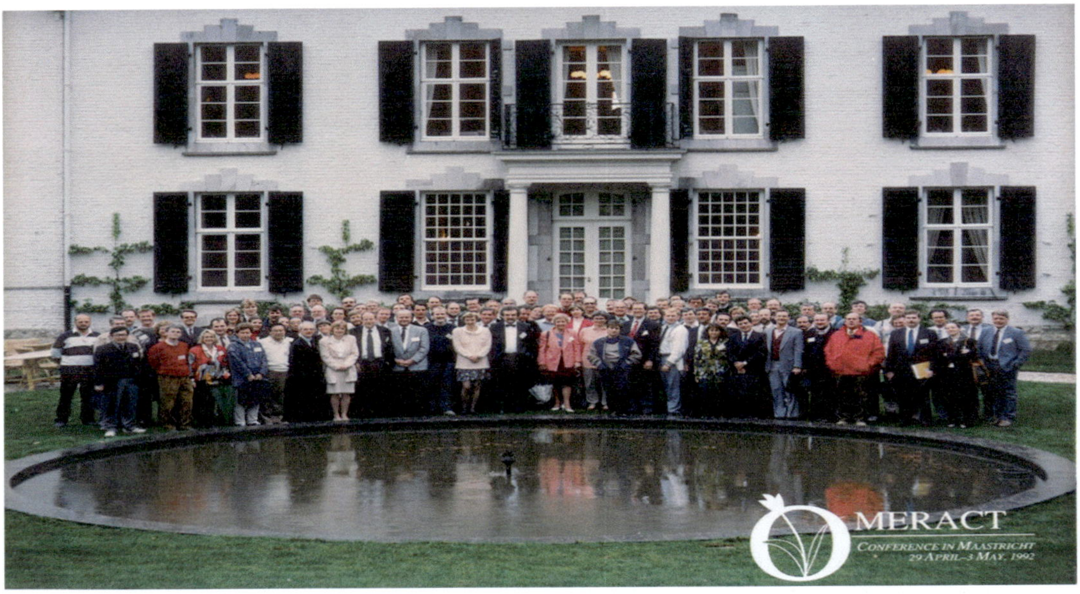

Fig. 4.1 First OMERACT conference held in the Netherlands. *(Source: with permission from Professor Rasker JJ, University of Twente, The Netherlands)*

1. Reaching a consensus regarding the minimal quantity of outcome measures required for all RA clinical trials.
2. Examining the spectrum of changes in magnitude that experts and clinical investigators deem clinically significant.
3. To review the extent to which experienced clinicians and clinical investigators feel that aggregate measures (indices) are useful in the assessment of trials and individual patients.

4.2 Ultrasound OMERACT

The use of ultrasound as a diagnostic method for musculoskeletal disorders has increased over the years [6]. Starting with investigating larger joints and soft tissue structures such as Baker's cysts (BCs), technological improvements in image resolution and tissue contrast have allowed the modality to be used for visualizing much smaller anatomical structures [6]. Inflammatory rheumatic conditions with bone erosions, synovitis, tendon disease, and enthesopathy can be assessed with ultrasound [6]. Ultrasound has several advantages over magnetic resonance imaging (MRI), such as assessment at the point-of-care, no radiation, prompt scanning of several joints in a limited time, and comparison of findings with those in other joints; dynamic scanning; being patient-friendly; being a less expensive alternative; and being a great tool for guiding injections to a body target [6]. Despite the obvious leverage that ultrasound is able to offer, concerns such as its lack of accuracy have spooked investigators for a long time, as it is operator-dependent and findings vary widely across sonographers depending on the expertise and uniformity of scanning methods, making the outcome less valid or reliable [7].

The above considerations drove a group of investigators interested in the use of ultrasound in rheumatology to gather and propose a set of criteria for defining pathological lesions in rheumatic diseases (Table 4.1) (Figs. 4.2, 4.3, and 4.4) [6]. Furthermore, these investigators decided to

Table 4.1 Ultrasound definitions are used in rheumatic disease [6] (Fig. 4.2)

Pathologies	Description
Synovial fluid	An abnormal hypoechoic or anechoic intra-articular material (relative to subdermal fat, but sometimes may be isoechoic or hyperechoic) is identified, which possesses the ability to be displaced and compressed, but does not display any Doppler signal.
Synovial hypertrophy	Anomalous hypoechoic intra-articular tissue characterized by its nondisplaceable and poorly compressible nature, potentially displaying a Doppler signal.
Tenosynovitis	The tendon sheath shows hypoechoic or anechoic thickening with or without fluid, visualized in two perpendicular planes and potentially displaying a Doppler signal.
Enthesopathy	Unusual hypoechoic characteristics (lacking normal fibrillar structure) and/or thickened tendon or ligament at its bony insertion point (potentially showing hyperechoic areas indicating calcification), observed in two perpendicular planes that may exhibit Doppler signal and/or bone alterations such as enthesophytes, erosions, or irregularities.
Bone erosion	An intra-articular discontinuity of the bone surface that is visible in two perpendicular planes.

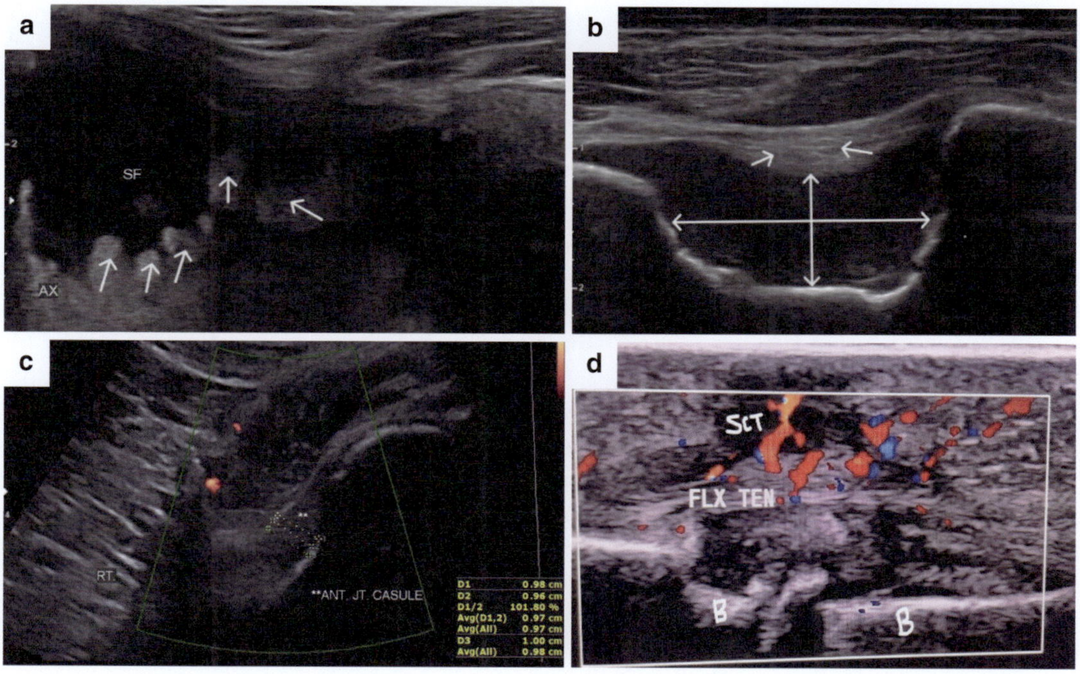

Fig. 4.2 Ultrasound in inflammatory arthritis. (**a**) Short axis gray-scale scan of anterior knee reveals villous synovium in undifferentiated inflammatory synovitis. (**b**) Short axis gray-scale scan of posterior flexed elbow joint depicts synovial hypertrophy in rheumatoid arthritis. (**c**) Oblique longitudinal scan of anterior hip explores synovial hypertrophy in ankylosing spondylitis. (**d**) Longitudinal scan of volar aspect of the finger unveils flexor tenosynovitis (Doppler spots around the FLX TEN) in psoriatic dactylitis. *AX* axial, *B* bone, *FLX TEN* flexor tendon, *SF* synovial fluid, *SCT* subcutaneous tissue

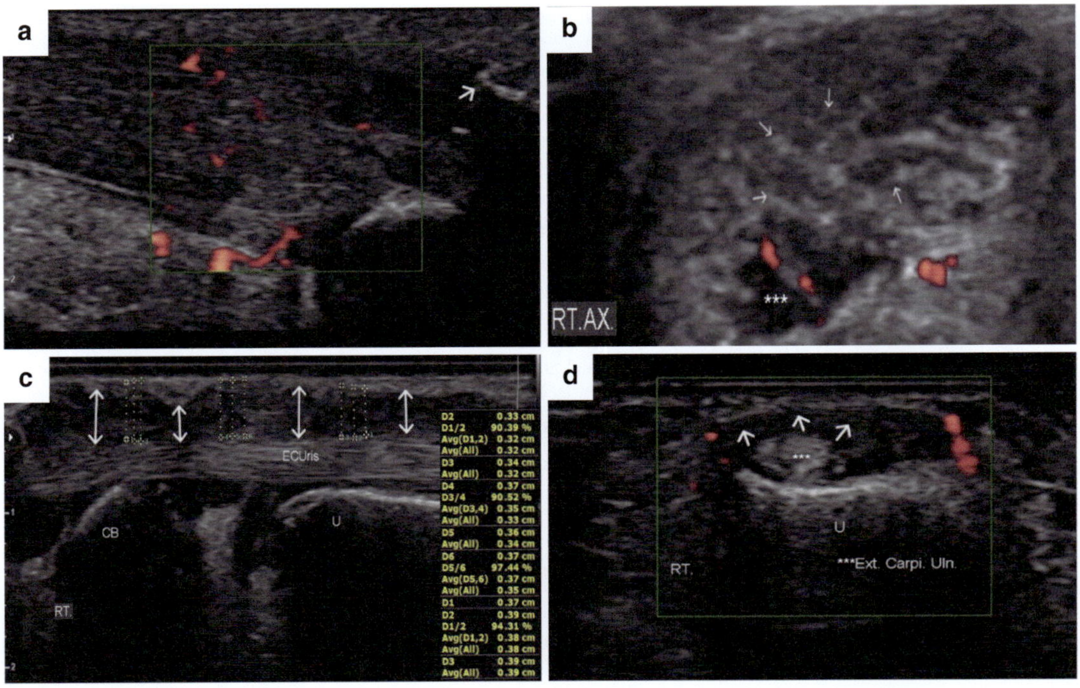

Fig. 4.3 Tendinopathy. (**a**, **b**) Long and short axes, scans of posterior heel and lower leg, respectively, reveal a thick and hypoechoic Achilles tendon with increased Doppler signals (**b**) and calcaneal spur (**a**) (white arrow). (**c**, **d**) Long and short axes, respectively, explore a thick and hypoechoic ECUris tenosynovial sheath (double and single arrows) around fibrillar tendon with increased Doppler signal. *AX* axial, *CB* carpal bone, *ECUris* Extensor Carpi Ulnaris, *RT* right, *U* ulna

create an ultrasound working group (WG) under the umbrella of OMERACT, an informal international network that strives to improve outcome measures through a data-driven, iterative consensus process [5, 6]. Subsequently, repetitive validation exercises by this working group have consistently demonstrated the validity and reliability of ultrasound in identifying both reversible and irreversible pathophysiological alterations, such as synovitis, tenosynovitis, or erosions in RA [8]. The OMERACT-ultrasound WG has so substantiated the utility of ultrasound

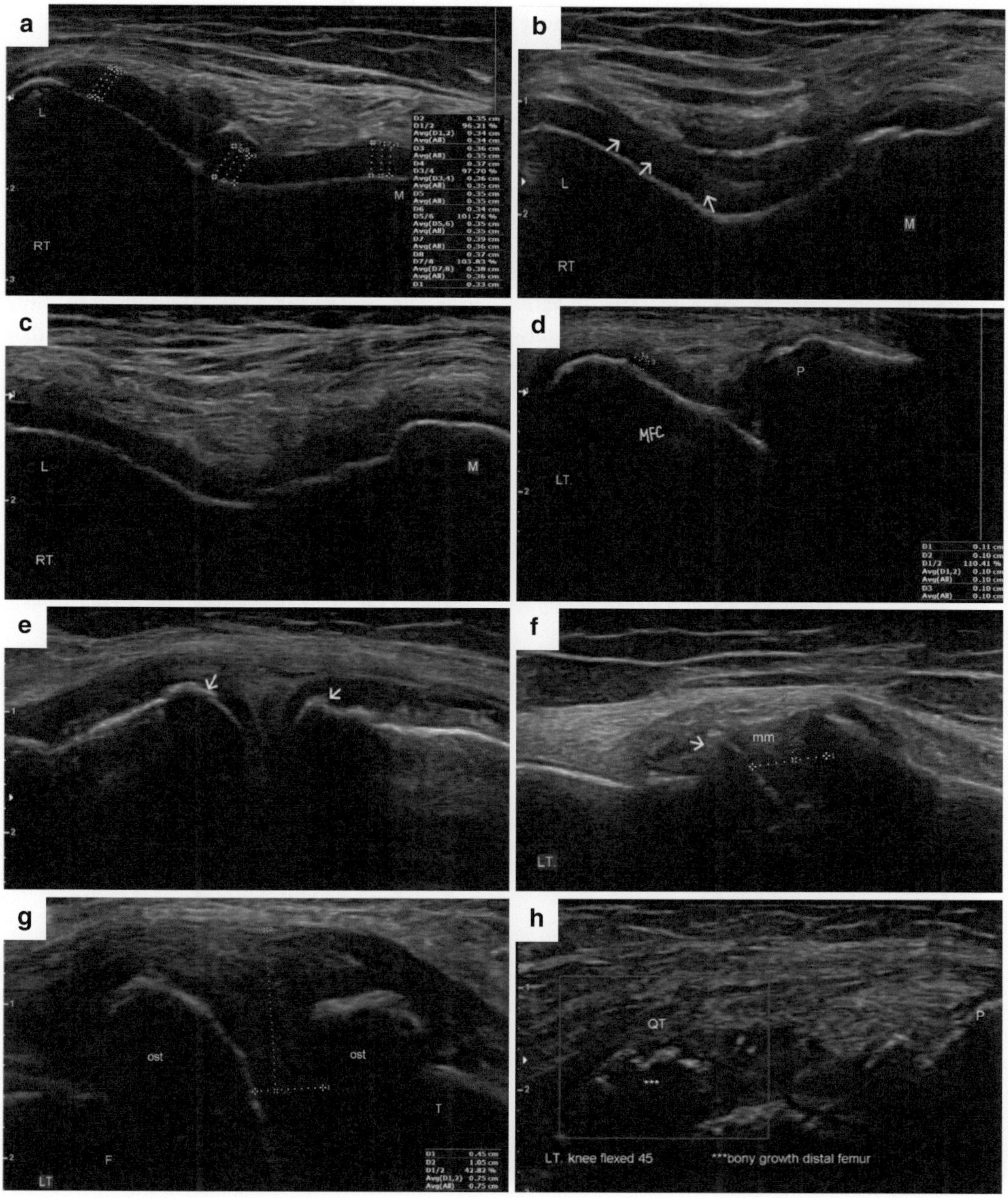

Fig. 4.4 Ultrasound in osteoarthritis. (**a**) Transverse scan of semi-flexed knee reveals preserved femoral cartilage thickness. (**b**, **c**) Transverse scan of the semi-flexed knee reveals reduced femoral condylar cartilage sharpness (arrows) and thickness. (**d**) Long axis scan of flexed knee shows MFC reduced cartilage thickness. (**e**–**g**) Longitudinal medial knee scans depict mild, moderate, and large osteophytes (arrows), respectively arise from the tibia and femoral condyles. (**h**) Longitudinal scan of anterior knee explores impacted loose body in the hypertrophied synovium in anterior joint recess with increased Doppler signal in knee OA. *F* femur, *LT* left, *L* lateral, *LT* left, *M* medial, *MFC* medial femoral condyle, *Ost* osteophyte, *P* patella, *QT* quadricep's tendon, *RT* right, *T* tibia

in various inflammatory and noninflammatory disorders [8].

4.3 Modification of the OMERACT-Ultrasound Measures

The OMERACT ultrasound-WG is actively involved in conducting research activities to validate the use of ultrasound as an outcome measuring instrument [8]. The OMERACT-ultrasound tool has been recognized as a valid method for evaluating RA [8]. The WG has made significant contributions by introducing new definitions and scoring systems for synovitis (including pediatric synovitis), enthesitis, tenosynovitis, and tendon damage [8]. In the most recent update in 2019, the OMERACT ultrasound WG redefined ultrasound pathology (Table 4.2) and elementary lesions (Table 4.3), along with scoring systems that have been widely utilized in clinical trials since its inception [8]. Furthermore, the OMERACT-WG is actively engaged in validating the use of ultrasound in other rheumatic conditions, including OA, SpA, psoriatic arthritis

Table 4.2 OMERACT definitions of ultrasound pathologies[#]

Pathologies	Description	Grading
1. Synovitis	Hypoechoic synovial hypertrophy (SH) regardless of the presence of synovial effusion or Doppler signal.	**Grading:** Normal: Only synovial effusion, no SH Grade 1 (mild): Minimal hypoechoic SH (up to the imaginary horizontal line connecting the two joint edges) Grade 2 (moderate): Moderate hypoechoic SH (protruding over the joint line along with a concave surface) Grade 3 (severe): Severe hypoechoic SH (protruding beyond the joint line with a convex surface) **EULAR-OMERACT combined score:** Normal: No SH & PD Grade 1: Grade 1 SH and/or ≤ grade 1 PD Grade 2: Grade 2 SH and/or ≤ grade 2 PD; or grade 1 SH and grade 2 PD Grade 3: Grade 3 SH and/or ≤ grade 3 PD; or grade 1 or grade 2 SH and grade 3 PD
2. Enthesitis	Hypoechoic and/or thickened insertion of the enthesis close to the bone (within 2 mm from the bony cortex) exhibiting active Doppler signal with structural damage, including erosions, enthesophytes, or calcifications.	**OMERACT combined grading:** **Gray-scale (GS) features:** Hypoechogenicity: 0/1 Thickened enthesis: 0/1 Calcification/enthesophytes: 0/1 Bone erosion: 0–1 **Doppler grading:** Grade 0: No Doppler signal Grade 1: <2 punctiform Doppler signals or 1 confluent Doppler signal Grade 2: 2–4 punctiform Doppler signals or 1 confluent Doppler signal Grade 3: >4 punctiform Doppler signals or 1 confluent Doppler signal

(continued)

Table 4.2 (continued)

Pathologies	Description	Grading
3. Tenosynovitis	Abnormal anechoic and/or hypoechoic (relative to tendon fibers) tendon sheath widening, due to either tenosynovial abnormal fluid and/or hypertrophy. Doppler signal can be considered within the widened peritendinous synovial sheath on B-mode, excluding synovial sheath normal feeding vessels.	**Combined grading (GS & Doppler signal)** Grade 0 (normal): No tenosynovial widening (either due to hypertrophy or effusion); no Doppler signal Grade 1 (mild): Minimal amount of anechoic or hypoechoic material within the tenosynovial sheath, either localized or displaceable; peritendinous focal Doppler signal within the widened synovial sheath (signals in only one area of the widened sheath), excluding normal feeding vessels Grade 2 (moderate): Moderate amount of anechoic or hypoechoic material within the tenosynovial sheath; peritendinous multifocal Doppler signals within the widened synovial sheath (i.e., signals in more than one area of the widened sheath), excluding normal feeding vessels Grade 3 (severe): Severe amount of anechoic or hypoechoic material within the tenosynovial sheath; peritendinous diffuse Doppler signals within the widened synovial sheath, excluding normal feeding vessels (if abnormal intrasheath and abnormal intratendinous signals are present in two perpendicular planes (excluding intratendinous feeding vessels on ultrasound), then grades 1 and 2 would be increased by one point)
4. Tendon damage	Internal and/or peripheral focal tendon defect (i.e., the absence of fibers) in the region enclosed by the tendon sheath, seen in two perpendicular planes; the grade of tendon damage should be assessed in both planes.	Tendon damage is a structural lesion and is solely defined in B mode because this mode allows the evaluation of the morphology.
5. Bone erosion	Intra- and/or extra-articular discontinuity of bone surface (visible in 2 perpendicular planes).	No new change
6. Pediatric synovitis	Presence of hypoechoic SH or of abnormal synovial effusion.	**Grading:** Grade 0 (normal): No signs of synovial effusion or SH (no joint recess enlargement/capsular distension); no Doppler signal within SH with or without detection of normal physiological Doppler signals. Grade 1 (mild): Synovial effusion and/or SH with mild joint recess enlargement/capsular distension. Detection of up to 3 single Doppler signals within the area of SH with or without normal physiological Doppler signals. Grade 2 (moderate): Synovial effusion and/or SH with moderate joint recess enlargement/capsular distension with detection of >3 single Doppler signals but <30% of the area of SH with or without normal physiological Doppler signals. Grade 3 (severe): Synovial effusion and/or SH with severe joint recess enlargement/capsular distension with detection of Doppler signals >30% of the area of SH with or without normal physiological Doppler signals.

All the features should be assessed in two perpendicular planes. *PD*, power Doppler; *SH*, synovial hypertrophy
Modified from Bruyn et al. [8]

Table 4.3 OMERACT ultrasound elementary lesions

Pathology	Inflammatory Elementary Lesions	Structural Elementary Lesions
Synovitis	Hypoechoic SH within the capsule that is not displaceable and poorly compressible and may exhibit Doppler signals	
Enthesitis	Hypoechoic increased thickness of anatomical enthesis (i.e., tendon insertion <2 mm from the bony surface) that exhibits Doppler signal	Calcifications/enthesophytes at enthesis, erosions at enthesis
Tenosynovitis	Abnormal hypoechoic tendon hypertrophy within the synovial sheath that is not displaceable and poorly compressible and seen in two perpendicular planes may exhibit Doppler signals	
OA osteophytes		Step-up bony prominence at the bony margin (visible in 2 perpendicular planes)
OA hyaline cartilage damage		Loss of anechoic structure and/or thinning of the cartilage layer, and irregularities and/or sharpness of at least 1 cartilage margin Grade 0 (normal): Normal cartilage Grade 1 (minimal): Loss of anechoic structure and/ or focal thinning of cartilage layer OR irregularities and/or loss of sharpness of at least one cartilage margin Grade 2 (moderate): Loss of anechoic structure and/or focal thinning of cartilage layer AND irregularities and/or loss of sharpness of at least one cartilage margin Grade 3 (severe): Focal absence or complete loss of cartilage layer
Gout DC		Abnormal hyperechoic band over the superficial margin of the articular hyaline cartilage, independent of the angle of insonation, which may be either irregular or regular, continuous or intermittent, and can be distinguished from the cartilage interface sign
Gout tophus		Circumscribed, inhomogeneous, hyperechoic, and/ or hypoechoic aggregation (which may or may not generate posterior acoustic shadow), which may be surrounded by a small anechoic rim
Gout aggregates		Heterogeneous hyperechoic foci that maintain their high degree of reflectivity, even when the gain setting is minimized or the insonation angle is changed and which occasionally may generate posterior acoustic shadow
CPPD fibrocartilage		Hyperechoic deposits of variable shape, localized within the fibrocartilage structure, that remain fixed or move along with the fibrocartilage during dynamic assessment
CPPD hyaline cartilage		Hyperechoic deposits of variable size and shape, without posterior shadowing, localized within the hyaline cartilage, that remain fixed and move along with the hyaline cartilage during dynamic assessment

(continued)

Table 4.3 (continued)

Pathology	Inflammatory Elementary Lesions	Structural Elementary Lesions
CPPD tendon		Hyperechoic, linear structure(s) generally without posterior shadowing, localized within the tendon and remaining fixed and moving along with the tendon during dynamic assessment
CPPD synovial fluid		Hyperechoic deposits of variable size, localized within the synovial fluid, without posterior shadowing, and mobile along with joint movement and probe pressure
Halo sign	Homogeneous, hypoechoic wall thickening, well delineated toward the luminal side, is visible in two perpendicular planes, most commonly concentric in transverse scan	
Compression sign	Thickened arterial wall remains visible under compression, i.e., the echogenicity contrasts hypoechogenic because of vasculitic vessel wall thickening in comparison to mid/hyperechoic surrounding tissue	

CPPD calcium pyrophosphate dihydrate, *DC* double contour, *OA* osteoarthritis
Modified from Bruyn et al. [8]

(PsA), crystalline arthropathies, large vessel vasculitis (LVV), Sjögren syndrome (SS), SLE, and juvenile inflammatory arthritis [8].

4.4 OMERACT Ultrasound Validity and Reliability in Rheumatic Diseases

Since inception, the OMERACT ultrasound has undergone reliability and validity tests for various rheumatic disorders [5]. In the subsequent sections, we demonstrate how recent rheumatology research has validated the OMERACT ultrasound outcome measures [8–32]. Table 4.4 shows the reliability of ultrasound in recent rheumatology research.

(i) **Rheumatoid arthritis:** Reliability assessment of the EULAR-OMERACT combined ultrasound score for SH and the power Doppler (PD) signal in the RA demonstrated moderate to good agreement [13]. A systematic review revealed that ultrasound assessment, specifically PD-positive synovitis, is more reliable than clinical examination in predicting relapse and radiographic progression in RA [14]. Ultrasound could be especially advantageous in cases of moderately active disease, where composite indices may have limitations [14]. High-frequency ultrasound can successfully distinguish between seronegative RA and OA [15]. There were significant differences between RA and OA regarding GS scores, PD scores of joints and tendons, and bone erosion scores ($P < 0.05$) [15]. The cumulative scores of the ultrasound variables were positively correlated with C-reactive protein, erythrocyte sedimentation rate, and the disease activity score (DAS28) ($P < 0.05$), unlike those of the OA group ($P > 0.05$) [15]. Ultrasound forecasting clinical response to treatment has also been studied [16, 17]. In a study with real-life data of baricitinib in RA, OMERACT-ultrasound components (except tendon PD) were confirmed to be useful in monitoring disease activity and treatment response. Further studies on larger cohorts and longer follow-up observations are needed [16]. Moreover, RA patients treated with tofacitinib for

Table 4.4 Ultrasound reliability and validity in rheumatic diseases [7, 13, 16, 20, 23, 25, 28, 29]

Rheumatic conditions	Ultrasound reliability (kappa, *k* value)
Rheumatoid arthritis [13]	Overall score: In MCP joints (static images), substantial IOR, good to excellent IRR. IOR–SH (0.87), PD (0.79), and the EULAR-OMERACT combined score (0.86) (using "standardized" scan). Other joints (static images), the IOR excellent for all scores (0.8–0.97) and IRR marginally lower. Standardized scanning in patients, IOR good (0.64 for SH and the EULAR-OMERACT combined score, 0.66 for PD), and IRR for PD good (0.41–0.92).
Psoriatic arthritis [7]	IRR (without adjustment) for enthesophytes (0.6), Doppler signal at insertion (0.4), lowest value for thickened enthesis 0.1 (95% CI 0–0.7). IOR (without adjustment) for erosion, hypoechogenicity at the enthesis, Doppler at the enthesis and outside, and for bursitis ranged between 0 and 1.0. The lowest value was seen for bone irregularities, calcifications, and enthesophytes (−0.1 to 0.5); 0.1–0.5; and 0.1–0.5, respectively. Adjusted for low prevalence—k for Doppler signal at insertion (0.9) and for bursitis (0.8).
Osteoarthritis [20]	Substantial IOR and IRR for inflammatory OA features (κ > 0.64). In the patient-based exercise, IOR and IRR (k values), respectively: SH, 0.73 and 0.45; joint effusion, 0.70 and 0.55; power Doppler PABAK, 0.90 and 0.88; PIP joint cartilage, 0.56 and 0.45; and STT osteophytes, 0.62 and 0.36. Percentage close agreement was high for all features (>85%).
Gouty arthritis [25]	IRR is good for all three ultrasound gout lesions (range 0.61–0.67). The lowest value for aggregates (0.61) and the highest value for tophi (0.67). IOR is good for all lesions, and IOR is 0.74–0.80.
CPPD [23]	IOR and IRR (static images) of CPPD deposit grades are perfect (0.90 and 0.84, respectively); in patients substantial (0.72 and 0.66, respectively).
Sjögren syndrome [28]	Vascular signal (static images), IOR, and IRR excellent (for all salivary glands together) (0.90 and 0.80, respectively). In patients, the IOR and IRR (all four salivary glands together) are 0.84 and 0.70, respectively.
GCA [29]	IRR for normal ultrasound findings, halo sign, and compression sign in preliminary exercise fair to moderate overall diagnosis of GCA (light κ 0.29–0.51) and poor to fair for identifying vasculitis in the respective anatomical segments (light κ 0.02–0.46). IOR moderate (Cohen κ 0.32–0.64). In the main exercise, IRR (good to excellent) (light κ 0.76–0.86) for the overall diagnosis of GCA, and moderate to good (light κ 0.46–0.71) for vasculitis diagnosis in the respective anatomical segments. IOR is excellent for GCA diagnosis (Cohen κ 0.91) and good (Cohen κ 0.71–0.80) for the anatomical segments.
JIA [16]	IOR is good (0.62, range 0.47–0.75) for synovitis and synovial hypertrophy; excellent for Doppler signals (quadratic weighted k 0.77, 0.66–0.86; 0.76, 0.61–0.84; and 0.87, 0.77–0.94, respectively); and moderate for effusion (0.55). IRR is good for synovitis (light k 0.68) and SH (0.63), excellent for Doppler signals (0.85), and moderate for effusion (0.49). Best score observed in knee (0.71, 0.54–0.85) except for Doppler signals, with reliability higher for MCP-II.

CPPD calcium pyrophosphate dihydrate, *EULAR-OMERACT* European Alliance of Associations for Rheumatology-Outcome Measures in Rheumatology, *GCA* giant cell arteritis, *IRR* inter-rater reliability, *IOR* intra-observer reliability, *JIA* juvenile idiopathic arthritis, *MCP-II* second metacarpophalangeal, *OA* osteoarthritis, *PABAK* prevalence-adjusted bias-adjusted kappa, *PIP* proximal interphalangeal, *STT* scaphotrapeziotrapezoid

12 weeks improved ($P < 0.0001$) in terms of clinical, imaging (including ultrasound), and biomarker endpoints. Baseline ultrasound (with the exception of PD score) and multibiomarker disease activity scores are predictive of clinical improvement at follow-up [17]. In real-life scenarios, the Global EULAR and OMERACT Synovitis Score (GLOESS) for MCPs 2–5 emerged as a valuable measure of RA activity [18]. The optimal cutoff for distinguishing remission/low disease activity from moderate/high disease activity was determined to be a GLOESS score ≤ 3, with all MCP joints exhibiting both GS and PD scores of ≤ 1 [18].

(ii) **Spondyloarthritis (SpA):** Reliability of consensus-based ultrasound definitions of elementary components of enthesitis (Fig. 4.3) in SpA and PsA performed among sonographers [10]. The prevalence of detected lesions was quite low except for enthesophytes (55%) and bone irregularities (54%) [10]. The reliability ranged from poor to good (the lowest for thickened enthesis), and the highest reliability was reported for enthesophytes [10]. When adjusted for low prevalence, reliability scores increased for all lesions, with the best result observed for detecting the Doppler signal at insertion and for bursitis [10]. The first large randomized controlled trial revealed that OMERACT ultrasound synovitis (GLOESS) and enthesitis scores over 12 months (GLOESS) improved following secukinumab therapy in PsA [18–19]. Another study revealed that interleukin (IL-17A) inhibition with secukinumab leads to a rapid and significant reduction in GLOESS synovitis in PsA patients [20, 21]. Further studies should implement this score in clinical trials and practice [10].

(iii) **Osteoarthritis:** The use of ultrasound has been studied in patients with knee (Fig. 4.4) and hand OA. OMERACT-ultrasound scores are associated with clinical symptoms and radiographic and MRI severity in OA [22]. Greater ultrasound SH, PD signal in SH, and meniscal extrusion (ME) scores are associated with worse numerical rating scales for pain [22]. All higher ultrasound scores, with the exception of cartilage grade, were significantly associated with worse Knee Injury and Osteoarthritis Outcome Score (KOOS) symptoms (other than pain), whereas only PD and ME were associated with worse KOOS pain [21]. All ultrasound scores, except for PD, were significantly correlated with Kellgren-Lawrence radiological grading [22]. Ultrasound pathologies (except for cartilage change) revealed moderate to good correlation with their MRI-OA knee score (MOAKS) counterparts, with ultrasound synovitis having the greatest correlation with MOAKS [22]. The OMERACT-WG ultrasound focused on structural abnormalities in hand OA and produced a dichotomous and a four-grade semiquantitative score for cartilage damage and osteophytes, respectively, that needs to be checked for validity and reliability in other joints [8]. In hand OA, ultrasound revealed substantial to excellent intra-reader reliability for inflammatory features (SH, joint effusion, and PD signals). However, inter-reader reliability varied widely; moderate for SH, effusion, and cartilage thickness; and the lowest for scapho-trapezio-trapezoid osteophytes [23].

OMERACT ultrasound measures of the inflammatory features of knee OA have shown moderate-substantial reliability and low-to-moderate sensitivity to change, whereas measures of structural OA features are less reliable [25]. The use of quantitative measures of synovitis and effusion has demonstrated good test-retest reliability [25]. Ultrasound measures of synovitis and effusion demonstrated low-to-moderate sensitivity to changes [10]. The associations between changes in ultrasound measures and KOOS pain scores over time appeared weak [24].

(iv) **Calcium pyrophosphate dihydrate deposition (CPPD):** definitions of the ultrasound characteristics of CPPD at the level of the fibrocartilage of the knee menisci, triangular fibrocartilage complex of the wrist, hyaline cartilage, tendons, and synovial fluid of the knee are provided in Table 4.3; these characteristics are reliable and valid [7, 8]. Ultrasound accurately demonstrates CPPD; however, it cannot differentiate CPPD in OA with or without inflammation [25]. The overall diagnostic accuracy of ultrasound for CPPD is 75%, with a sensitivity of 91% (range 71–87% at single sites) and a specificity of 59% (range 68–92%) [25].

The CPPD-subgroup of the OMERACT-WG ultrasound developed a validated semiquantitative scoring tool for CPPD crystals in joints [26]:

grade 0 (no findings consistent with CPPD), grade 1 (≤3 single spots or 1 small deposit), grade 2 (>3 single spots or > 1 small deposit or ≥ 1 larger deposit occupying ≤50% of the structure under examination in the reference image, i.e., the scanning view with the highest grade of depositions), and grade 3 (deposits that occupy more than 50% of the structure under examination in the reference image) [26]. The instrument was assessed on the knee (menisci and hyaline cartilage) and the triangular fibrocartilage complex of the wrist, demonstrating high levels of reliability among readers both within and between, as evidenced by nearly perfect to substantial agreement in static images and clinical evaluations. These findings suggest that the score could serve as a valuable instrument for monitoring the effectiveness of pseudogout treatment [26].

(v) **Gout:** Four elementary lesions in gout, namely, double contour (DC), aggregates, tophus, and erosions (Fig. 4.5), were found to be reliable for testing [8]. The reliability of ultrasound definitions for gout aggregate, DC, and aggregates has been assessed through intra- and inter-reader reliability tests conducted among rheumatologists [27]. In a clinical setting, the ultrasound revealed a statistically significant decrease in DC and tophus sum scores at the 3- and 6-month follow-ups, whereas the aggregate sum score only significantly decreased from 3 to 6 months [28]. The erosion sum score remained relatively unchanged [28]. All four structural lesions are most commonly found in metatarsophalangeal (MTP) 1 joints (>1 lesion bilaterally), and MTP 2–4 and knee joints are common

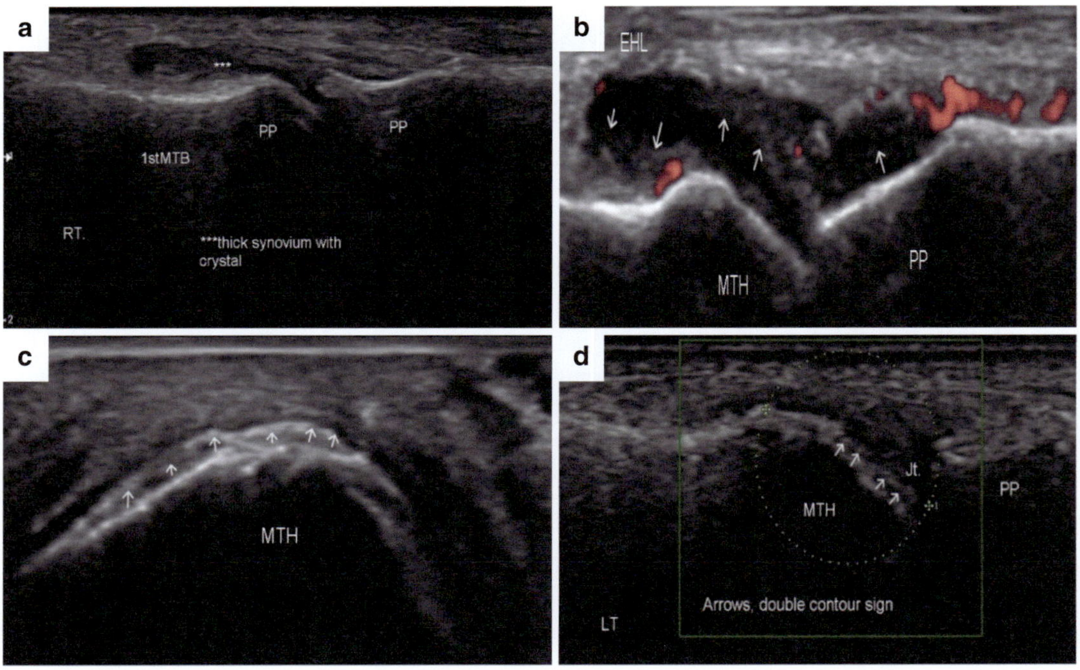

Fig. 4.5 Ultrasound in gout. (**a**, **b**) Longitudinal scans of anterior aspect of first metatarsophalangeal joint reveal thick and hypoechoic synovial hypertrophy (asterisks) with increased Doppler activity (red spots) (**b**) (**c**, **d**) Short and long axes scans, respectively explore the Double contour sign (arrows) over the first metatarsal head. *EHL* extensor hallucis longus, *LT* left, *MTB* metatarsal bone, *MTP* metatarsophalangeal, *MTH* metatarsal head, *PP* proximal phalanx, *RT* right

sites, especially for DC [28]. The recent EULAR recommendation suggests the use of ultrasound in the diagnosis and treatment of crystal-induced arthritis, including gout [29].

(vi) **Sjögren syndrome (SS) and salivary glands (SGs):** Ultrasound homogeneity assessment of the SGs has proven to be a valuable tool for differentiating between healthy and abnormal parenchyma [30]. The OMERACT ultrasound scoring system, which considers structural damage, presents a novel and comprehensive approach to diagnosing patients with primary SS (pSS) and has the potential to be readily adopted by sonographers for clinical use [30]. Construct validity of the OMERACT-ultrasound semiquantitative (0–3, GS) scoring system for morphological lesions in major SGs (parotid glands, PGs, and submandibular glands [SMGs]) compared with that of MRI and unstimulated whole salivary flow rates (U-WSFRs) demonstrated in primary SS (pSS) [31]. The agreement between U-WSFRs and imaging structural lesions (ultrasound and MRI) was determined [31]: a score ≥ 2 for both ultrasound and MRI was defined as gland pathology. The percentage of ultrasound morphological lesions with a score ≥ 2 was 58% for PGs, 76% for SMGs, and 46% and 41% for PGs and SMGs, respectively, for MRI. The agreement between OMERACT-ultrasound scores and MRI scores was 73–91% in the right PG, 73–91% in the left PG, 55–91% in the right SMG, and 55–82% in the left SMG [31]. The associations between hypo-salivation and ultrasound score ≥ 2 were 91–100% in both PGs and 55–91% in both SMGs [27]. There is moderate to strong agreement between the OMERACT-ultrasound and MRI scores for major SGs, between the higher OMERACT ultrasound scores and the presence of hyposalivation [31]. OMERACT-ultrasound color Doppler (CD) reliability was further tested in SGs in pSS [32]. Consensus-based semiquantitative CD ultrasound scoring in pSS showed good to excellent inter- and intra-rater reliability performed based on static images and in the clinical setting [32].

(vii) **Large vessel vasculitis (LVV)/giant cell arteritis (GCA):** Ultrasound features of the LVV, including the "halo sign" and the "compression sign" in GCA, have been well-documented (Table 4.3) [8]. A recent study compared the reliability of OMERACT consensus-based ultrasound definitions for normal and vasculitic temporal and axillary arteries in patients with GCA and in controls [33]. The study revealed that OMERACT-derived definitions of halo and compression signs of temporal and axillary arteries are reliable in recent-onset GCA, provided that experienced sonographers with prior training examined patients for an appropriate time (15–20 min) [33]. An investigation was conducted to compare the diagnostic discriminant validity of ultrasound-intima-media thickness (IMT) between GCA and atherosclerosis. The study revealed that IMT values were notably greater in LV-GCA than in atherosclerosis, with an IMT ≥ 1 mm being deemed pathological [34]. Furthermore, the suggested count of the ultrasound halo (OMERACT feature) exhibited an accuracy of more than 95% in distinguishing between LVV-GCA and atherosclerosis [34].

(viii) **Cardiovascular risk in GCA:** The impact of cardiovascular risk (CVR) on the diagnostic accuracy of the ultrasound-halo score in GCA patients has been measured [35]. Extracranial artery IMT was significantly greater in patients with high/very high CVRs than in those with low/moderate CVRs, but only among patients without GCA [35]. Non-GCA patients with high/very high CVRs also had significantly higher halo scores than did those with low/moderate CVRs [34]. Higher IMT values may be found in cranial and extracranial arteries in subjects with high/very high CVR without GCA [35].

(ix) **Juvenile idiopathic arthritis (JIA):** In contrast to the definition of synovitis in adults (Table 4.2), the ultrasound definition in children includes SH and/or synovial effusion and PD activity [8, 19]. The combined scoring system for synovitis using B-mode and PD mode is presented in Table 4.2 [8]. In JIA, the reliability of the OMERACT ultrasound score for synovitis, SH, effusion, and Doppler signals has been validated in five joints, namely, the second metacarpophalangeal, wrist, elbow, knee, and ankle joints [8, 19].

Intra-reader reliability has demonstrated satisfactory outcomes for binary scoring, synovitis, and synovial hypertrophy [20]. Doppler signals exhibit excellent reliability [19]. Effusion, on the other hand, has shown moderate reliability [19]. Inter-reader reliability was good for synovitis and synovial hypertrophy, excellent for Doppler signals, and moderate for binary scoring and effusion [19]. The knee region generally yielded the best scores, except for Doppler signals, where the MCP 2 showed higher reliability [19]. Older children tend to have better results [19]. The tenosynovitis diagnosis criteria in adults can be modified for children with minor adjustments on the basis of a Delphi consensus, as suggested by research [36].

In conclusion, ultrasound is regarded as an affordable, noninvasive diagnostic option that is beneficial for the diagnosis of rheumatic diseases and monitoring the effectiveness of treatments. While MRI is considered the gold standard in rheumatology practice and research, recent studies have shown that ultrasound is a valid and reliable outcome measurement tool in this field. Advancements in ultrasound technology, such as superb microvascular imaging and contrast-enhanced ultrasound, are valuable for examining low blood flow in inflamed tissues and predicting the effectiveness of treatments. Additionally, ultrasound guidance has been shown to increase the accuracy of guided interventions. It is hoped that future research will delve into the limitations of ultrasound and explore ways to overcome them, further solidifying its role in the diagnosis and management of rheumatic diseases.

Conflict of Interest MAB is supported by a Faculty of Medicine and Health Executive Dean Stipend scholarship, University of Sydney, Australia, for his PhD course.

References

1. Brooks P, Hochberg M, For ILAR and OMERACT. Outcome measures and classification criteria for the rheumatic diseases. A compilation of data from OMERACT (Outcome Measures for Arthritis Clinical Trials), ILAR (International League of Associations for Rheumatology), regional leagues and other groups. Rheumatology. 2001;40:896–906.
2. Smith TO, Hawker GA, Hunter DJ, et al. The OMERACT-OARSI Core domain set for measurement in clinical trials of hip and/or knee osteoarthritis. J Rheumatol. 2019;46:981–9.
3. Nielsen W, Strand V, Simon LS, OMERACT SLE Working Group, et al. OMERACT 2023 systemic lupus erythematosus special interest group: winnowing and binning preliminary candidate domains for the core outcome set. Semin Arthritis Rheum. 2024;65:152380.
4. White DK, Master H. Patient-reported measures of physical function in knee osteoarthritis. Rheum Dis Clin N Am. 2016;42:239–25.
5. Tugwell P, Boers M, Brooks P, et al. OMERACT: an international initiative to improve outcome measurement in rheumatology. Trials. 2007;8:38.
6. Wakefield RJ, Balint PV, Szkudlarek M, OMERACT 7 Special Interest Group, et al. Musculoskeletal ultrasound including definitions for ultrasonographic pathology. J Rheumatol. 2005;32:2485–7.
7. Kang T, Horton L, Emery P, Wakefield RJ. Value of ultrasound in rheumatologic diseases. J Korean Med Sci. 2013;28:497–507.
8. Bruyn GA, Iagnocco A, Naredo E, OMERACT Ultrasound Working Group, et al. OMERACT definitions for Ultrasonographic pathologies and elementary lesions of rheumatic disorders 15 years on. J Rheumatol. 2019;46:1388–93.
9. D'Agostino MA, Terslev L, Aegerter P, et al. Scoring ultrasound synovitis in rheumatoid arthritis: a EULAR-OMERACT ultrasound taskforce-part 1: definition and development of a standardised, consensus-based scoring system. RMD Open. 2017;3:e000428.
10. Balint PV, Terslev L, Aegerter P, et al. Reliability of a consensus-based ultrasound definition and scoring for enthesitis in spondyloarthritis and psoriatic arthritis: an OMERACT US initiative. Ann Rheum Dis. 2018;77:1730–5.
11. Naredo E, D'Agostino MA, Wakefield RJ, et al. Reliability of a consensus-based ultrasound score

for tenosynovitis in rheumatoid arthritis. Ann Rheum Dis. 2013;72:1328–34.
12. Lin CT, Lai KL. Ultrasound scoring systems for evaluation of synovitis and tenosynovitis in patients with rheumatoid arthritis. J Med Ultrasound. 2022;30:3–5.
13. Terslev L, Naredo E, Aegerter P, et al. Scoring ultrasound synovitis in rheumatoid arthritis: a EULAR-OMERACT ultrasound taskforce-part 2: reliability and application to multiple joints of a standardised consensus-based scoring system. RMD Open. 2017;3:e000427.
14. Silvagni E, Callegher SZ, Mauric E, et al. Musculoskeletal ultrasound for treating rheumatoid arthritis to target – a systematic literature review. Rheumatology. 2022;61:4590–602.
15. Wang J, Wang M, Qi Q, et al. High-frequency ultrasound in patients with seronegative rheumatoid arthritis. Sci Rep. 2022;12:21372.
16. Tesei G, Cometi L, Nacci F, et al. Baricitinib in the treatment of rheumatoid arthritis: clinical and ultrasound evaluation of a real-life single-centre experience. Therapeutic Adv Musculoskelet Dis. 2021;13 https://doi.org/10.1177/1759720X211014019.
17. Razmjou AA, Brook J, Elashoff D, et al. Ultrasound and multi-biomarker disease activity score for assessing and predicting clinical response to tofacitinib treatment in patients with rheumatoid arthritis. BMC Rheumatol. 2020;4:L55.
18. de Andrade NPB, Brenol CV, da Silva Chakr RM. How does ultrasound Global OMERACT-EULAR Synovitis Score (GLOESS) for Rheumatoid Arthritis (RA) activity assessment perform in real-life? J Ultrasound Med. 2024;43:1313–8.
19. Rossi-Semerano L, Breton S, Semerano L, et al. Application of the OMERACT synovitis ultrasound scoring system in juvenile idiopathic arthritis: a multicenter reliability exercise. Rheumatology (Oxford). 2021;60:3579–87.
20. D'Agostino MA, Schett G, López-Rdz A, et al. Response to secukinumab on synovitis using power Doppler ultrasound in psoriatic arthritis: 12-week results from a phase III study, ULTIMATE. Rheumatology. 2022;61:1867–76.
21. Conaghan PG, D'Agostino MA, Schett G, et al. P253 ultrasound demonstrates continued improvement in psoriatic arthritis synovitis and enthesitis with secukinumab: 52-week results from a phase 3 study. Rheumatology. 2022;61:keac133.252.
22. Oo WM, Linklater JM, Bennell KL, et al. Are OMERACT knee osteoarthritis ultrasound scores associated with pain severity, other symptoms, and radiographic and magnetic resonance imaging findings? J Rheumatol. 2021;48:270–8.
23. Mathiessen A, Hammer HB, Terslev L, OMERACT Ultrasound Working Group, et al. Ultrasonography of inflammatory and structural lesions in hand osteoarthritis: an outcome measures in rheumatology agreement and reliability study. Arthritis Care Res (Hoboken). 2022;74:2005–12.
24. Philpott HT, Birmingham TB, Dima R, Pinto R, Bryant D, Appleton CT. Test-retest reliability and sensitivity to change of ultrasound-based methods of measuring synovial inflammation in knee osteoarthritis. Arthritis Care Res (Hoboken). 2023;75:902–10.
25. Filippou G, Scanu A, Adinolfi A, et al. Criterion validity of ultrasound in the identification of calcium pyrophosphate crystal deposits at the knee: an OMERACT ultrasound study. Ann Rheum Dis. 2021;80:261–7.
26. Sirotti S, Terslev L, Filippucci E, et al. OMERACT ultrasound working group-CPPD subgroup. Development and validation of an OMERACT ultrasound scoring system for the extent of calcium pyrophosphate crystal deposition at the joint level and patient level. Lancet Rheumatol. 2023;5:e474–82.
27. Christiansen SN, Filippou G, Scirè CA, et al. Consensus-based semi-quantitative ultrasound scoring system for gout lesions: results of an OMERACT Delphi process and web-reliability exercise. Semin Arthritis Rheum. 2021;51:644–9.
28. Christiansen SN, Østergaard M, Slot O, et al. Assessing the sensitivity to change of the OMERACT ultrasound structural gout lesions during urate-lowering therapy. RMD Open. 2020;6:e001144.
29. Mandl P, D'Agostino MA, Navarro-Compán V, et al. 2023 EULAR recommendations on imaging in diagnosis and management of crystal-induced arthropathies in clinical practice. Ann Rheum Dis. 2024;83:752–9.
30. Inanc N, Jousse-Joulin S, Abacar K, et al. The novel OMERACT ultrasound scoring system for salivary glands changes in patients with Sjögren's syndrome is associated with MRI and salivary flow rates. J Rheumatol. 2024;51:263–9.
31. Hočevar A, Bruyn GA, Terslev L, et al. Development of a new ultrasound scoring system to evaluate glandular inflammation in Sjögren's syndrome: an OMERACT reliability exercise. Rheumatology (Oxford). 2022;61:3341–50.
32. Quéré B, Saraux A, Carvajal-Alegria G, et al. Reliability exercise of ultrasound salivary glands in Sjögren's disease: an international web training initiative. Rheumatol Ther. 2024;11:411–23.
33. Schäfer VS, Chrysidis S, Dejaco C, et al. Assessing vasculitis in giant cell arteritis by ultrasound: results of OMERACT patient-based reliability exercises. J Rheumatol. 2018;45:1289–95.
34. Monjo-Henry I, Fernández-Fernández E, Mostaza JM, et al. Ultrasound halo count in the differential diagnosis of atherosclerosis and large vessel giant cell arteritis. Arthritis Res Ther. 2023;25:23.
35. Molina-Collada J, López Gloria K, Castrejón I, et al. Impact of cardiovascular risk on the diagnostic accuracy of the ultrasound halo score for giant cell arteritis. Arthritis Res Ther. 2022;24:232.
36. Collado P, Martire MV, Lanni S, et al. OMERACT international consensus for ultrasound definitions of tenosynovitis in juvenile idiopathic arthritis: systematic literature review and Delphi process. Arthritis Care Res. 2023;75:2277–84.

Artifacts in Musculoskeletal Ultrasound Practice

5

Md Abu Bakar Siddiq and Patricia van der Meijde

5.1 Introduction

Ultrasound artifacts are frequently encountered during imaging procedures, and having a good understanding of them can help prevent misdiagnoses [1, 2]. In certain situations, these artifacts can actually provide valuable diagnostic clues. It is essential to differentiate between artifacts and ultrasound probe defects. Ultrasound probe defects refer to hardware failures of the transducers that result in abnormalities in the scan images, such as complete signal loss [1, 2]. Therefore, being able to recognize signs of equipment damage, monitoring the in-air reverberation pattern of ultrasound probes, and assessing long-term transducer wear are all important practices [1, 2].

Ultrasound artifacts are reflections observed on a sonogram that do not accurately represent tissue interfaces in terms of location or intensity [3–5]. Identifying artifacts is essential to avoid misinterpretation or incorrect findings [3–5]. It is often mistakenly believed that artifacts are synonymous with pitfalls, biases, or errors. A pitfall refers to a hidden risk or challenge that may occur during image acquisition or interpretation [3–5]. The Doppler ultrasound operator must understand the factors that generate a Doppler signal, whether it is vascular, motion-related, or an artifact [3–5]. Color or power Doppler artifacts can be recognized by their atypical spectral waveform [3–5]. Doppler artifacts are extremely useful for diagnostic purposes [3–5]. Ultrasound probe defects and quality assessment are detailed in Chap. 2. In this chapter, a brief discussion of probe malfunction artifacts is presented, followed by an examination of ultrasound artifacts.

5.2 Electrical Interference and Probe Malfunction Artifacts

Electrical interference artifacts typically arise when an ultrasound machine is positioned too near unshielded electrical devices, such as ventilators, resulting in arc-like moving bands within

M. A. B. Siddiq (✉)
Department of Rheumatology, Royal North Shore Hospital, Northern Clinical School, Faculty of Medicine and Health, The University of Sydney, Sydney, NSW, Australia

Sydney Musculoskeletal Health, The University of Sydney, Sydney, NSW, Australia

Kolling Institute of Medical Research, St Leonards, NSW, Australia

School of Health Sports and Professional Practice (Rheumatology), University of South Wales, Pontypridd, United Kingdom

Department of Physical Medicine and Rehabilitation, Brahmanbaria Medical College, Brahmanbaria, Bangladesh
e-mail: msid8426@uni.syndey.edu.au

P. van der Meijde
SonoCare, Apeldoorn, The Netherlands

M. A. B. Siddiq (ed.), *Musculoskeletal Ultrasound in Rheumatic Diseases*,
https://doi.org/10.1007/978-981-96-5298-3_5

the ultrasound images [6]. Additionally, this type of artifact may also occur due to malfunctions in the ultrasound probe itself. In addition to testing phantoms and specialized electronic equipment, visual evaluation is a precise technique for detecting probe damage [1, 2]. Obvious visual damage, such as cracks in the probe casing or marks on the delicate lens, can greatly affect the quality of images. Therefore, it is advisable to examine the probe in question via the preset most frequently utilized in real-world scenarios, such as the musculoskeletal preset for a linear transducer [1, 2]. The reverberation pattern in the air typically manifests as multiple parallel bright lines in the near field. Common indicators of probe damage include the following [1, 2]:

- Dropout: disrupting the reverberation pattern and potentially extending toward the lens. This is probably the result of a defective piezo-element (PZT) caused by either damage or a flaw in the manufacturing process.
- Delamination: a modified reverberation pattern that results in a partial loss of signal. This alteration, although sometimes subtle, can serve as an indicator of underlying issues such as damage, a weakened PZT, or a defect in the manufacturing process.
- Nonuniformity: Reverberation lines are not aligned in a parallel manner. This distortion in the images highlights the necessity for prompt replacement of the probe.
- Lens wear: The reverberation depth along the edges may gradually shift when lenses are worn for an extended period. It is important to stay vigilant for any changes and to contemplate replacing them promptly.

5.3 Practical Points to Assess Probe Defects

The ultrasound system is equipped with integrated features designed to enhance image quality. By selecting appropriate presets, verifying the depth, utilizing the correct frequency, fine-tuning the gain, modifying the time-gain compensation, and adjusting the focus, the quality of ultrasound images can be significantly improved [7]. The paper-clip method has been suggested as a straightforward yet sensitive tool for monitoring the quality of probes [1]. By moving a paper clip along the surface of the probe lens, with the assistance of a small amount of ultrasound acoustic gel, this technique can highlight smaller interruptions in the echo pattern [2]. However, this method is less effective for evaluating phased array transducers since small failures in the elements of these probes can affect the entire scanning field, thereby concealing minor damage. For phased array transducers, a modified paper-clip test utilizing the M-mode has been proposed [2]. In this chapter, ultrasound gray scale and Doppler artifacts are detailed.

Ultrasound Artifacts Musculoskeletal structures such as bone, nerve, tendon, and muscle typically have similar appearances on B-mode (brightness mode) gray scale ultrasound. Doppler imaging aids in identifying blood flow in tissues and distinguishing between solid and cystic masses. Ultrasound operates under the assumption that echoes are detected from the main ultrasound beam, which travels in a straight line, and that sound attenuation in tissue is uniform with constant speed across all tissue types [3, 4]. Each reflector is expected to produce only one echo, and the depth of the imaged object is directly proportional to the time taken for the sound to return to the transducer [3]. Deviations from these ideal assumptions can result in artifacts, such as misinterpretation of normal findings as pathologies, imaging of structures appearing in the wrong location or size, nonvisualization of an actual structure, or visualization of a nonexistent structure [3, 5]. Ultrasound artifacts are commonly encountered [1]. In certain situations, specific artifacts can provide valuable diagnostic information [3]. However, by comprehending the causes and timing of artifact development, clinicians can effectively minimize the risk of misinterpreting the clinical significance of these artifacts [3]. In the subsequent sections, gray scale ultrasound artifacts associated with the focal zone, beam attenuation, path of the beam, side lobe of the beam, speed of sound, and range ambiguity have been demonstrated. Doppler artifacts are also highlighted.

5.4 Gray Scale Artifacts

1. **Improper focal zone (FZ) adjustment**: This can lead to FZ or beam width artifacts influenced by the section thickness and lateral resolution of the ultrasound beam (Fig. 5.1a-c) [3, 4]. In the FZ, both the section thickness and beam width are minimized, resulting in high-resolution images that can separate two objects perpendicular to the direction of ultrasound wave propagation (Fig. 5.1c) [3, 4]. If the distance between two adjacent targets is smaller than the width of the ultrasound wave, their images may overlap on the screen. A lesion with poor resolution can blend with nearby structures, leading to diminished image resolution in the near or distant zones (Fig. 5.11b) [3].

2. **Attenuation of Ultrasound Signals**

Posterior Enhancement Scattering, reflection, or absorption can diminish the strength of ultrasound wave energy [5]. Compared with nearby tissues, structures with low attenuation, such as joint effusions, hematomas, ganglion cysts, or abscesses, can increase in intensity as the ultrasound beam travels through them (Fig. 5.2a) [3–5]. For example, Baker's cyst (BC) is a fluid-filled cystic mass that arises between the semimembranosus tendon and the medial gastrocnemius muscle and communicates with the knee joint in meniscal tears and inflammatory or degenerative arthritis [3]. On ultrasound, the tissues deep within Baker's cyst appear hyperechoic due to posterior acoustic enhancement (Fig. 5.2b). Similarly, a complete tear of the supraspinatus tendon with effusion with significant acoustic impedance between the effusion and humeral cartilage contributes to enhanced reflection of the ultrasound beam deep to the effusion, referred to as the "cartilage interface sign" [6, 8, 9] (Fig. 5.2c).

Excessive compensation for tissue attenuation via the time-gain control feature of the ultrasound machine may further contribute to posterior sound amplification [3], which could be improved by adjusting the gain to a low level at the deeper region of a low-attenuation structure (Fig. 5.3a–b).

Acoustic Shadowing When ultrasonic waves pass through a structure with significant attenuation, such as calcification, bone, metal, or gas, the echo beyond the structure is greatly reduced, resulting in a clean, partial, or dirty acoustic shadow (Fig. 5.4) [4].

Ultrasound beams cannot penetrate air but instead are reflected in different directions within

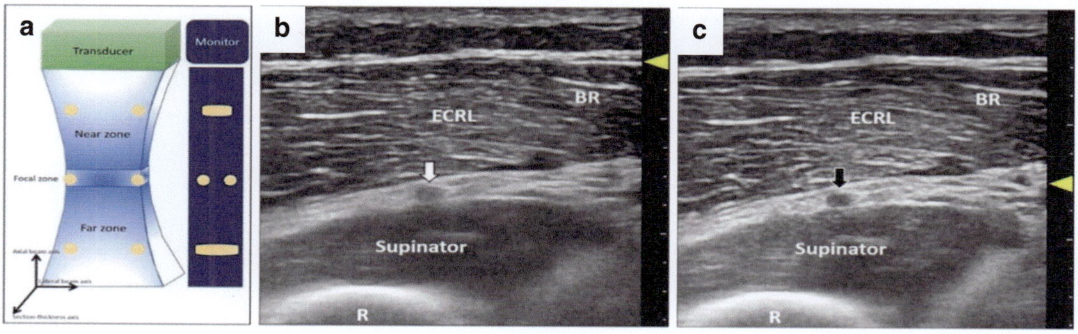

Fig. 5.1 Artifacts due to improper focal zone adjustment. (**a**) The schematic diagram shows the ultrasound beam width and best image resolution at the focal zone. (**b**) The deep radial nerve appears blurred (white arrow) when the focal zone is set far away. (**c**) Blurred radial nerve resolution improves (black arrow) when the focus (yellow) is adjusted to the target focal zone. *ECRL* extensor carpi radialis longus muscle, *BR* brachioradialis muscle, *R* radius [3]. (Source: with permission from Chang KV et al. Diagnostics (Basel) 2020; 10:645)

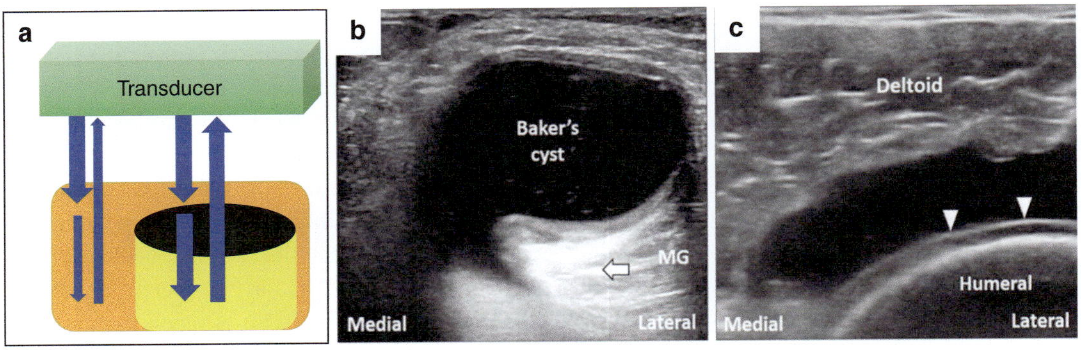

Fig. 5.2 Posterior acoustic enhancement. (**a**) The schematic diagram of an ultrasound beam passing through a low-attenuating structure, and the signals reflected from the deep structure are greater than those from the surrounding tissues. (**b**) Posterior acoustic enhancement (white arrow) in Baker's cyst. (**c**) Posterior acoustic enhancement in complete tear of the supraspinatus tendon with effusion and a hyperechoic humeral head cartilage (arrowheads, cartilage interface sign). *MG* medial gastrocnemius muscle [3]. (Source: with permission from Chang KV et al. Diagnostics (Basel) 2020; 10:645)

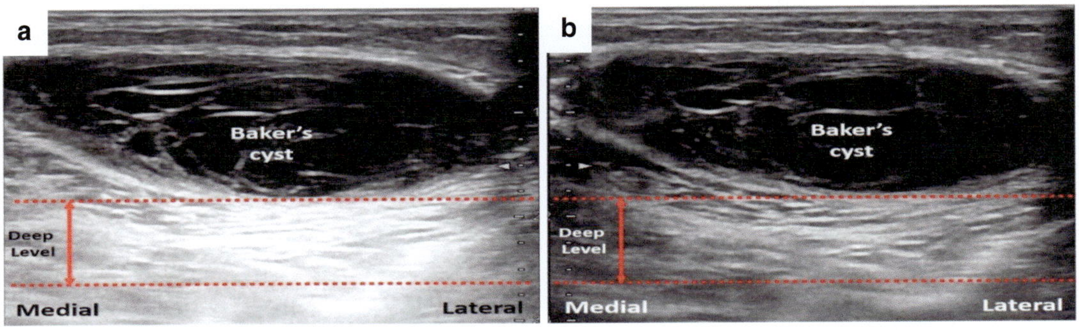

Fig. 5.3 Posterior acoustic enhancement. (**a**) Hyperechoic posterior acoustic enhancement beneath Baker's cyst. (**b**) Reduced gain improves posterior enhancement. The red dashed line indicates the depth below the target, whereas the red double arrow represents the extent of the depth affected by the artifact [3]. (Source: with permission from Chang KV et al. Diagnostics (Basel) 2020; 10:645)

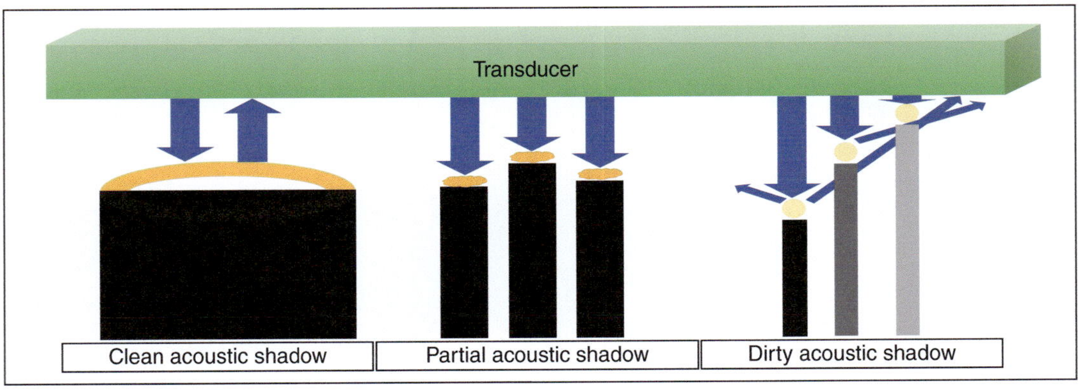

Fig. 5.4 The schematic diagram illustrates the impact of a high-attenuation structure on the passage of an ultrasonic wave. The blue arrows represent the projected and reflected ultrasound beams, and the dark yellow circles indicate high-attenuation objects. The gas bubbles are denoted by light yellow circles [3]. (Source: with permission from Chang KV et al. Diagnostics (Basel) 2020; 10:645)

gas bubbles, causing the formation of a contaminated acoustic shadow [4]. Acoustic shadowing can manifest as a clean anechoic acoustic band deep within a calcification in the tendon (Fig. 5.5a), a partial hypoechoic acoustic region deep within fragmented calcifications in heterotrophic ossification (Fig. 5.5b), or dirty acoustic shadowing with heterogeneous echoes within a region of low signal intensity with gas bubbles (Fig. 5.5c). To improve the visibility of the target within a high-attenuation structure, scanning through the lateral aspect of the structure may help avoid acoustic shadowing [3].

Reverberation Passing ultrasound waves through two closely positioned reflective planes results in multiple reflections between the reflectors (Fig. 5.6a) [1, 3]. Some of the signals travel back to the transducer, whereas others bounce back and forth between the surfaces, creating parallel lines extending into the target (Fig. 5.6b) [3]. As these lines penetrate deeper into the target, they become shorter and less echogenic, resembling the tail of a comet [3, 10]. This is due to energy attenuation away from the reflective surfaces [3, 10]. The comet tail artifact is a type of reverberation artifact, resulting in a short train

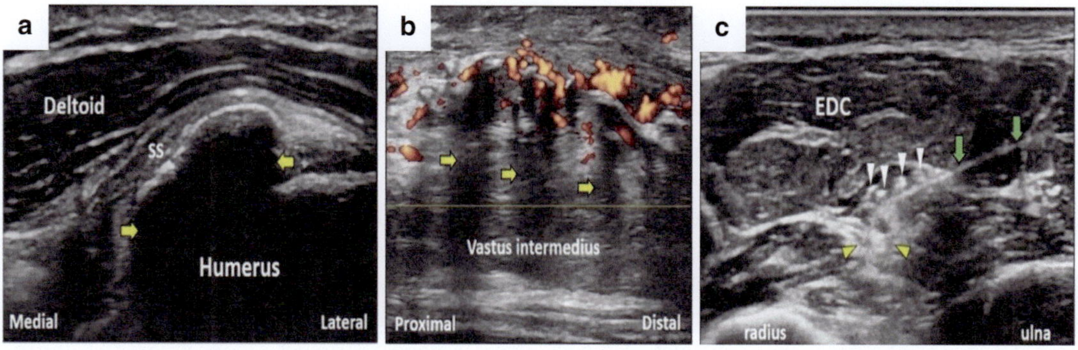

Fig. 5.5 Posterior acoustic shadowing. (**a**) Clean acoustic shadowing is visible below the egg-shelled calcifications. (**b**) Partial acoustic shadowing is observed deep to fragmented calcifications in heterotrophic ossification in muscle. (**c**) Dirty acoustic shadowing is observed in the gas bubbles during ultrasound-guided injection. The yellow arrow indicates the acoustic shadowing artifact, the white arrowhead points to the gas bubbles, the yellow arrowhead highlights the dirty acoustic shadowing, and the green arrow represents the needle. *SS* supraspinatus tendon, *EDC* extensor digitorum communis muscle [3]. (Source: with permission from Chang KV et al. Diagnostics (Basel) 2020; 10:645)

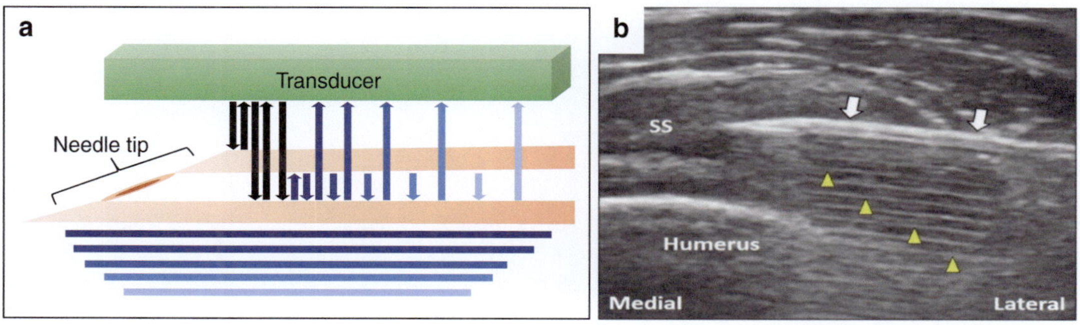

Fig. 5.6 Reverberation artifacts. (**a**) The shematic diagram of an ultrasound beam passing through multiple acoustic reflectors. (**b**) The comet tail appearance (yellow arrowhead) is visible below the needle (white arrows). *SS* supraspinatus tendon. The blue and black arrows indicate the projected and reflected ultrasound beams, respectively [3]. (Source: with permission from Chang KV et al. Diagnostics (Basel) 2020; 10:645)

of reverberations from an echogenic focus with strong parallel reflectors within it [3]. In the case of comet tail artifacts, the space between two strong parallel reflectors may be less than half the spatial pulse length, causing the echoes to be displayed as triangular lines [3]. The later echoes attenuate and have a decreased amplitude, resulting in a decreased width on the display [3].

Ring-Down Artifact As the ultrasound beam travels through air bubbles, sound waves vibrate within the bubbles, creating continuous waves that are reflected back to the transducer, leading to the ring-down artifact. The ultrasonic streaks decrease in intensity as they move away from the designated target (Fig. 5.7a) [1, 3, 11]. This artifact is specifically associated with gas bubbles and occurs when an ultrasound pulse encounters a fluid collection that has a "horn" or "bugle" shape and is trapped between four bubbles arranged in an inverted tetrahedron formation (with three bubbles on top and one nestled deep beneath them). The trapped fluid resonates and emits a continuous signal back to the transducer. Unlike the broad spectrum of the transducer pulse, the returning signal consists of one or more distinct resonant frequencies. The interaction between these frequencies creates the varying appearance of the ring-down artifact. This artifact can be eliminated by adjusting the angle of the ultrasound probe [1]. Ring-down artifacts are frequently observed in the bowel during the examination of an inguinal hernia with gas within the lumen (Fig. 5.7b) [1]. In cellulitis, ring-down artifacts are observed in anaerobic bacterial infections [11]. During intercostal nerve block [12], pleural movement can exhibit ring-down artifacts (Fig. 5.7c). The ring-down artifact is occasionally mistaken for the ladder-like reverberation associated with the comet-tail artifact [13]. However, comet-tail artifacts arise when ultrasound waves interact with small calcific, crystalline, or highly reflective objects, representing a distinct type of reverberation artifact [3].

Mirror Image Artifacts When sound waves pass through an object, the primary image is formed through reflection. However, sometimes, a portion of the sound waves encounters another structure in its path and is reflected back to the highly reflective surface instead of reaching the transducer directly (Fig. 5.8a) [3]. This leads to a false assumption by the ultrasound machine that the returning echo has been reflected and returned from a deeper structure. Consequently, a mirror artifact appears on the opposite side of the reflective surface (Fig. 5.8a) [3]. To avoid this artifact, one can adjust the position and angle of scanning

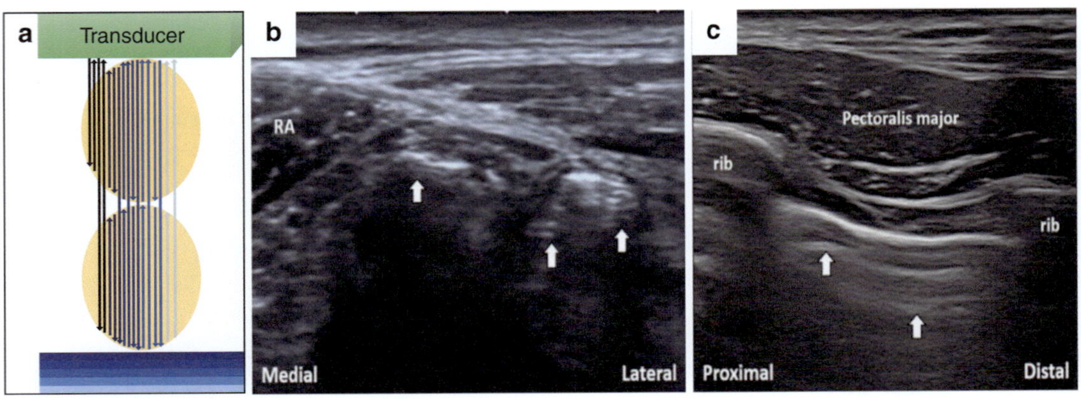

Fig. 5.7 Ring-down artifacts. (**a**) The black and blue arrows represent the projected and reflected ultrasound beams, respectively. (**b**) The presence of ring-down artifacts (white arrows) was observed in the bowels of the inguinal hernia. (**c**) During intercostal block, ring-down artifacts (white arrows) are visible deep to the pleura. *RA* rectus abdominis. The black and blue arrows represent the projected and reflected ultrasound beams, respectively [3]. (Source: with permission from Chang KV et al. Diagnostics (Basel) 2020; 10:645)

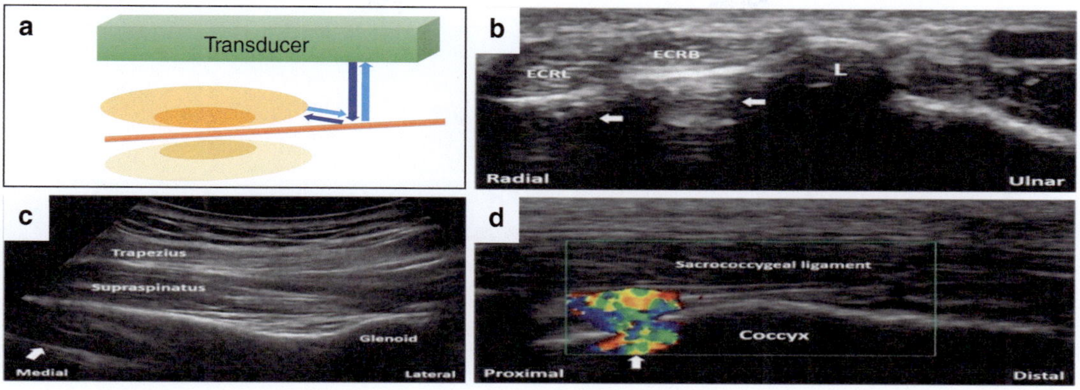

Fig. 5.8 Mirror image artifacts. (**a**) The schematic diagram illustrating the mirror artifact. The blue arrows represent the ultrasound beams. The brown pillar signifies the reflective interface. (**b–d**) These mirror artifacts (white arrows) are visible in various body regions, such as the forearm (**b**), supraspinatus fossa (**c**), and coccyx (**d**) with Doppler signals. *ECRL* extensor carpi radialis longus tendon, *ECRB* extensor carpi radialis brevis tendon, *L* Lister's tubercle [3]. (Source: with permission from Chang KV et al. Diagnostics (Basel) 2020; 10:645)

to change the angle of insonation of the primary ultrasound beam [1]. For example, when the extensor carpi radialis longus and brevis tendons in the short axis at the distal forearm are examined, two echogenic reflections can be observed within the underlying cortical bone (Fig. 5.8b) [3]. Similarly, during a suprascapular nerve block procedure [14], mirror artifacts of the supraspinatus muscle may symmetrically appear on the opposite side of the scapular spine (Fig. 5.8c) [3]. Additionally, artifacts may be visualized when the Doppler mode is activated to track a vessel that overlays a bony cortex (Fig. 5.8d) [3]. Notably, reducing the gain below the reflective surface can help minimize artifacts [3].

Anisotropy The presence of anisotropy in an artifact is influenced by the angle of examination, especially when fibrous linear structures such as tendons, ligaments, and nerves are scanned [3]. If the ultrasound beam is not aligned perpendicularly to the target, signals may deflect away from the transducer, resulting in a hypoechoic appearance (Fig. 5.9a) [15]. For example, the Achilles tendon (AT) might appear hypoechoic during long-axis scanning, but applying slight compression at the transducer's distal end can enhance echogenicity and reduce this artifact (Fig. 5.9b) [15]. To prevent misinterpretation, the transducer should be tilted perpendicular to the bicipital groove when the long head of the biceps tendon is scanned (Fig. 5.9c, d) [3].

Side Lobe Artifacts Most of the energy in ultrasound is carried through the central beam (Fig. 5.10a) [3]. Owing to the radial expansion and compression of the crystal elements in the transducer, lateral dispersion of residual off-axis beams (side and grating lobes) can be observed (Fig. 5.10b) [3]. When the ultrasound beam interacts with an object and then reflects back to the transducer, the signals from the side lobes are mistakenly interpreted by the ultrasound machine as waves originating from the main beam, resulting in a "ghost image" on the main axis, a side lobe artifact [16, 17]. Echogenic, linear, or curvilinear artifacts are observed as side lobe artifacts. Examples of strong reflectors include bowel gas adjacent to the gallbladder or urinary bladder [1]. Sometimes, when a cystic lesion is analyzed, hyperreflective images from structures located on the side lobes can be observed within the cyst. This can lead to the misunderstanding that these images are the desired targets along the main axis of the ultrasound beams (Fig. 5.10c) [3]. Adjusting the transducer position could improve this.

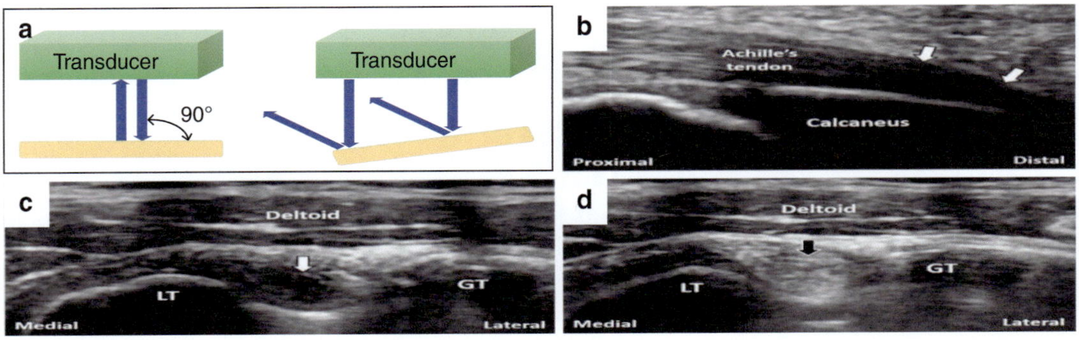

Fig. 5.9 Anisotropy. (**a**) The schematic diagram reveals ultrasound beam reflection (blue arrows) depending on the angle. (**b**) Anisotropy (white arrows) is observed at the Achilles tendon insertion point. (**c**) A normal long head of the biceps may be mistaken for tendinopathy due to anisotropy (white arrow). (**d**) The transducer was adjusted to align perpendicularly with the bicipital groove to remove the artifact (black arrow). *GT* greater tubercle, *LT* lesser tubercle [3]. (Source: with permission from Chang KV et al. Diagnostics (Basel) 2020; 10:645)

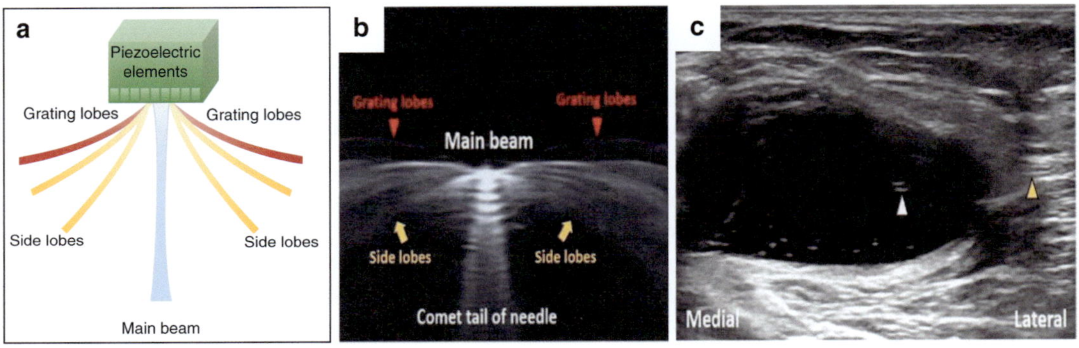

Fig. 5.10 Side lobe artifact. (**a**) The schematic diagram reveals the lateral dispersion of the ultrasound beams. (**b**) The yellow arrow indicates the side lobe, the red arrowheads represent grating lobes, and the white arrowhead points to the nail plate. (**c**) Ghost image (white arrowhead) on the main axis of the ultrasound beam, the yellow arrowhead signifies a side lobe artifact [3]. (Source: with permission from Chang KV et al. Diagnostics (Basel) 2020; 10:645)

3. **Artifact in Connection with Sound Speed**

Refraction Artifacts Variations in the acoustic impedance of tissues lead to differences in the speed of sound [3]. As the ultrasound beam travels through an area with high impedance, there is a delay in the return of the ultrasound signals to the transducer [3]. This delay causes an overestimation of the object's depth. Conversely, if the target is located in an area with low acoustic impedance, the object displayed on the monitor appears shallower than its actual depth (Fig. 5.11a) [3, 18]. The bayonet artifact is a type of refraction artifact that occurs during ultrasound-guided injections, particularly when the needle traverses areas with varying acoustic impedance [19], for example, in procedures such as deep peroneal (fibular) nerve block, where the needle moves across the interface between the tibialis anterior muscle [3, 19, 20] and the surrounding fatty tissue of the nerve [3]. This interaction can lead to an inaccurate assessment of the depth of the targeted structure (Fig. 5.11b) [3].

Edge Artifact When the ultrasound beam reaches the edge of a curved surface, most of it is redirected away from the transducer [3]. This redirection appears as hypoechoic lines running parallel to the target's boundaries (Fig. 5.12a) [3]. This

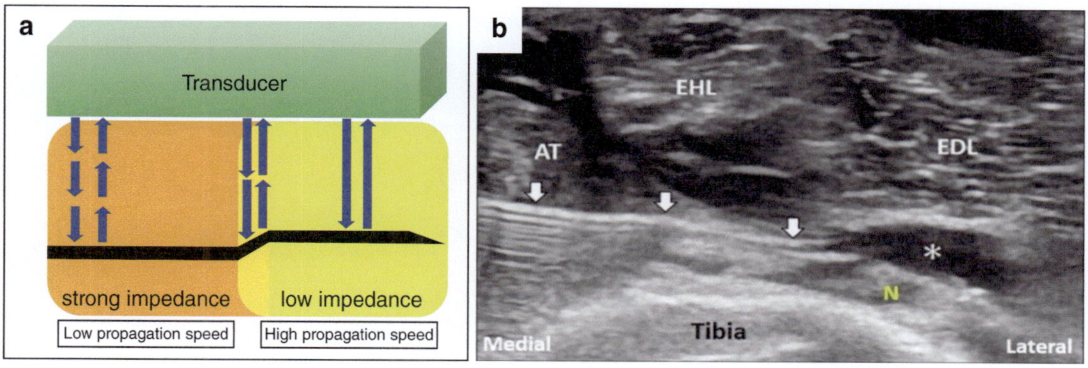

Fig. 5.11 Refraction artifacts. (**a**) The schematic diagram reveals the projected and reflected ultrasound waves (blue arrows). (**b**) The difference in ultrasound tissue impedance between muscle and fat tissues causes the needle to bend (white arrows) toward the tibia (refraction artifacts) during peroneal nerve block (asterisks, injectate). *EHL* extensor hallucis longus tendon, *AT* anterior tibialis tendon, *EDL* extensor digitorum longus tendon [3]. (Source: with permission from Chang KV et al. Diagnostics (Basel) 2020; 10:645)

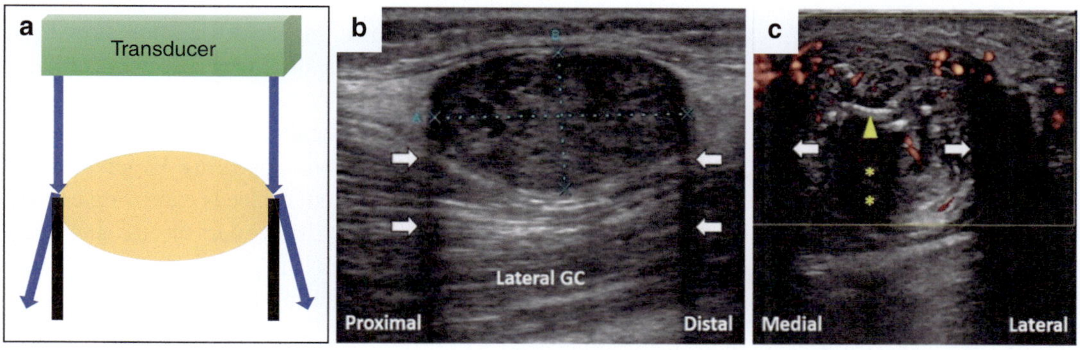

Fig. 5.12 Lateral edge shadowing artifacts. (**a**) The schematic diagram of edge artifact. (**b**) Edge artifact (white arrows) at the edge of a schwannoma of the lateral sural cutaneous nerve. (**c**) Lateral edge shadowing (arrows) in the Achilles paratenon, the yellow arrowhead (**c**) points to the sutures, and the yellow asterisk (**c**) represents acoustic shadowing caused by the sutures. *GC* gastrocnemius muscle [3]. (Source: with permission from Chang KV et al. Diagnostics (Basel) 2020; 10:645)

phenomenon can be observed on the periphery of circular structures, such as BCs or schwannomas of the lateral sural cutaneous nerve (Fig. 5.12b) [3]. Additionally, during axial scanning of the AT (Fig. 5.12c) [3], lateral edge shadowing may be misinterpreted as a thickened paratenon, but this can be corrected by adjusting the angle of insonation with the heel-toe maneuver.

Range Ambiguity Artifact The initial ultrasound pulse emitted by the machine hits an object and then reflects it back to the transducer [3]. Owing to an error in identification, the machine mistakes the first returning pulse for the second returning pulse, leading to the creation of a false object at a shallower depth than the actual object location (Fig. 5.13a) [3]. For example, when a large BC is scanned, the transducer takes longer to receive the echo reflected from the deep wall of the cyst [3]. As a result, by the time the first pulse from the posterior wall returns to the transducer, the second pulse has already been emitted, causing the appearance of multiple parallel lines near the cyst surface that resemble intracystic septa (Fig. 5.13b) [3].

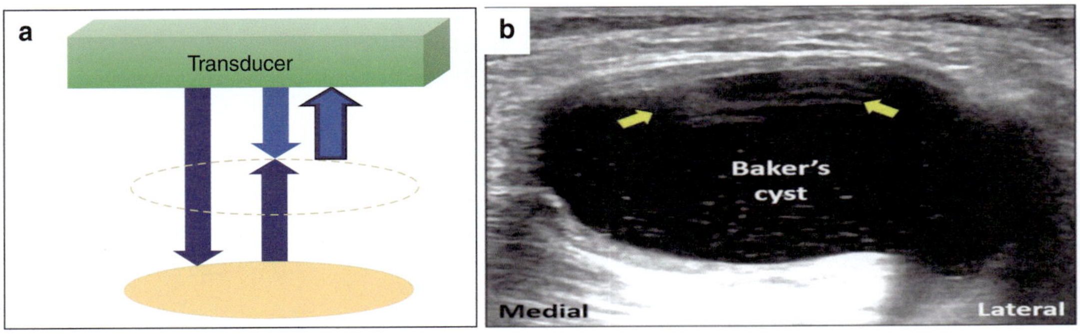

Fig. 5.13 Range ambiguity artifact. (**a**) The schematic diagram reveals how the ultrasound pulse (dark blue arrow) interacts with the object and travels back to the transducer following the emission of the subsequent pulse (bright blue arrow). (**b**) Ultrasound imaging of a large Baker's cyst revealed artifacts such as intracystic septae (yellow arrows) [3]. (Source: with permission from Chang KV et al. Diagnostics (Basel) 2020; 10:645)

5.5 Doppler Artifacts

Doppler artifacts such as motion, blooming, background noise, reverberation, mirror imaging, and aliasing can lead to falsely increased vascularity and inflammation [21–25]. The following sections illustrate various Doppler artifacts in relation to rheumatic disorders [21–25].

Motion (Flash or Clutter Artifacts) Two potential factors contribute to motion artifacts (Fig. 5.14) [21]: (i). Movement of the patient and/or investigator while holding the probe, (ii). Ultrasound is used to set the wall filter too high. In an ideal scenario, erythrocytes in blood vessels act as both moving receivers and sources and reflect the ultrasound beam back to the transducer, resulting in a Doppler shift. Doppler shift helps visualize the colors and vascular contour in the ultrasound image [21]. However, during the examination, there are also slower movements from the patient, probe, and surrounding tissue, generating lower-frequency Doppler shifts obscuring the true flow vascular image [21, 22]. Motion artifacts are easily distinguishable from the true flow and cannot be replicated in the same location, resembling fireworks (Fig. 5.14) [21].

Random Noise and Blooming Random interference persists until the settings are accurately adjusted. This interference is impacted by the actions of the examiner and can be readily identified; for instance, high-gain configurations lead to multiple color spots in the ultrasound image, which shift upon gain modification (Fig. 5.15). The blooming phenomenon resembles peony blooms, with lesions appearing larger than the actual size due to color bleeds extending beyond the vessel wall [23]. Color bleeds are often observed in cases of partial occlusion from thrombus formation in larger vessels [21]. High gain settings may lead to overestimation of arthritis activity, and reducing gain can help minimize artifacts but may also eliminate genuine flow signals [21]. Therefore, it is crucial to prioritize the optimization of random noise to accurately evaluate the true flow [21].

Reverberation Misinterpretation of ultrasound findings in vessels could be due to reverberation artifacts [21, 26] (Fig. 5.16). Possible reasons for misinterpretation of ultrasound findings in vessels due to reverberation artifacts include the following: (i) Superficial vessel signals may be mistaken for reflection toward the synovium, mimicking its activity [21], (ii) Distinct foci resembling vessel size or a cluster of raindrops may be observed [24], and (iii) Large-diameter vessels situated deep within the joint cavity may reflect a signal toward the bone, creating a cascade of color [21, 26]

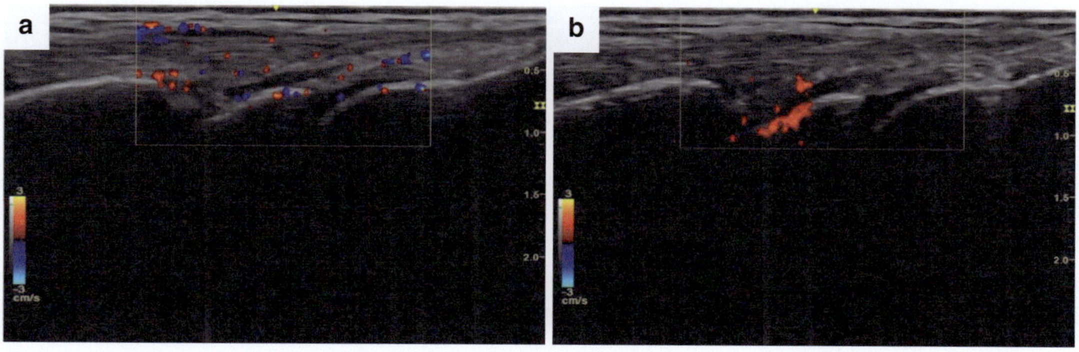

Fig. 5.14 Motion artifacts. (**a**, **b**) Detection of motion artifact from transducer and the tissue movements. (Source: with permission from Patricia van der Maijde, SonoCare Apeldoorn, The Netherlands)

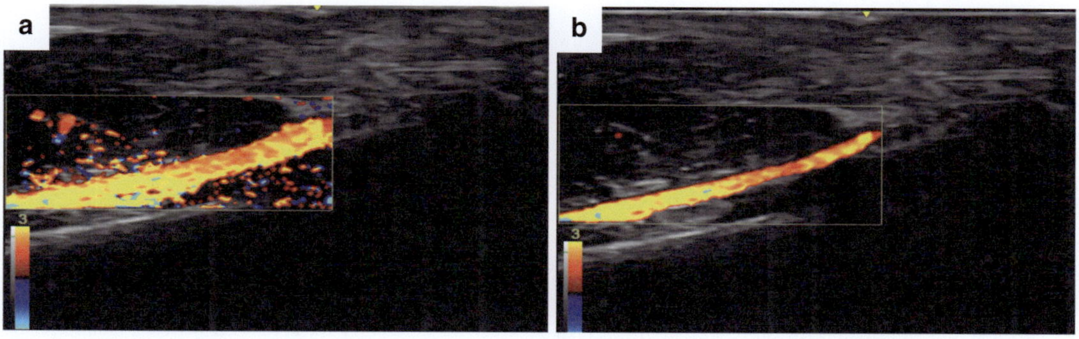

Fig. 5.15 Random noise and blooming. (**a**) Random noise simulates turbulent flow, resulting in the visual effect of small, randomly colored pixels scattered around the vessel wall. (**b**) Blooming mimics obstruction by producing color overflow beyond the actual vessel wall boundaries. (Source: with permission from Patricia van der Maijde, SonoCare Apeldoorn, The Netherlands)

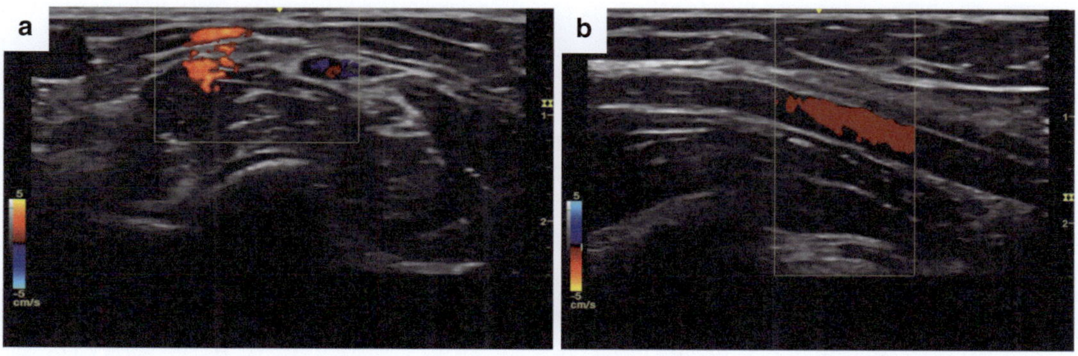

Fig. 5.16 Reverberation Doppler artifact. (**a**,**b**) Complex reverberation artifact in the brachial artery. The superficial vessel displays reverberation as a showering of color below the vessel (Source: with permission from Patricia van der Maijde, SonoCare Apeldoorn, The Netherlands)

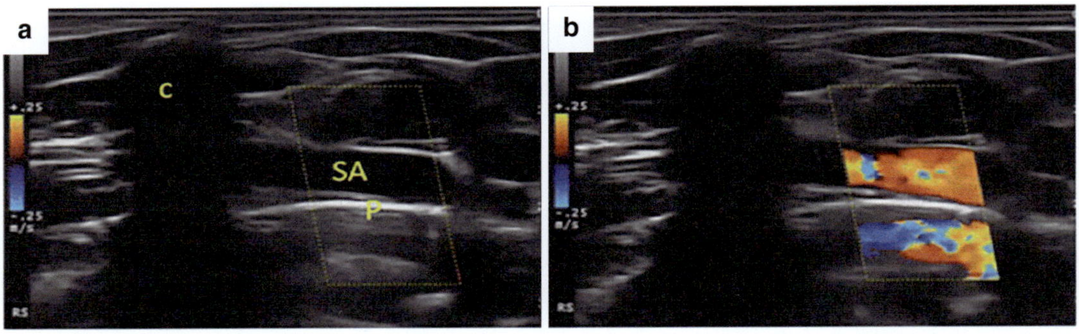

Fig. 5.17 Mirror artifacts. The pleura is a smooth surface with air behind it that may serve as an acoustic mirror. On the left image (**a**) The subclavian artery (SA) is visible, with the pleura appearing as a white line (p) below. On the right image (**b**) The SA is mirrored beneath the pleura. The clavicle (c) is observed creating an acoustic shadow. (Source: with permission from Terslev et al. Arthritis Res Ther 2017; 19:167)

Mirror Artifacts Mirror artifacts are rare in larger vessels, as the mirror surface is usually filled with air (Fig. 5.17). The mirror artifact is easily recognizable when the actual image, mirror, and mirror image are all visible. However, it may be more difficult to identify when only the mirror and mirror images are present. When examined via spectral Doppler, the artifact will display true flow, as it mirrors the actual flow [27]. Adjustments cannot prevent mirror artifacts. When using spectral Doppler, the entire Doppler spectrum may be reflected in the posterior vessel wall, causing an arterial Doppler spectrum to appear on both sides of the baseline [27] (Fig. 5.17).

Aliasing Aliasing occurs when the Doppler shift of the moving blood exceeds half of the PRF (Nyquist limit), causing signals to be displayed incorrectly in terms of direction and velocity [27]. This phenomenon is visible as a change in color hue, with red appearing blue and vice versa (Fig. 5.18) [27]. Aliasing is specifically observed in CD and spectral Doppler, and while it may not be significant in arthritic conditions, it plays a crucial role in identifying stenosis areas with high blood velocities in large vessel vasculitis [27]. Adjusting the PRF can help prevent aliasing and improve the accuracy of diagnosing stenotic areas within the blood flow [27].

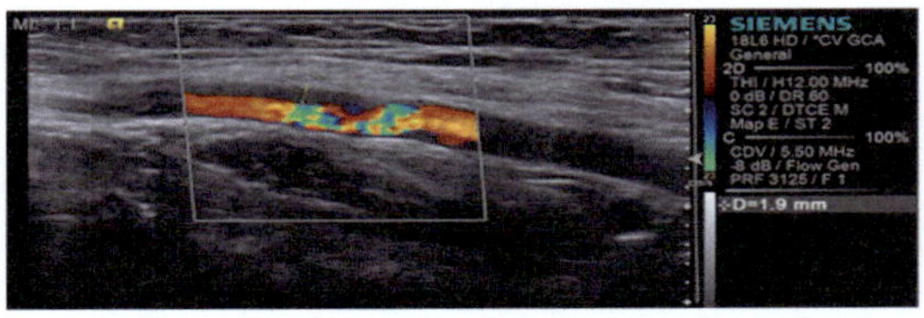

Fig. 5.18 Aliasing. The aliased signal in the axillary artery helps identify the area with stenosis, characterized by the highest blood velocities. The flow is shown with an incorrect direction (red instead of blue and vice versa) and velocity (the hue of the color). (Source: with permission from Terslev et al. Arthritis Res Ther 2017; 19:167)

Conflict of Interest MAB is supported by a Faculty of Medicine and Health Executive Dean Stipend scholarship, University of Sydney, Australia, for his PhD course.

References

1. Degefu D. Radiopaedia. 2023. Available at: https://radiopaedia.org/articles/ultrasound-artifacts-3. Accessed on 24 April 2024.
2. Bálint Botz. Ultrasound probe defect. Available at: https://radiopaedia.org/articles/ultrasound-probe-defect?lang=us. Accessed on 23 Jun 2024.
3. Wu WT, Chang KV, Hsu YC, Hsu PC, Ricci V, Özçakar L. Artifacts in musculoskeletal ultrasonography: from physics to clinics. Diagnostics (Basel). 2020;10:645.
4. Baad M, Lu ZF, Reiser I, Paushter D. Clinical significance of US artifacts. Radiographics. 2017;37:1408–23.
5. Gimber L, Melville DM, Klauser A, Witte RS, Arif-Tiwari H, Taljanovic MS. Artifacts at musculoskeletal US: resident and fellow education feature. Radiographics. 2016;36:479–80.

6. Jassim D, Patel M, Moore C. Electrical interference artifact (ultrasound). Reference article, Radiopaedia.org Accessed on 14 Sep 2024. https://doi.org/10.53347/rID-73101
7. Sassaroli E, Crake C, Scorza A, Kim DS, Park MA. Image quality evaluation of ultrasound imaging systems: advanced B-modes. J Appl Clin Med Phys. 2019;20:115–24.
8. Blome A, Harrigan R, Goett H, Costantino T, Gibbons R. Ultrasonographic characteristics of Baker's cysts: the sonographic Foucher's sign. J Emerg Med. 2017;53:753–5.
9. Griffith JF. Top-ten pitfalls in rotator cuff ultrasound. Semin Musculoskelet Radiol. 2019;23:429–35.
10. Rubin JM, Adler RS, Bude RO, Fowlkes JB, Carson PL. Clean and dirty shadowing at US: a reappraisal. Radiology. 1991;181:231–6.
11. Oh SH, Han HY, Kim HJ. Comet tail artifact on ultrasonography: is it a reliable finding of benign gallbladder diseases? Ultrasonography. 2019;38:221–30.
12. Avruch L, Cooperberg PL. The ring-down artifact. J Ultrasound Med. 1985;4:21–8.
13. Gaillard F, Ranchod A, Bell D, et al. Comet tail artifact. Reference article, Radiopaedia.org. Accessed on 14 Sep 2024. https://doi.org/10.53347/rID-9930
14. Magazzeni P, Jochum D, Iohom G, Mekler G, Albuisson E, Bouaziz H. Ultrasound-guided selective versus conventional block of the medial brachial cutaneous and the Intercostobrachial nerves: a randomized clinical trial. Reg Anesthesia Pain Med. 2018;43:832–7.
15. Aydın T, Şen EI, Yardımcı MY, Kesiktaş FN, Öneş K, Paker N. Efficacy of ultrasound-guided suprascapular nerve block treatment in patients with painful hemiplegic shoulder. Neurol Sci. 2019;40:985–91.
16. Van Holsbeeck MT, Soliman S, Van Kerkhove F, Craig J. Advanced musculoskeletal ultrasound techniques: what are the applications? Am J Roentgenol. 2021;216:436–45.
17. Ricci V, Soylu AR, Özçakar L. Artifacts and artistic facts. Am J Phys Med Rehabil. 2019;98:521–5.
18. Paul Y, Barthez D, Léveillé R, Peter V, Scrivani D. Side lobes and grating lobes artifacts in ultrasound imaging. Veter-Radiol Ultrasound. 1997;38:387–93.
19. Bönhof J, McLaughlin G. Artifacts in sonography-part 3. Ultraschall der Med Eur J Ultrasound. 2018;39:260–83.
20. Reusz G, Sarkany P, Gal J, Csomos A. Needle-related ultrasound artifacts and their importance in anesthetic practice. Br J Anaesth. 2014;112:794–802.
21. Seskute G, Montvydaite M, Butrimiene I. Power Doppler artifacts in evaluating inflammatory arthritis of small joints: comparison with a superb microvascular imaging technique. J Ultrasound. 2022;25:765–71.
22. Hata J. Seeing the unseen. New techniques in vascular imaging. Otawara: Toshiba. Med Rev. 2014:1–8. https://www.toshiba-medical.eu/eu/wpcontent/uploads/sites/2/2014/09/WP_OI_MOIUS0070EA_SMI_Hata_03_2014.pdf
23. Franceschini E, Yu FT, Destrempes F, Cloutier G. Ultrasound characterization of red blood cell aggregation with intervening attenuating tissue-mimicking phantoms. J Acoust Soc Am. 2010;127:1104–15.
24. Yokota K, Wada TT, Akiyama Y, Mimura T. Detection of synovial inflammation in rheumatic diseases using superb microvascular imaging: comparison with conventional power Doppler imaging. Mod Rheumatol. 2018;28:327–33.
25. Yu X, Li Z, Ren M, Xi J, Wu J, Ji Y. Superb microvascular imaging (SMI) for evaluating hand joint lesions in patients with rheumatoid arthritis in clinical remission. Rheumatol Int. 2018;38:1885–90.
26. Kokhanovsky N, Nachtigal A, Reindorp N, Zeina AR. Superior mesenteric artery-related aortic pseudomass as a form of reverberation artifact in a 10-year-old boy. J Clin Imaging Sci. 2014;4:73.
27. Terslev L, Diamantopoulos AP, Døhn UM, et al. Settings and artifacts relevant for Doppler ultrasound in large vessel vasculitis. Arthritis Res Ther. 2017;19:167.

6 Ultrasound Documentation Principles in Rheumatology Practice and Research

Md Abu Bakar Siddiq, George A. W. Bruyn, and Johannes J. Rasker

6.1 Introduction

To ensure optimal patient care, thorough and precise documentation as well as effective communication within the diagnostic ultrasound healthcare team are essential [1]. A comprehensive record of the ultrasound procedure, along with its analysis and accompanying images displaying relevant normal and abnormal findings, must be documented and stored in a manner that allows easy retrieval [1]. It is imperative that ultrasound images and reports align with clinical necessities and comply with legal and institutional healthcare standards [1]. Additionally, the interaction between the individual interpreting the report and the referring healthcare provider should be unambiguous, prompt, and devoid of potential errors [1]. In situations where the referring, performing, and interpreting physician are the same individual, this fact should be clearly indicated in the documentation to avoid any confusion [1]. Patient confidentiality is paramount throughout this process, and healthcare professionals are encouraged to consult the relevant practice guidelines for specific ultrasound examinations to ensure that all documentation requirements are met [1]. The use of ultrasound without generating a separate report is not in accordance with the aforementioned guidelines [1].

M. A. B. Siddiq (✉)
Department of Rheumatology, Royal North Shore Hospital, Northern Clinical School, Faculty of Medicine and Health, The University of Sydney, Sydney, NSW, Australia

Sydney Musculoskeletal Health, The University of Sydney, Sydney, NSW, Australia

Kolling Institute of Medical Research, St Leonards, NSW, Australia

School of Health Sports and Professional Practice (Rheumatology), University of South Wales, Pontypridd, United Kingdom

Department of Physical Medicine and Rehabilitation, Brahmanbaria Medical College, Brahmanbaria, Bangladesh
e-mail: msid8426@uni.sydney.edu.au

G. A. W. Bruyn
Department of Rheumatology, Reumakliniek Lelystad, Lelystad, The Netherlands

Tergooi MC Hospital, Hilversum, The Netherlands

J. J. Rasker
Faculty of Behavioral Science, Psychology, Health and Technology, University of Twente, Enschede, The Netherlands

6.2 Requirements for Ultrasound Examination

Ultrasound examinations with archiving of (still frame and dynamic) images should include the following information [1]:

- Patient identity
- Facility identity
- Date and time of the ultrasound examination

M. A. B. Siddiq (ed.), *Musculoskeletal Ultrasound in Rheumatic Diseases*,
https://doi.org/10.1007/978-981-96-5298-3_6

- Output display standard (thermal index and mechanical index)
- Label of the anatomic location and laterality (when appropriate)
- Image orientation (when appropriate)
- Clinical information

(**Note:** For digitally stored data, the information should be contained in the metadata and readable while reviewing images. For analog records, identifiers should be contained in the image.)

6.3 Reporting of Nonroutine Results

In cases where immediate patient care is needed, a preliminary ultrasound report may be shared with the patient's referring healthcare provider(s) prior to the final report [1]. This preliminary report must contain the patient's identification, details of the referring physician, contact information for the interpreting provider, relevant clinical data, the date of the procedure, and examination specifics [1]. However, it may not include all the results. The preliminary report should be stored, as it contributes to clinical decisions [1]. Any significant differences between the preliminary and final reports should be communicated to the patient's provider and noted in the final report, along with the date, time, and method of communication. If the interpreting provider believes that a delay in the ultrasound results could negatively impact the patient's outcome, they must inform the patient's healthcare provider while adhering to privacy laws [1]. This communication should take place as soon as possible after the examination results are interpreted [1].

6.4 Ultrasound Final Report

A signed final report from the interpreting provider should include a) demographic data, b) key ultrasound findings in body parts, and c) concluding statements (Box 6.1) [1]:

(a) **Demographic data:**
  - Patient identification information (name, age, sex, etc.).
  - Name of the ordering provider.
  - Location of the ultrasound facility and contact information.
  - Relevant clinical information, including the indication for the examination and/or the current version of the appropriate *International Classification of Diseases* code (https://www.who.int/standards/classifications/classification-of-diseases), was obtained.
  - Date and time of the ultrasound examination.
  - Specific ultrasound examination performed (e.g., ultrasound of wrist in rheumatoid arthritis patients).
  - If endocavitary techniques are applied, the method should be specified.

(b) **Body of the report:**
  - A description of the diagnostic or guided procedures performed, for example, synovial effusion and synovial hypertrophy, is given for knee osteoarthritis, or intra-articular (IA) ultrasound-guided injection of hyaluronic acid has been performed via an in-plane technique.
  - Components of the examination as outlined in the relevant practice parameter(s) (please check the joint-specific ultrasound examination section below).
  - All contrast media (normally no contrast media will be introduced during an ultrasound examination) and/or pharmaceuticals used (including route and dose) (e.g., IA ultrasound-guided injection of hyaluronic acid (4 mg/2 ml) and triamcinolone acetonide (40 mg/ml) has been given via the in-plane technique).
  - Additional medications, catheters, or devices used (needle size used for joint aspiration or injection of IA local anesthetics or platelet-rich plasma during intervention).
  - Any significant patient reaction or complication from contrast, medicines, or

Box 6.1 Sample ultrasound examination report in knee osteoarthritis

Feni Clinic, SSK Road, Feni, Post box 3900, Bangladesh

ID: xxxxx

Date: dd/mm/yyyy

Name of Patient: Mr. AH **Sex**: Male **Age**: 60 years
Referred By: Physical medicine outpatient door
Name of examination: Ultrasound of knee
Clinical data: A 60-year-old woman presented with complaints of pain and restricted range of motion in her right knee, which had hindered her daily physical activities for several months. She reported no significant morning stiffness. Clinical examination did not indicate the presence of joint effusion. Radiographic assessment revealed advanced osteoarthritis in the medial tibiofemoral compartment, characterized by diminished joint space, subchondral cyst formation, sclerosis, osteophyte development, and bony end deformity. Additionally, there was an increase in soft tissue opacity on the knee back, accompanied by a distinct area of well-defined opaque mass. Further scrutiny under ultrasound was performed.

Ultrasound findings: Examination of the anterior joint recess revealed no signs of anechoic, compressible accumulation (Fig. 6.1a). Additionally, there was an absence of a noncompressible, hyperechoic, pliable mass within this recess. The synovial membrane did not display any thickening, and it was neither branched nor villous in appearance. Severe medial femoral condylar osteophyte was noted. The medial meniscus appeared hyperechoic but was torn and extruded from its normal position (Fig. 6.1b). The thickness of the cartilage on the medial femoral condyle was diminished (positive chondral print sign), measuring an average of 0.8 mm (0.6–0.9 mm) (Fig. 6.1c), whereas the articular cartilage thickness remained intact in the intercondylar region. A posterior view of the knee revealed beak-shaped Baker's cyst (BC) with compressible, anechoic collection and increased Doppler flow in its wall (Fig. 6.1d-f). Additionally, a noncompressible, hyperechoic, non-mobile mass with irregular surface and posterior acoustic shadowing was identified within the BC. The semitendinosus tendon appeared fibrillar.

Impression: Reduced medial femoral condylar cartilage thickness, medial femoral condylar osteophyte, medial meniscal tear and extrusion and loose body in Baker's cyst

DD: Knee osteoarthritis with complicated Baker's cyst
(Images are attached herewith the report.)

(Dr.) MABS
MBBS, FCPS, MSc (Rheumatology)
RMSK, POCUS (MSK), FACR

intervention should be documented (e.g., immediate injection site bruising or bleeding).
   - Anatomic measurements of abnormal structures should be documented, for example, any presence of and measurement of the diameter of a Baker's cyst on the back of the knee in arthritis. .
   - A description of examination findings, using appropriate anatomic and ultrasound terminology (e.g., at the attachment to the calcaneus, Achilles tendon loss of fibrillar pattern, appearing thick and hypoechoic).

(c) **Concluding statements:**
   - A specific diagnosis or differential diagnosis.
   - Any follow-up studies (if appropriate) (e.g., an IA steroid injection is performed at baseline and is recommended at a 3-month follow-up visit to document any changes in baseline ultrasound biomarkers, effusion, Doppler signals, etc.).
   - For any failure to include standard views or other necessary components (e.g., in advanced knee osteoarthritis (OA), sometimes, a deroute of needle penetration for IA injection from the lateral to the medial side) is needed.
   - If prior relevant imaging studies are available, a statement of comparison (at follow-up, ultrasound biomarkers could be compared with baseline features to assess the treatment effect), and.
   - Details of provider-to-provider communication in cases where a delay in communication may have adversely affected the patient's outcome.

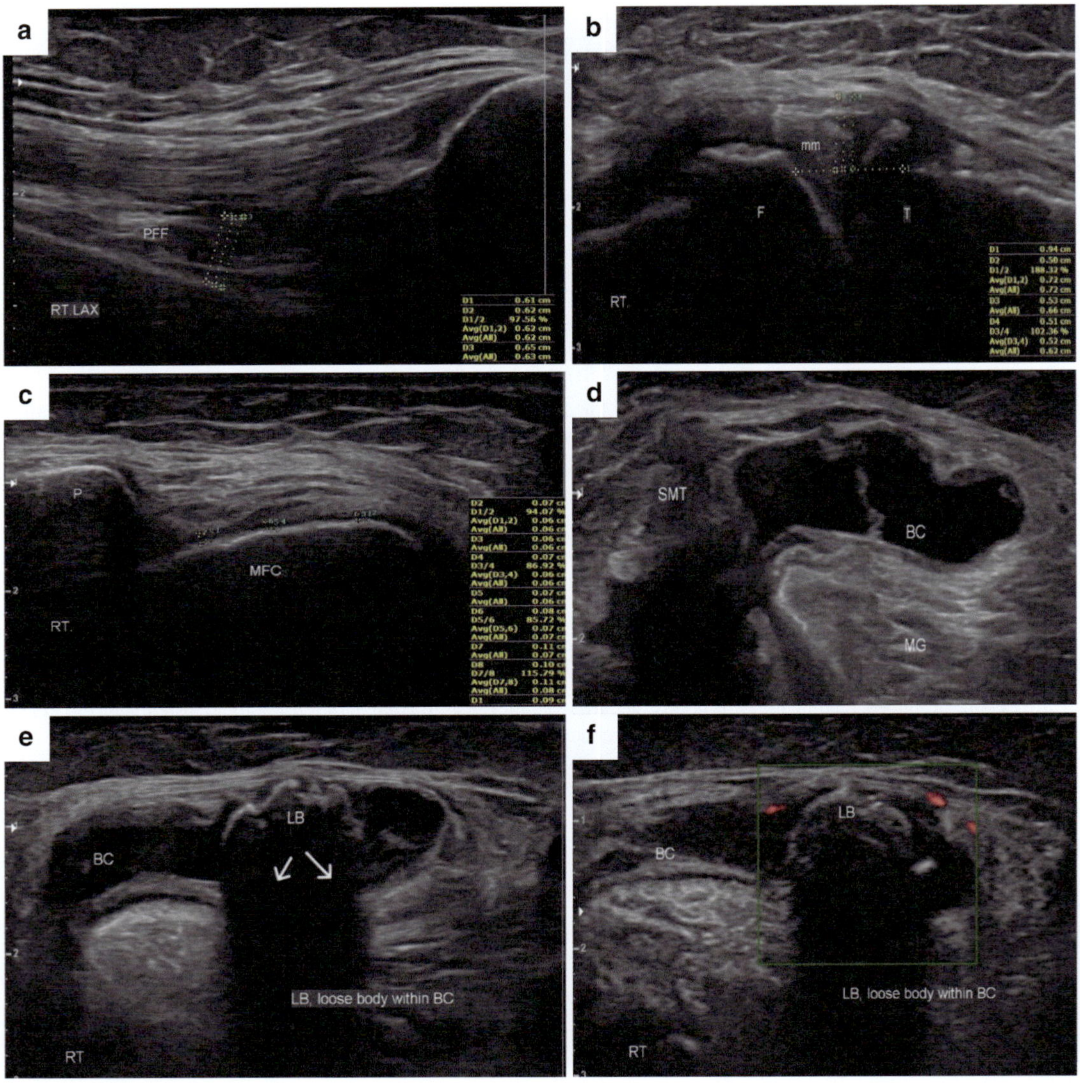

Fig. 6.1 Osteoarthritis of the knee. (**a**) Anterior, longitudinal scan of the suprapatellar area reveals no anechoic, compressible accumulation in the anterior joint recess. (**b**) Longitudinal scan revealing medial joint line osteophytes and MME. (**c**) Short axis scan of medial knee explores reduced MFC cartilage thickness. (**d–f**) Short axis scans of posterior knee unveil BC, BC with LB (**e, f**), and increased cyst wall Doppler activity (**f**) (red spots). *BC* Baker's cyst, *F* femur, *LB* loose body, *MG* medial gastrocnemius, *MM* medial meniscus, *MFC* medial femoral condyle, *RT* right, *SMT* semimembranosus tendon, *T* tibia

The interpreting provider should make the final report available to the ordering provider, who is responsible for reviewing the report. A retrievable copy should be included in the patient's medical record, which is accessible to the requesting provider. Archiving methods and communication of reports and images must comply with local, state, and federal regulations. Box 6.1 shows a sample knee ultrasound report in an osteoarthritis patient.

6.5 Ultrasound Documentation in Guided Procedures

Ultrasound-guided procedures should be documented in accordance with the Joint Commission (https://www.jointcommission.org/standards/universal-protocol/) [1]. A final report, signed and dated by the performing physician, should be made available within 24 h of completion of the examination or, for nonemergency cases, by the next business day [1]

Information Should Include Indications for ultrasound-guided procedures

- Documentation of compliance in line with the TJC universal protocol
- Documentation of the procedure site
- Description of the target and relevant associated structures (normal and abnormal)
- The essential elements related to the procedure are as follows:
  1. An approach (e.g., in knee OA, IA injection via a superolateral or superomedial approach).
  2. Needle and device type and gauge (e.g., aspiration from the knee OA performed with an 18 G needle).
  3. The number of passes performed during the procedure should be clearly documented.
  4. Deviations from standard techniques should be described and justified.
  5. Medications names and amounts (e.g., in knee OA, IA injection of 2 ml of triamcinolone acetonide and 1–2 ml of 2% lidocaine sodium is used to relieve pain).
  6. Type of specimen and amount removed (e.g., a 25 ml pale-yellow fluid is aspirated from the knee OA).
  7. Complications (or lack thereof) (e.g., accidental injury to the popliteal vessels during Baker's cyst aspiration and injection, if appropriate).
  8. Patient response to the procedure (increased pain during injection, immediate pain relief, or loss of sensation during nerve block).
  9. Follow-up imaging recommendation (e.g., to register any change in synovial inflammation following IA corticosteroid injection).

6.6 Qualifications and Responsibilities of Personnel

Physicians interpreting or performing musculoskeletal ultrasound examinations should meet some specified qualifications [2]. Physicians may be qualified with the European Alliance of Associations for Rheumatology (EULAR), American Institute of Ultrasound in Medicine (AIUM), American College of Rheumatology (ACR), American Registry for Diagnostic Medical Sonography (ARDMS), or Alliance for Physician Certification and Advancement (APCA) endorsed musculoskeletal ultrasound certifications, such as, EULAR/AIUM sonography courses (basic, intermediate, and advanced), Musculoskeletal Ultrasound Certification in Rheumatology (RhMSUS), Registered Musculoskeletal Sonographer (RMSKS), Registered in Musculoskeletal Sonography (RMSK), and Point-of-Care Ultrasound (POCUS) (Musculoskeletal), respectively.

A physician must be available for consultation with the sonographer on a case-by-case basis. Ideally, the physician should be onsite and available to participate actively in the ultrasound examination when needed. The initial set of education and practice guidelines for ultrasound in rheumatology in the United Kingdom was formulated and approved by the British Society for Rheumatology Ultrasound Special Interest Group (BSRUSSIG) [3]. These recommendations are anticipated to serve to bolster and authenticate the practice of rheumatology ultrasound, as well as guide the evolution of forthcoming rheumatology training schemes and educational initiatives (Table 6.1) [3]. It is recognized, however, that geographic realities may not permit the presence of an onsite physician in all locations. In this case, a supervising physician should be available for quality assurance and sonographer supervision via a picture archiving and communication system (PACS) [1].

Table 6.1 The BSRUSSIG recommendations for ultrasound training and practice in rheumatology [3]

Recommendations
1. All future rheumatologists should know indications for ultrasound examination in rheumatology and be able to operate the ultrasound machine for basic procedures such as aspiration of the acute hot joint.
2. Independent musculoskeletal ultrasound scanning of the hands, wrists, ankles, and feet in patients with inflammatory arthritis is desirable for rheumatologists/AHPs (BSR level 1).
3. Independent musculoskeletal ultrasound scanning of other anatomical regions for other indications is appropriate for rheumatologists/AHPs (BSR level 2). For example, salivary glands and arteries. In that case, musculoskeletal ultrasound is much broader than just musculoskeletal.
4. A blended modular educational program will be developed and delivered by the BSRUSSIG to facilitate BSR level 1 and 2 rheumatology ultrasound training.
5. Mentors and trainers in rheumatology ultrasound will receive ongoing training and support through the BSRUSSIG (BSR level 3).
6. Rheumatologists/AHPs performing ultrasound scanning need to be able to demonstrate their ongoing training, practice, and competence.
7. Mentors and trainers should be able to demonstrate their ongoing training, practice, and competence in ultrasound scanning and teaching.

AHP Allied Health Professional, *BSR* British Society for Rheumatology, *SIG* special interest group, *BSRUSSIG* British Society for Rheumatology Ultrasound Special Interest Group

6.7 Ultrasound Documentation and Routine Quality Assessment (QA)

To ensure top-notch documentation quality, it is essential to conduct regular quality assurance checks that encompass cleanliness, safety, image display (Table 6.2) [4, 5], and performance (Table 6.3) [4, 5]. This includes inspecting for malfunctions and ensuring that all equipment functions at the expected level [5]. Any irregularities, whether physical or operational, should be promptly reported to the responsible personnel [5]. Collaboration with sonographers, physicians, medical physicists, and biomedical engineers is crucial in carrying out these procedures effectively [4, 5].

It is crucial to ensure that equipment and scan rooms are thoroughly cleaned and disinfected [4, 5]. Regular checks for cracks, dead elements, or lens delamination in transducers are essential [4, 5]. By maintaining cleanliness and promptly detecting any malfunctions in the scanner, transducer, or display, image quality and safety can be significantly enhanced [5]. The manuals provided by ultrasound equipment manufacturers offer valuable insights into equipment operation, safety protocols, and effective cleaning techniques [4, 5].

Regular QA tests involve checking transducers and connecting cables for any signs of damage, partially detached lenses, reduced performance in specific electrical circuits, and testing for element drop-out, grayscale and Doppler imaging performance, as well as shear-wave elastography [4, 5]. It is crucial for sonographers, physicists, and engineers to be knowledgeable about these tests to ensure the proper functioning of the equipment [4, 5]. In the event of a nonfunctional transducer, it is recommended to conduct a check by imaging a uniform section of a phantom and inspecting the B-mode image, either subjectively or by using image analysis techniques, before using it [4, 5]. Furthermore, the Food and Drug Administration guidelines suggest that ultrasound equipment manufacturers should utilize transducer test software for routine QA checks [4, 5]. It is also beneficial for sonographers to familiarize themselves with routine QA tasks, which can be facilitated by medical physicists, biomedical engineers, or trained personnel onsite [4, 5].

6.8 ALARA (As Low As Reasonably Achievable)

Adhering to ALARA principles is essential for keeping ultrasound energy at a safe level to prevent any potential bioeffects while still preserving the necessary diagnostic information [6]. It

Table 6.2 Cleanliness and safety [1]

Ultrasound cleanliness and safety check	When
Clean any spill of bodily fluids or hazardous materials	Immediately
Clean gel from transducers and ultrasound machine control panels	After the procedure
Disinfect transducer	After the procedure
Check transducer cables for damage	Daily
Check the transducer for cracks, separations, and discolorations	Daily
Clean monitors and inspect for cracks	Daily
Check for any damage to power cords or PACS connections	Daily
Identify and report improper operation of switches or knobs on the machine console	Daily
Identify and report any burned-out indicator lights	Daily
Clean rooms for dust, dirt, and infection control	Daily
Clean dust from machine console air filters	Weekly
Check the machine for dents and other damage	Weekly
Thoroughly clean the ultrasound machine console and other equipment in the examination room	Monthly
Inspect keyboards, control knobs, monitors, and air filters for cleanliness, operation of indicator lights, and functioning of trackball	Yearly
Inspect the mechanical integrity of the system, including wheels and wheel locks and the security of attached accessories and cords	Yearly

PACS picture archiving and communication system

Table 6.3 Image display and performance [1]

Ultrasound image display and performance check	When
During routine scanning, visually assess images for vertical shadows and streaks commonly caused by dead elements or a delaminated lens in the transducer	Daily
Check brightness and contrast controls	Annually
Confirm machine monitor settings are at calibration points used for setting up primary image display workstations (i.e., PACS displays) and/or hard copy devices	Annually

PACS picture archiving and communication system

is important to be mindful of the acoustic output when adjusting controls and to consider the transducer dwell time and overall scanning time [4, 5]. Users must follow all the necessary measures [7–9]:

Guidelines to Ensure that ALARA Is Practiced Effectively

(a) Ensure that the appropriate examination presets are applied and take the time to review the manufacturer's default presets to ensure that they are suitable for the procedure.
(b) Always adjust the power to the lowest available level that still allows for high-quality diagnostic images, and remember to decrease the power at the conclusion of each examination so that the next user can begin with the lowest acoustic output setting.
(c) Keep a close eye on the mechanical index and thermal index, being aware of the recommended upper limits for each and any duration restrictions that apply to the specific type of examination being conducted.
(d) When scanning, the transducer should be moved and lifted to minimize exposure time to any one anatomic structure, avoiding areas that contain sensitive tissues such as the eyes, lungs, intestines, and fetal calcified structures such as the skull and spine.
(e) Last, an effort is made to minimize the overall scanning time to gather the necessary diagnostic information efficiently and effectively.

6.9 Infection Control

The quality assessment program includes steps to minimize the spread of infection. The AIUM guidelines for the cleaning of ultrasound transducers, safe handling, and use of ultrasound coupling gel have been demonstrated [1].

General Guidelines for Transducer Preparation and Cleaning (Fig. 6.2) [9] are as follows:

(a) The external transducers should be cleaned after every use.
(b) External transducers that come into contact with contaminated skin must be protected by a disposable transducer cover.
(c) For procedures involving percutaneous needle or catheter placement, such as vascular access or lumbar puncture, transducers should undergo low-level disinfection (LLD) and be paired with a single-use transducer cover to prevent the transmission of clinically significant human viruses.
(d) On the other hand, internal transducers should also be shielded by a single-use transducer cover, with the level of sterility of the cover dependent on the sterility requirements of the procedure, categorizing these transducers as semi-critical devices.

Ultrasound Transducer Cleaning and Preparation Below are the AIUM's recommendations to follow for the cleaning and preparation of all ultrasound transducers [6, 9].

(a) **Cleaning of transducers**: Cleaning is the process of eliminating visible soil, whether organic or inorganic, from surfaces and objects, typically done through manual or mechanical means using water, soap, or enzymatic cleaners. Any leftover residue can be wiped away with a damp cloth and mild soap or wiped. For more stubborn debris, a small brush can be used to remove bulk gel, especially in hard-to-reach areas. It is crucial to thoroughly clean instruments before they are subjected to high-level disinfection (HLD) and sterilization to ensure the effectiveness of these processes by removing any material that could interfere with the disinfection and sterilization methods [9].
(b) **Disinfection**: A process that eliminates many or all pathogenic microorganisms, except bacterial spores.
   - *Low-level infection* (LLD) [10] involves the sterilization of external transducers, such as interventional percutaneous procedures that may be contaminated with blood or bodily fluids, to eliminate mycobacteria and bloodborne pathogens (including hepatitis B virus, hepatitis C

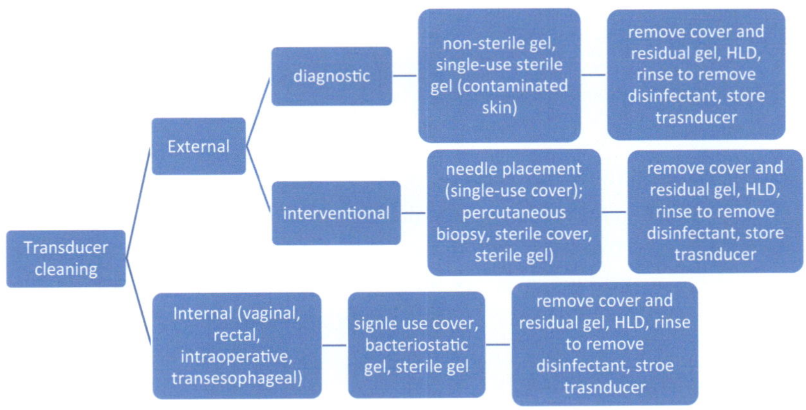

Fig. 6.2 Flowchart illustrating transducer cleaning procedures

Table 6.4 Chemical sterilants and high-level disinfectants [9, 10]

Name of the chemicals	Mechanism of action
Glutaraldehyde	The antimicrobial agent causes cell death by forming cross-links between cellular proteins. This results in the disruption of essential cellular functions and ultimately leads to the demise of the affected cells
Hydrogen peroxide	Antiseptic and antibacterial (a very strong oxidizer)
Peracetic acid	Antimicrobial (high oxidation potential)
Ortho-phthalaldehyde	This antimicrobial agent has a high affinity for the outer cell wall of contaminant organisms, resulting in a strong binding effect. This binding helps to effectively neutralize and eliminate the harmful microorganisms, preventing their growth and spread
Hypochlorous acid	Antimicrobial (myeloperoxidase-mediated peroxidation of chloride ions)
Iodine cleaning solution	Effective broad-spectrum bactericide, and is also effective against yeasts, molds, fungi, viruses, and protozoans
Phenol/phenolate	Antimicrobial
Hibidil	Antiseptic

virus, and HIV). Hands were thoroughly cleaned with LLD and then covered with gloves. LLD consists of the use of soap, water, transducer covers, medical gloves, or other physical barriers (compatible medical dressings) [6]. LLD is effective in destroying most bacteria, some viruses, and some fungi, but it does not deactivate *Mycobacterium tuberculosis* or bacterial spores.

- *High-level disinfection* (HLD) (Table 6.4) involves various physical and chemical sterilization methods. The primary sterilizing agents utilized in healthcare settings include steam under pressure, dry heat, ethylene oxide gas, hydrogen peroxide gas plasma, and liquid chemicals known as chemical sterilants [9]. Certain medical devices, such as internal transducers (e.g., transvaginal, transrectal, and transesophageal) and intraoperative transducers, necessitate HLD before being used on another patient. Importantly, even if there is an obvious disruption in the integrity of the transducer cover, the protocol for HLD remains unchanged. Owing to the risk of barrier sheath disruption, HLD with chemical agents becomes essential [6, 9]. Additionally, drying the transducer before being subjected to HLD with chemical disinfectants is recommended [9]. A comprehensive list of HLD chemical agents can be found in Table 6.4 [9].

(c) **Rinsing:** A transducer should be thoroughly rinsed and dried after disinfection [9].

(d) **Storing:** Transducers need to be stored in accordance with their disinfection level [9].

(e) **Gloves and hand washing**: The gloves should be discarded properly after use, and then the hands should be washed thoroughly [9].

6.10 Infection Control Policy for Ultrasound-Coupled Gel

Sterile Gel Sterile single-use gel packets are preferred when infection is a concern [9], for example,

- Invasive procedures involve passing a needle through a tissue for aspiration and tissue biopsy.
- Ultrasound examinations were performed on neonates.
- All ultrasound procedures were performed on nonintact skin or near fresh surgical sites.
- Sterile or bacteriostatic gels should be considered for endocavitary examinations performed on intact mucous membranes (e.g., esophageal, gastric, rectal, and vaginal).

Nonsterile Gel single-use gel packets or multidose containers may be used. The use of multidose containers should follow [9]:

- Discard and replace multidose containers when empty; these should not be refilled.
- The container should be appropriately sealed when not in use.
- Direct contact between the gel container dispensing tip and any person or instrument, including the ultrasound transducer, was avoided. If gel is to be used on a patient who is under droplet or contact precautions (such as COVID-19), the multidose container should be discarded after use, or a single-use gel packet should be used.

Gel Warming Dry heat should be the only method used to warm gel. Gel warmers should be cleaned and disinfected regularly according to the manufacturers' and infection-control policy requirements [9].

6.11 Practical Ultrasound-Guided Procedures: General Requirements and Hygiene

General Requirements
The procedure must comply with patient consent and involve thorough counseling about the possible adverse effects linked to the intervention [11]. It is essential to evaluate the coagulation time prior to the procedure and implement necessary measures to reduce the risk of bleeding [11]. For example, if the platelet count is low, a platelet transfusion should be administered before proceeding, whereas patients with an international normalized ratio (INR) exceeding 1.5 may need fresh plasma [11]. Before performing a needle puncture, a local anesthetic should be given, and both the needle and injection site must be adequately sterilized [11, 12]. It is important to choose the appropriate ultrasound mode or consider alternative options; for example, when dealing with deeply located lesions or structures, the use of 3.5- or 5-MHz curved array probes may be needed. The lesion that needs treatment should subsequently be identified. Selecting the right technique and becoming familiar with the relevant anatomy can help minimize the risk of damaging vital structures [11, 12]. Additionally, adjusting the probe angle or choosing the correct focal zone can improve the visualization of the needle during intervention [11, 12].

6.12 Ultrasound Puncture Technique and Better Visualization of the Needle

Needle Puncture Freehand ultrasound-guided punctures can be performed in two ways: by marking the skin while using ultrasound and then inserting the needle without ultrasound guidance or by guiding the needle with direct sonographic visualization [12]. The first method is effective for larger structures that are close to the skin, such as Baker's cysts, which contain significant fluid [12]. To identify the optimal puncture site, applying pressure to the skin with a finger can be helpful; additionally, a metal paper clip can create two bright echo lines that assist in pinpointing the exact location for needle insertion [12]. The technique chosen often depends on the specific anatomy involved [9, 12].

Better Needle Visualization In certain areas, the needle can be positioned parallel to the ultrasound probe, which enhances the visibility of both the needle's tip and its entire length (Fig. 6.3) [11, 12]. In some anatomical regions, such as between the toes, the needle can be introduced opposite the probe, again resulting in only the tip being visible. Alternatively, the sonographer may opt for a transverse approach, where the needle is positioned transversely to the probe, appearing as a spot on the ultrasound image when located beneath the probe, which can also be observed if the probe is moved. Identifying the precise location of the needle tip can be challenging. During ultrasound-guided injections, the needle should be visible on the ultrasound image corresponding to its anatomical position; for example, if the needle is inserted from the right side of the probe, it should be seen on the right side of the image. Typically, right-handed sonographers hold an ultrasound probe [11, 12].

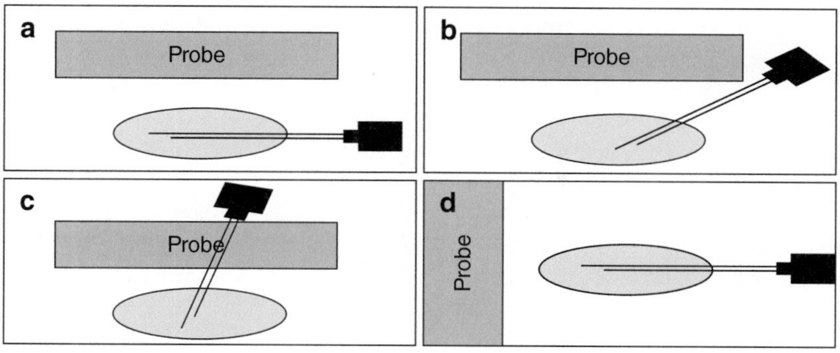

Fig. 6.3 Diagram illustrating four configurations of a probe relative to an oval object

6.13 Hygiene

Skin and Probe Preparation Skin preparation should involve either a 70% alcohol solution or a chlorhexidine solution. However, this method may obscure visibility in certain areas of the skin, and using a safe and cost-effective iodinated solution can help mitigate this issue [10, 12]. Additionally, the specific skin area and the probe could be covered with sterile gel.

Hygiene for the Proceduralist It is advisable for the examiner to wear sterile gloves during the puncture while maintaining direct vision, and they should also be vaccinated against hepatitis B. Gloves should remain on throughout the procedure. Instead of using sterile gloves, some authors recommend thoroughly washing hands with surgical soap and applying a chlorhexidine solution to the fingertips before beginning the procedure [9, 10, 13].

Hygiene for Aspirated Materials Any aspirated materials must be placed in suitable containers, and all items that may have been contaminated with blood or synovial fluid should be disposed of properly. Importantly, procedures performed under indirect vision do not necessitate the use of sterile gel. The area should be outlined with an indelible marker [12].

Hygiene for Contrast Agent and Medications To collect medications from sterile vials, sterile syringes and needles must be utilized [12]. The sterile air found in a capped vial of corticosteroid or lidocaine can be employed for air sonography, allowing the air to be visible within the joint capsule when the injection is administered and the needle is correctly positioned [12]. This technique is particularly beneficial for accessing challenging joints such as the hip [12]. In certain areas, the needle can be positioned parallel to the ultrasound probe, which enhances the visibility of both the needle's tip and its entire length. This parallel alignment also allows for improved hygiene, as the needle can be inserted away from the probe [12]. Conversely, if the needle is angled at approximately 45 degrees to the probe, only the tip will be visible as a hyperechoic spot, complicating localization and hygiene since the needle and probe are in close proximity [12]. Similar challenges arise when the needle is inserted next to the midpoint of the probe [12].

6.14 Ultrasound Documentation Principles in Rheumatology Research

The updated OMERACT ultrasound definitions used in rheumatic diseases were released in 2019 [13]. OMERACT ultrasound is detailed in Chap. 3. The EULAR task force developed a checklist of 23 items (including 21 mandatory items) organized into 13 categories to ensure transparent and comprehensive reporting of aspects of ultrasound in rheumatic disease research, as detailed in Table 6.5 [14]. Research addressing

Table 6.5 Recommendation checklist for reporting studies using ultrasound in RMDs [14]

Topic	Items to report
Objective	1. Objective of the ultrasound measurement in the study (e.g., *description, prediction, diagnosis, validation,* etc.)
Design	2. Study design (e.g., *cross-sectional, case–control, cohort, and randomized clinical trial*) 3. Prospective or retrospective data collection*
Participants	4. Informed consent procedure (written, oral) 5. Source, selection criteria, and sampling of the participants (including controls where appropriate)
Blinding	6. Procedures for blinding of sonographers and participants
Ultrasound features	7. (a) Broad domain* of interest (e.g., *inflammation or structural damage*), (b) target domain* with corresponding theoretical ultrasound definition(s)* (e.g., synovitis: Synovial hypertrophy plus increased synovial blood flow), (c) domain components (i.e., elementary lesions)* with corresponding operational definitions* (e.g., *synovial hypertrophy: Increased thickness of synovium with hypoechoic appearance*)
Scanning/acquisition procedures	8. (a) Anatomical region(s)* or structure(s)* that were studied, (b) rationale for choosing these anatomical region(s)/structure(s), 9. (a) Patient position (e.g., prone, supine, etc.), (b) anatomical region position (e.g., neutral, etc.), (c) surfaces scanned (e.g., volar, dorsal), (d) transducer position (e.g., transverse, longitudinal), (e) whether the examination was dynamic*
Ultrasound scoring system	Scoring system used: 10. (a) Type (e.g., *quantitative, semiquantitative, binary*), (b) level (e.g., *patient level, joint/anatomical region level*)
	11. For existing scoring systems: (a) references or results of previous validity and reliability studies, (b) score range (minimum–maximum), and meaning of the score (e.g., *higher is* ...), (c) rationale for any thresholds or cut-offs, (d) training session details if performed, (e) the reliability* of the scoring system in the hands of the study sonographers/readers
	12. For new scoring systems: (a) rationale for developing a new scoring system, (b) detailed description of the scoring system, (c) reliability assessment: (i) type of reliability: Interreader, other, (ii) Training session if performed, (iii) The reliability of the scoring system as applied by the study sonographers/readers, (iv) Whether reliability was assessed on static images, video clips, or real-time examination of patients, (v) sample size of the reliability study, vi. Reliability results (e.g., kappa or ICC with 95% CI and type of kappa or ICC, prevalence of observed lesions, smallest detectable change, SE of measurement)
Sonographer(s)*/ reader(s)*	13. (a) whether acquisition and reading were performed at the same time, (b) whether acquisition and reading were performed by the same person, (c) number of sonographers or readers, d. in longitudinal studies, whether the same sonographer scanned the same patient at each assessment
	14. Optional: Information about the experience of sonographer(s) and reader(s) (e.g., *numbers of scans performed, certification, qualification,* etc.)
Equipment	15. (a) Brand and model of the ultrasound device, (b) type and model of the transducer, (c) whether the ultrasound device (or software) was changed during the study
	16. Ultrasound modalities* and settings: (a) grayscale, (b) Doppler, (c) other
Images (pictures and drawings)	17. For images included in the manuscript, verify that: (a) information identifying the patient is deleted, (b) essential targets in the image(s) are clearly labeled, (c) images match the content of the manuscript, (d) quality of the images is adequate
Contextual factors	18. Duration of ultrasound examination when relevant for the study question *19.* Optional: *(a) whether ambient conditions* (e.g., *temperature, time of day*) *were kept stable during the study, (b). potential confounding factors* (e.g., *exercise, alcohol, caffeine, smoking*)
Statistical analysis	20. (a) Existence of a prespecified statistical analysis plan and specification of post hoc analyses, (b) analyses performed, (c) whether the analyses were performed at patient or at joint/region level, (d) extent of missing data, e. handling of missing data
Disclosure	21. Potential conflicts of interest, including those related to ultrasound

ICC intraclass reliability, *RMDs* rheumatic and musculoskeletal diseases

Table 6.6 Definition of ultrasound terminologies [14]

Terminology	Definition
Prospective data collection	Data collection that starts before the outcome has occurred.
Retrospective data collection	Data collection that starts after outcome status has been determined and refers to information up to that moment.
Broad domain	A pathological (or pathophysiological) manifestation we are interested in assessing/measuring. For example, current broad domains in rheumatic and musculoskeletal diseases measured by ultrasound are "inflammation" and "structural damage."
Target domain	Further specification of the broad domain we are interested in assessing/measuring with ultrasound. For example, synovitis, enthesitis, and erosion.
Target domain component	An individual characteristic of the target domain that can be measured. All domain components together constitute the theoretical definition.For example, synovial hypertrophy and synovial hyperemia are the domain components that can be measured and together define the target domain of synovitis as assessed by ultrasound.
Operational definition of target domain component	The ultrasound definition of a target domain component (i.e., the "signal" that can be detected by ultrasound). For example, synovial hypertrophy is defined as hypoechoic thickening of the synovium and synovial hyperemia as increased Doppler signal within the synovial hypertrophy.
Anatomical region	The region of the body that is the focus of the ultrasound examination may include more than one related structure. For example, muscles, nerves and arteries, or joint cavity and tendons.
Anatomical structure	Isolated tissue(s) or organ(s) that is/are examined by ultrasound.For example, synovium, bone, tendon, and muscle.
Dynamic examination	Procedure in which the transducer is moved along the anatomical region under study, or the anatomical region is moved during the ultrasound examination, for example, through muscle contraction or tendon movement.
Reliability	The degree to which the measurement is free from measurement error.
Reader	The person who is reading (i.e., interpreting) the ultrasound images or the video clips of the examination. This interpretation may take place at the same time as the acquisition of the ultrasound images/video clips, or later. In the latter case, the reader may be the same person who performed the ultrasound examination and the acquisition of the images/video clips or a different person.
Sonographer	The person performing the ultrasound evaluation. Usually, the sonographer is a health professional with the appropriate skills to perform an ultrasound examination in RMDs.
Ultrasound modalities	The ultrasound technique(s) used, that is, grayscale mode (or B mode), Doppler (color, power, pulse), elastography, contrast-enhanced ultrasound, etc.

B-mode brightness mode, *RMDs* rheumatic and musculoskeletal diseases

these items could improve the interpretability of study development and assessment of ultrasound validity, generalizability, and applicability [9]. Table 6.6 further shows the relevant terminologies used in ultrasound clinical research [14]. The content validity of the recommendation checklist was confirmed by a panel of external experts [14].

Conflict of Interest MAB is supported by a Faculty of Medicine and Health Executive Dean Stipend scholarship, University of Sydney, Australia, for his PhD course.

References

1. AIUM. Practice parameter for documentation of an ultrasound examination. J Ultrasound Med. 2020;39:E1–4.
2. Page P, Manske RC, Voight M, Wolfe C. MSK ultrasound - an IJSPT perspective. Int J Sports Phys Ther. 2023;18:1–10.
3. Atchia I, Brown AK, Chitale S, et al. Recommendations for rheumatology ultrasound training and practice in the UK. Rheumatology (Oxford). 2021;60:2647–52.
4. Grazhdani H, David E, Ventura Spagnolo O, et al. Quality assurance of ultrasound systems: cur-

rent status and review of literature. J Ultrasound. 2018;21:173–82.
5. AIUM. Routine Quality Assurance of Clinical Ultrasound Equipment. http://aium.s3.amazonaws.com/resourceLibrary/rqa2.pdf. Accessed on 27 March, 2024.
6. Abramowicz JS, Barnett SB. The safe use of non-medical ultrasound. Ultrasound Obstet Gynecol. 2009;33:617–20.
7. American Institute of Ultrasound in Medicine. Recommended maximum scanning times for displayed thermal index (TI) values. American Institute of Ultrasound in Medicine website. https://www.aium.org/resources/official-statements. Approved October 30, 2016.
8. AIUM. As Low As Reasonably Achievable (ALARA) Principle. Available at: https://www.aium.org/resources/official-statements/view/as-low-as-reasonably-achievable-(alara)-principle. Accessed on July 10, 2024.
9. AIUM. Official statement: guidelines for cleaning and preparing external- and internal-use ultrasound transducers and equipment between patients as well as safe handling and use of ultrasound coupling gel. J Ultrasound Med. 2023;42:E13–22.
10. Abril A, Berianu F. Absence of infections in outpatient ultrasound guided musculoskeletal procedures performed at a rheumatology clinic using either sterile gel or iodine cleaning solution: are sterile ultrasound probe covers needed? Ann Rheum Dis. 2014;73:1113.
11. del Cura JL. Ultrasound-guided therapeutic procedures in the musculoskeletal system. Curr Probl Diagn Radiol. 2008;37:203–18.
12. Bruyn GA, Schmidt WA. How to perform ultrasound-guided injections. Best Pract Res Clin Rheumatol. 2009;23:269–79.
13. Bruyn GA, Iagnocco A, Naredo E, et al. OMERACT ultrasound working group. OMERACT definitions for Ultrasonographic pathologies and elementary lesions of rheumatic disorders 15 years on. J Rheumatol. 2019;46:1388–93.
14. Costantino F, Carmona L, Boers M, et al. EULAR recommendations for the reporting of ultrasound studies in rheumatic and musculoskeletal diseases (RMDs). Ann Rheum Dis. 2021;80:840–7.

Part II

Ultrasound Case Scenarios in Rheumatic Diseases

7 Clinical Cases

Md Abu Bakar Siddiq

Case Summary 1 A 70-year-old woman reported pain and swelling in her left knee for the past 3 days. She exhibited erythema and vesicular lesions that spread from the lower anterolateral thigh to the middle anterolateral leg (Fig. 7.1a), with the affected skin feeling warm and showing a localized rise in temperature. There was no prior history of diabetes mellitus. Upon physical examination, the knee joint was swollen, and flexion was restricted. There was notable joint effusion (aspirated under ultrasound guidance) (Fig. 7.1b); however, there was no medial joint line tenderness. X-ray of the knee revealed soft tissue swelling but no medial joint line osteophytes or reduced joint space width. A clinical diagnosis of cellulitis accompanied by knee osteoarthritis was made. An ultrasound of the knee was performed.

Ultrasound Findings The anterior joint recess was observed distended with compressible anechoic fluid collection. A noncompressible, hyperechoic mass was observed traversing the anterior joint cavity (Fig. 7.1c). The synovial membrane appeared thick, hypoechoic, and branched, exhibiting increased Doppler activity as well (Fig. 7.1d–e). There were no medial joint line osteophytes or cases of medial meniscal extrusion. The femoral condylar cartilage thickness was reduced, with a positive "*chondral print sign*." Moreover, an increase in subcutaneous tissue thickness was noted in the posterolateral leg, accompanied by heightened Doppler activity. Anechoic compressible fluid collection was identified surrounding the subcutaneous hyperechoic areolar tissue, which typically appears hypoechoic, creating a cobblestone-like appearance (Fig. 7.1f); however, the hyperechoic septum between the hypoechoic areolar tissue was not clearly defined. Posteriorly, fluid containing superficial (over the medial gastrocnemius) Baker's cyst or deep ganglion cysts (underneath the medial gastrocnemius) was not revealed. At the insertion of the semimembranosus tendon, no bursal swelling with anechoic, compressible collection was documented. The patient received effective treatment with both parenteral and oral flucloxacillin.

M. A. B. Siddiq (✉)
Department of Rheumatology, Royal North Shore Hospital, Northern Clinical School, Faculty of Medicine and Health, The University of Sydney, Sydney, NSW, Australia

Sydney Musculoskeletal Health, The University of Sydney, Sydney, NSW, Australia

Kolling Institute of Medical Research, St Leonards, NSW, Australia

School of Health Sports and Professional Practice (Rheumatology), University of South Wales, Pontypridd, United Kingdom

Department of Physical Medicine and Rehabilitation, Brahmanbaria Medical College, Brahmanbaria, Bangladesh
e-mail: msid8426@uni.sydney.edu.au

M. A. B. Siddiq (ed.), *Musculoskeletal Ultrasound in Rheumatic Diseases*,
https://doi.org/10.1007/978-981-96-5298-3_7

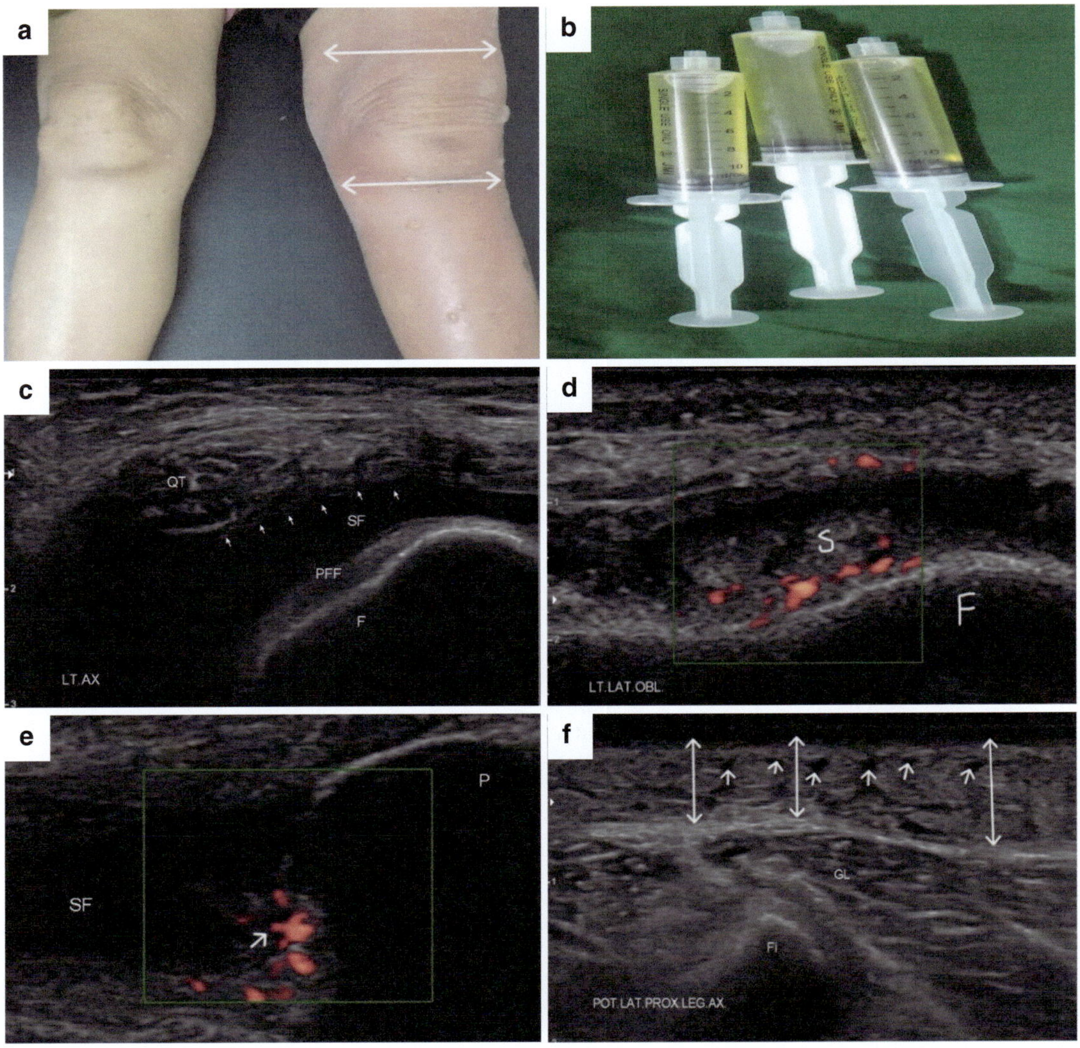

Fig. 7.1 Knee cellulitis in knee osteoarthritis. (**a**) Extension of vesicular skin lesions on the anterior thigh (double arrows). (**b**) Clear synovial fluid aspirated from the suprapatellar joint recess. (**c**) Short axis scan of the suprapatellar knee displaying the synovial fluid (SF) and synovial plica (white arrows). (**d, e**) Lateral oblique longitudinal (**d**) and anterior longitudinal (**e**) suprapatellar knee scans, respectively revealed SF (**e**) and thick synovial membrane (**d**) (arrows) with heightened Doppler activity (**d, e**). (**f**) Postero-lateral longitudinal scan of the proximal leg depicted thick subcutaneous fat with a cobblestone appearance (double arrows) and hypoechoic-anechoic compressible collection between the fat lobules (single arrows). *AX* short axis, *Fi* fibula, *F* femur, *GL* lateral gastrocnemius, *P* patella, *PFF* prefemoral fat, *QT* quadricep tendon, *SF* synovial fluid

Impression Knee cellulitis in knee osteoarthritis.

Case Summary 2 A 53-year-old man working as a restaurant chef complained of pain, swelling, and restricted movement in his right knee over several months. Clinical examination revealed tenderness along the joint line and moderate effusion, as indicated by a positive fluctuation test, along with genu varus deformity. Furthermore, a soft, cystic mass was detected at the posterior aspect of the knee. X-ray revealed narrowing of the medial tibiofemoral joint space width, medial femoral condyle osteophytes, subchondral cysts, sclerosis, and soft tissue swelling around the knee (Fig. 7.2a). Further assessment with ultrasound was performed.

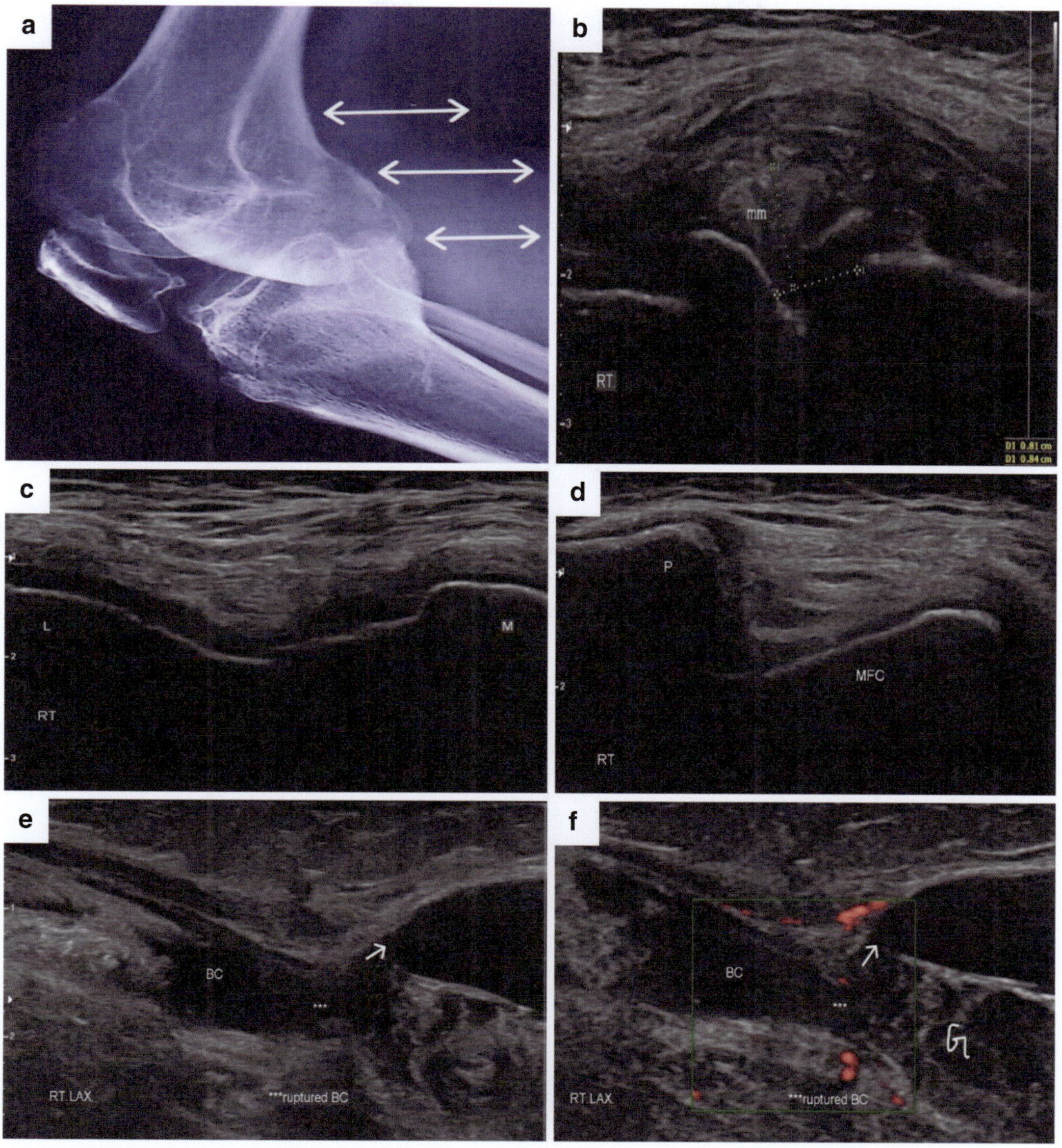

Fig. 7.2 Medial meniscal extrusion with ruptured Baker's cyst in knee osteoarthritis. (**a**) X-ray knee showing a radiopaque soft tissue mass on the knee back (double arrows). (**b**) Longitudinal scan of the medial knee explored severe medial meniscal extrusion. (**c, d**) Transverse suprapatellar scan of the femoral condyles (**c**) and short axis scan of the MFC (**d**) revealed reduced femoral condylar cartilage thickness (**c**), including MFC cartilage (**d**). (**e, f**) Posterior longitudinal scan of the proximal leg depicted ruptured Baker's cyst with fluid leakage (white arrows) over the gastrocnemius muscle (**f**) and increased Doppler signal (**f**) in the cyst wall. *BC* Baker's cyst, *G* gastrocnemius, *mm* medial meniscus, *MFC* medial femoral condyle, *RT* right

Ultrasound Findings The anterior joint recess was not distended, with compressible and anechoic fluid accumulation. The synovial membrane appeared normal. The thicknesses of the prefemoral fat were measured to be 4.6 mm and 6.6 mm in the long and short axes, respectively. Medially, there were moderate medial joint line osteophytes and medial meniscus extrusion (8.4 mm) (Fig. 7.2b). Moreover, the medial femoral condylar cartilage thickness was reduced (Fig. 7.2c–d), with a positive *"chondral print sign."* Posteriorly, a ruptured Baker's cyst with fluid leakage spread over the medial gastrocnemius (MG), and increased Doppler activity was noted (Fig. 7.2e–f). Anechoic compressible or noncompressible cystic masses were not observed beneath the MG or around the semimembranosus tendon.

Impressions Medial meniscal extrusion and ruptured Baker's cyst in knee osteoarthritis.

Case Summary 3 A 40-year-old woman complained of pain and a tingling sensation along the radial aspect of her right hand and fingers, with symptoms worsening at night and during her daily activities. She did not exhibit any radiating pain in her neck. She was nondiabetic and had no history of inflammatory arthritis with significant morning stiffness, and her thyroid function was normal. A thorough examination of her wrists and hands revealed no significant muscle wasting in the hypothenar or thenar regions. Phalen's and reverse Phalen's tests were positive.

Ultrasound Findings A detailed ultrasound examination of the volar wrist was performed. The median nerve was bifid. The hyperechoic epineurium surrounding the nerve remained intact. The nerve exhibited a transversely elongated shape (Fig. 7.3a), with total cross-sectional areas measuring 2.154 cm^2 and large and small segment measurements of 1.19 cm^2 and 0.95 cm^2, respectively (Fig. 7.3b). On longitudinal scan, a hyperechoic septum was observed between the nerve segments; a persistent median artery also exhibited pulsation within the nerve (Fig. 7.3d). Within the carpal tunnel, the nerve showed signs of constriction beneath the hyperechoic flexor retinaculum. The median nerve lost the fascicular pattern.

Impression Carpal tunnel syndrome with a bifid median nerve.

Case Summary 4 A 53-year-old male reported persistent pain and restricted range of motion in his left shoulder. The patient had sustained blunt trauma to the shoulder 6 months earlier, had a medical history of diabetes and hypertension,

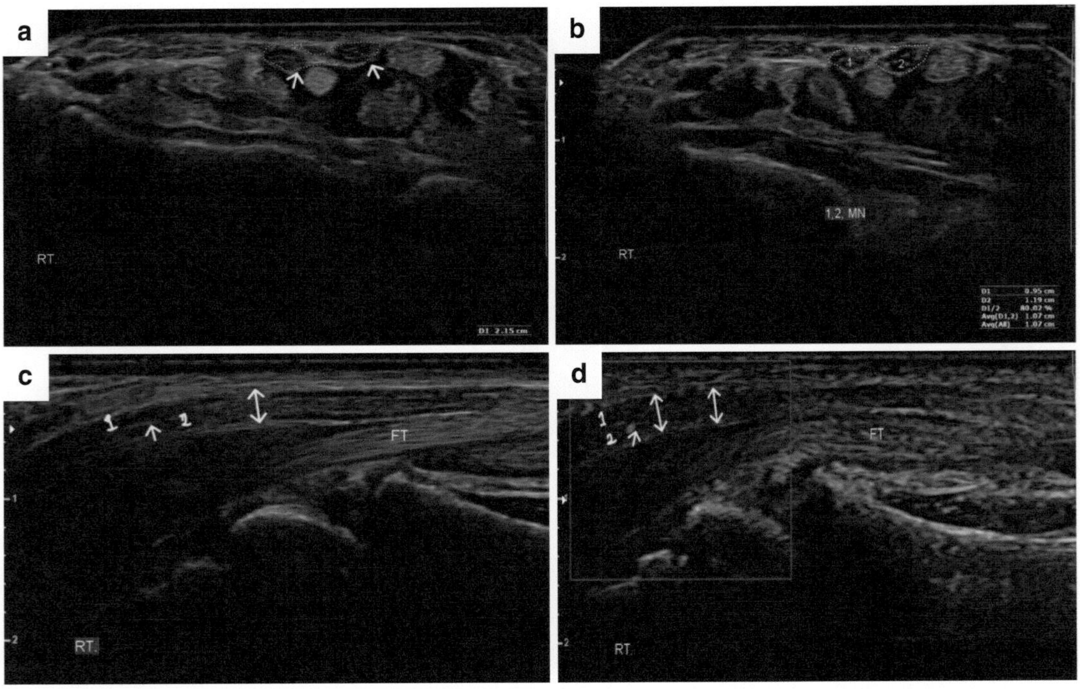

Fig. 7.3 Carpal tunnel syndrome with bifid median nerve. (**a**, **b**) Short axis scans of the volar wrist revealed increased cross-sectional area of the bifid median nerve (arrows)^2 and nerve segments (small and ^{2} large^2). (**c**, **d**) Longitudinal scans depicted a bifurcated median nerve segments (1, 2) (double arrows) (**c**) with a persistent median artery (**d**) (arrow). *FT* flexor tendon, *MN* median nerve, *RT* right

and was on medication for cardiogenic chest pain. He did not exhibit significant morning stiffness, headache, weight loss, or fever. During the physical examination, all movements of the shoulder were found to be restricted, with the most significant limitations observed in abduction and external rotation. Additionally, any attempt to scratch the back or shoulder intensified the pain. X-ray of the shoulder indicated increased radioopacity at the greater tuberosity and the tip of the acromion (Fig. 7.4a). A clinical diagnosis of frozen shoulder syndrome was made. On the basis of the patient's history of previous shoulder trauma, further examination via ultrasound was suggested.

Ultrasound Findings The long head of the biceps tendon (LHBT) exhibited a hypoechoic appearance, with loss of the fibrillar pattern; no peritendon compressible effusion was observed. The intra-articular LHBT was intact. A thick, hypoechoic synovial sheath (Fig. 7.4b–c) was noted anterior to the LHBT. The synovial capsule was also thick and hypoechoic. In the modified Crass shoulder position, the supraspinatus tendon (SST) appeared thick and hypoechoic, revealing a full-thickness incomplete tear (Fig. 7.4d–f). No aponeurotic expansion of the SST was visible over the LHBT. Fragments of the torn SST floated in anechoic compressible fluid. A mild anechoic compressible collection was identified in the subacromial-subdeltoid (SASD) bursa (Fig. 7.4g); however, the bursa did not extend over the thick, hypoechoic, and convex transverse humeral ligament (Fig. 7.4h). When the shoulder was abducted, the SASD bursa did not bunch under the acromion process. Furthermore, the subscapularis tendon (SuT) was noted to be thick and hypoechoic, with a loss of the fibrillar pattern. During the examination of the external rotation of the SuT, the subcoracoid bursa did not show any distension with anechoic, compressible fluid or thickening of the bursal wall. The coracoacromial ligament appeared hyperechoic and fibrillar (Fig. 7.4d). Articular cartilage thickness was reduced over the humeral head (Fig. 7.4g). The glenoid labrum appeared hypoechoic but was not torn on dynamic scanning. No posterior joint recess effusion was detected.

Impressions Long head biceps tendon tenosynovitis with incomplete full-thickness supraspinatus tendon tear.

Case Summary 5 A 10-year-old child complained of pain and a swollen left knee (Fig. A), with no concurrent neck or low back pain. His other joints appeared normal, and there were no silver scaly lesions on his skin. He denied any issues with bowel or bladder function and did not have a fever. The patient had a confirmed diagnosis of seronegative enthesitis arthritis (SEA) syndrome and was currently on a methotrexate regimen of 5 mg per week. Upon examination, the knee joint was swollen, with moderate effusion, and the thigh muscle was wasted. He tested negative for rheumatoid factor and antinuclear factor. Serum inflammatory biomarkers were elevated.

Ultrasound Findings The anterior joint recess displayed signs of swelling due to the presence of compressible anechoic fluid accumulation. The synovial membrane was hypoechoic and thickened (Fig. 7.5b), characterized by a branched or frond-like morphology along with increased Doppler activity (Fig. 7.5c–d). There was no osteophyte at the medial joint line. The medial meniscus was noted to have a triangular shape, remaining intact without any extrusion or anechoic cleft. Measurements of the articular cartilage thickness at the medial femoral condyle, intercondylar area, and lateral femoral condyle revealed that the cartilage was anechoic and maintained its thickness. Additionally, no anechoic compressible Baker's cyst was identified at the junction of the semimembranosus tendon (SMT) and the medial gastrocnemius muscle, and no hypo-anechoic compressible mass was observed surrounding the SMT tendon.

Impression Inflammatory knee synovitis.

Case Summary 6 A 60-year-old woman presented with complaints of pain and restricted

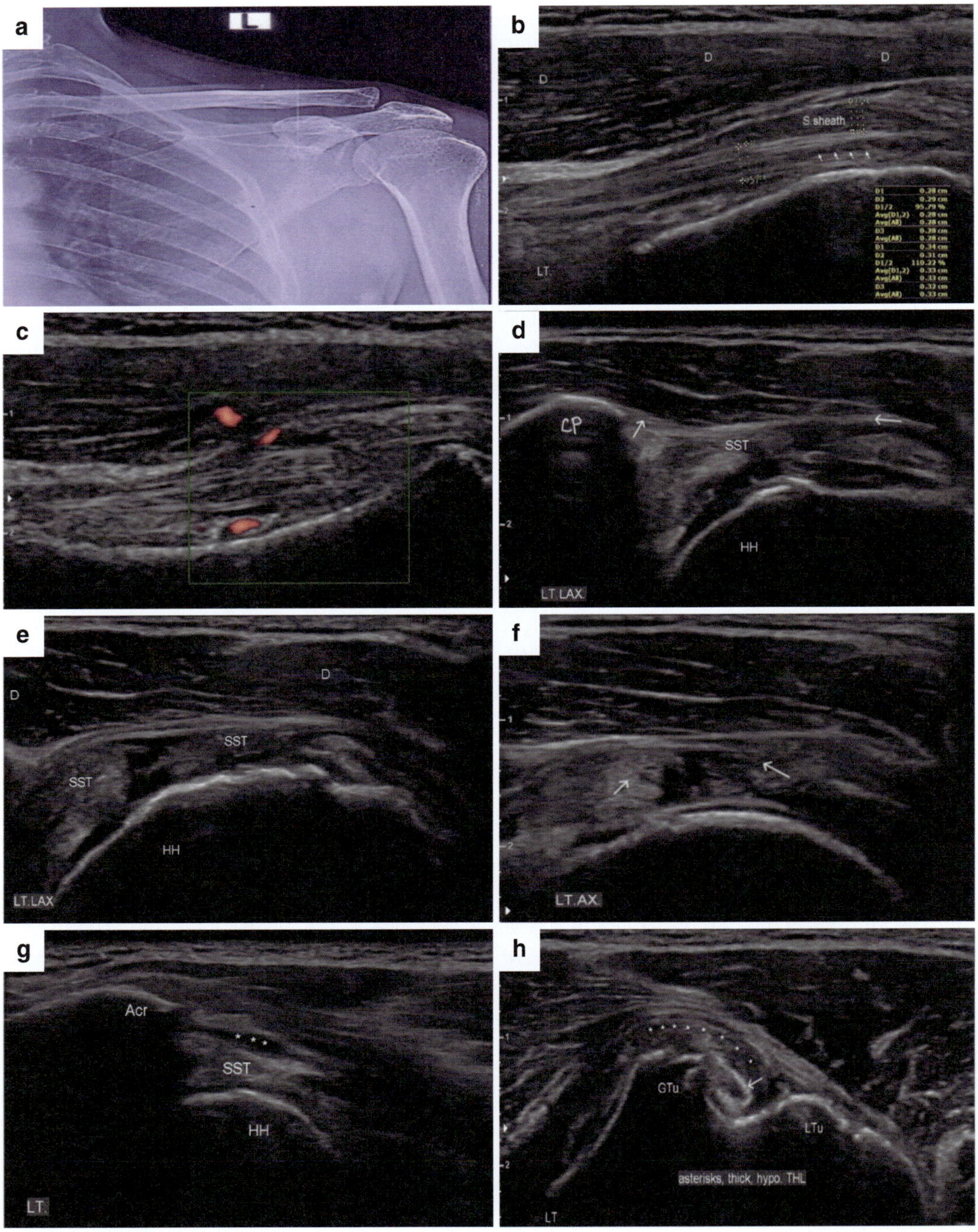

Fig. 7.4 Bicep's tenosynovitis and supraspinatus tendon tear. (**a**) X-ray shoulder revealing humeral head contour change. (**b, c**) Longitudinal scans of the anterior shoulder revealed synovial sheath thickening around the LHBT (**b**) with Doppler activity (red spots) (**c**), the LHBT lost fibrillar pattern (**c**). (**d–f**) Longitudinal (**d, e**) and short axes (**f**) scans explored SST tear. (**d**) Longitudinal scan unveiled SST tear under the CAL (white arrows). (**g**) Oblique, longitudinal scan of the lateral shoulder at the acromion process demonstrated mild, anechoic collection in the SASD bursa (asterisks). (**h**) Short axis scan of the anterior shoulder at the bicipital groove exposed thick, hypoechoic, and convex THL (asterisks) with cortical defect in GTu. *Acr* acromion, *CAL* calcaneoacromial ligament, *HH* humeral head, *GTu* greater tuberosity, *LTu* lesser tuberosity, *LHBT* long head biceps tendon, *SST* supraspinatus, *SASD* subacromial subdeltoid bursa, *THL* transverse humeral ligament

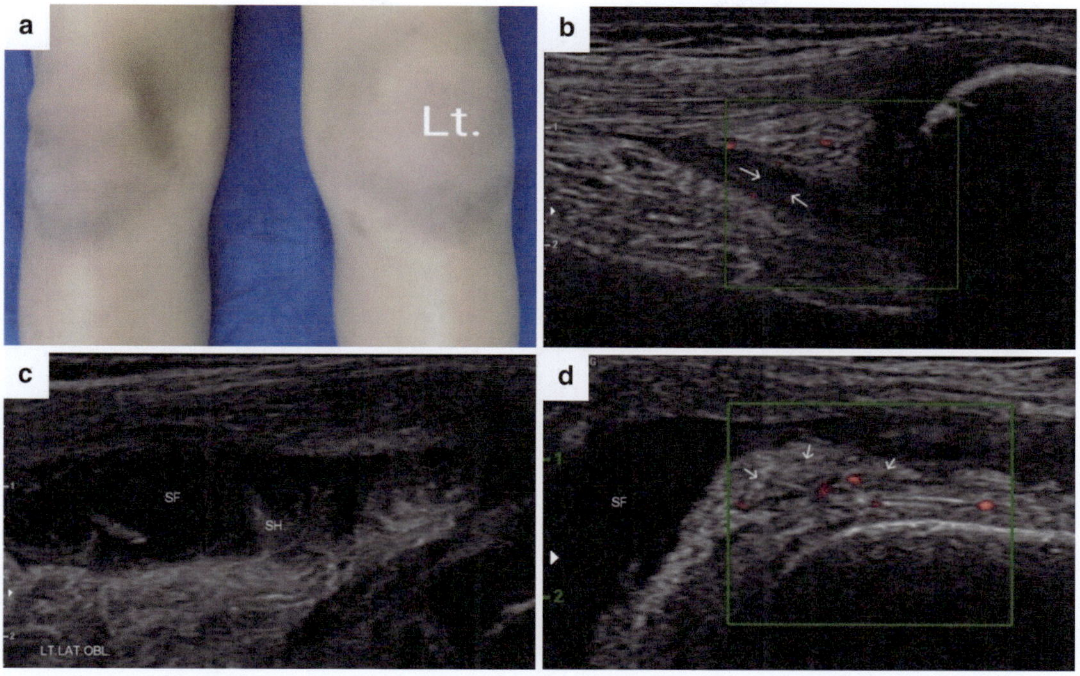

Fig. 7.5 Inflammatory knee synovitis. (**a**) Swollen left knee. (**b**) Longitudinal scan of the suprapatellar knee revealing a thick, hypoechoic synovium (white arrows) with an increased Doppler signal. (**c**) Oblique, longitudinal scan of the lateral knee depicted hypoechoic SH and anechoic synovial fluid (SF). (**d**) Short axis scan of the lateral knee demonstrated SH (arrows) with increased Doppler signal (red spots). *Lt* left, *SF* synovial fluid, *SH* synovial hypertrophy

range of motion in her right knee, which had hindered her daily physical activities for several months. She reported no significant morning stiffness. Clinical examination did not indicate the presence of joint effusion. Radiographic assessment revealed advanced osteoarthritis in the medial tibiofemoral compartment, characterized by diminished joint space, subchondral cyst formation, sclerosis, osteophyte development, and bony end deformity. Additionally, there was an increase in soft tissue opacity on the knee back, accompanied by a distinct area of well-defined opaque mass (Fig. 7.6a). Further scrutiny under ultrasound was performed.

Ultrasound Findings Examination of the anterior joint recess revealed no signs of anechoic or compressible accumulation. Additionally, there was an absence of a noncompressible, hyperechoic, pliable mass within this recess. The synovial membrane did not display any thickening, and it was neither branched nor villous in appearance. A moderate medial joint line osteophyte was noted. The medial meniscus appeared hyperechoic but was torn and extruded from its normal position (Fig. 7.6b). The thickness of the cartilage on the medial femoral condyle was diminished (positive chondral print sign), measuring an average of 0.8 mm (0.6–0.9 mm) (Fig. 7.6c), whereas the articular cartilage thickness remained intact in the intercondylar region. A posterior view of the knee revealed a compressible, anechoic, superficial septate Baker's cyst, which did not exhibit increased Doppler flow in its wall (Fig. 7.6d–f). Additionally, a noncompressible, hyperechoic mass with posterior acoustic shadowing was identified within the cyst. The semitendinosus tendon was fibrillar.

Impressions Articular cartilage degeneration, osteophyte formation, and loose body in Baker's cyst.

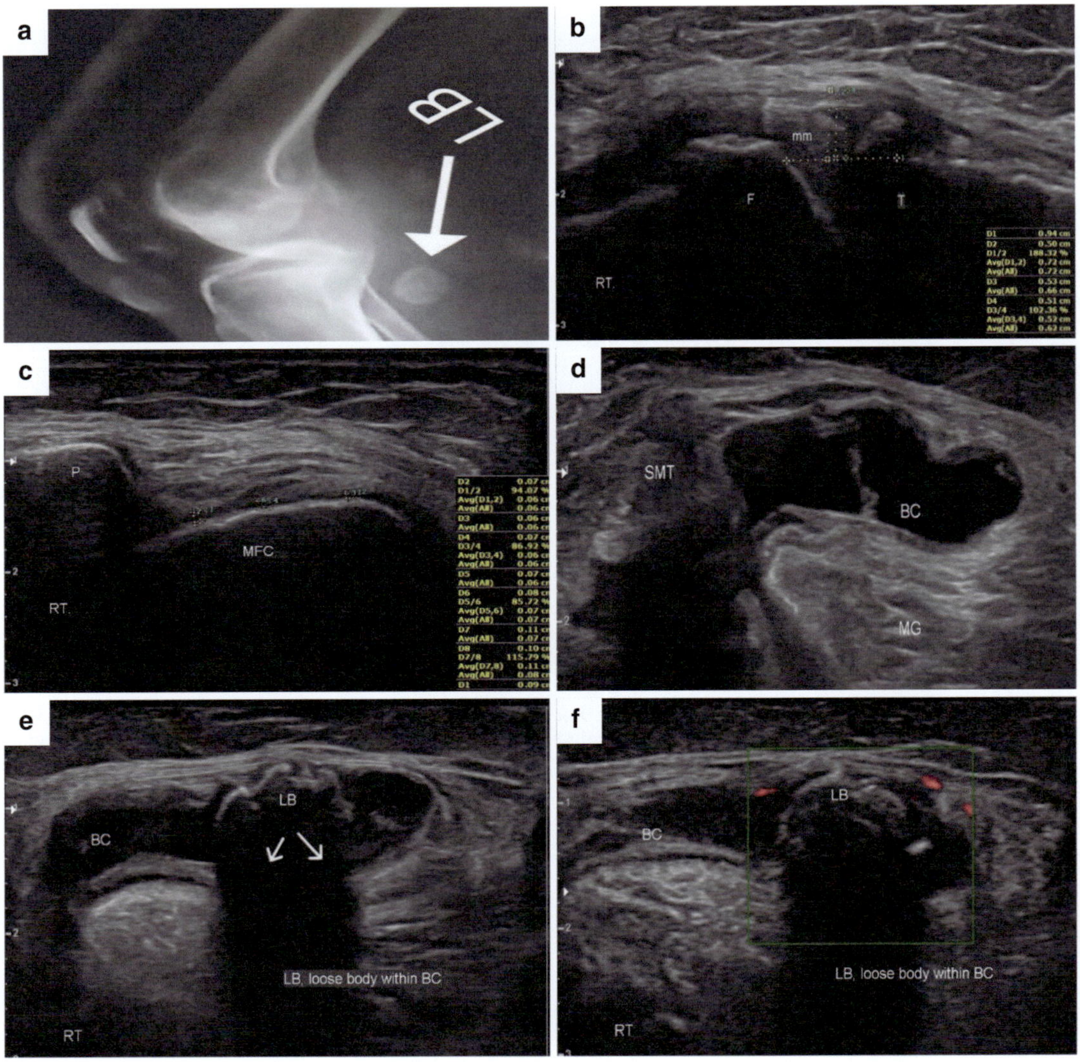

Fig. 7.6 Loose body in Baker's cyst in knee osteoarthritis. (**a**) X-ray image showing a radiopaque mass in the back of the knee. (**b**) Longitudinal scan of the medial knee revealing joint line osteophytes and MME. (**c**) Short axis scan of the MFC depicted reduced cartilage thickness. (**d–f**) Short axis scans of the posterior knee explored beak-shaped BC (**d**), BC with LB (**e**), and BC with LB and increased Doppler activity of cyst wall (**f**). *BC* Baker's cyst, *F* femur, *LB* loose body, *MG* medial gastrocnemius, *MM* medial meniscus, *MME* medial meniscal extrusion, *MFC* medial femoral condyle, *SMT* semimembranosus tendinitis, *T* tibia

Case Summary 7 A 65-year-old female patient reported bilateral shoulder pain and restricted mobility, with difficulty in extending her arm backward for several months. Notably, the discomfort and limitations were more pronounced on the left side, and scratching her back was painful. External rotation was significantly restricted. The patient had sustained trauma to her left shoulder a few months earlier but had no prior history of diabetes mellitus or hypertension. Hawkin's and Empty can tests were also negative. She did not report any significant morning stiffness, headache, weight loss, or low-grade fever. Shoulder abduction did not provoke pain. Radiographic examination of both shoulders indicated subchondral sclerosis and the presence of osteophytes in the humeral head. Further examination via ultrasound was performed.

Ultrasound Findings The long head of the biceps tendon (LHBT) exhibited a fibrillar echotexture, with no evidence of peritendinous compressible anechoic collection. A hypoechoic and thickened synovial sheath surrounding the LHBT bilaterally was noted (Fig. 7.7a–b). The intra-articular LHBT remained intact, whereas both the joint capsule and supraspinatus tendon (SST) displayed thickening and hypoechoic characteristics. The SST appeared hypoechoic and thick but not torn. The subacromial-subdeltoid (SASD) bursa was bilaterally thickened (Fig. 7.7c–d), yet it did not appear to bunch under the acromion during shoulder abduction. Neither the SASD nor the subcoracoid bursa showed signs of distension with anechoic and compressible fluid collection. A bony protrusion from the lesser tuberosity was identified, which was

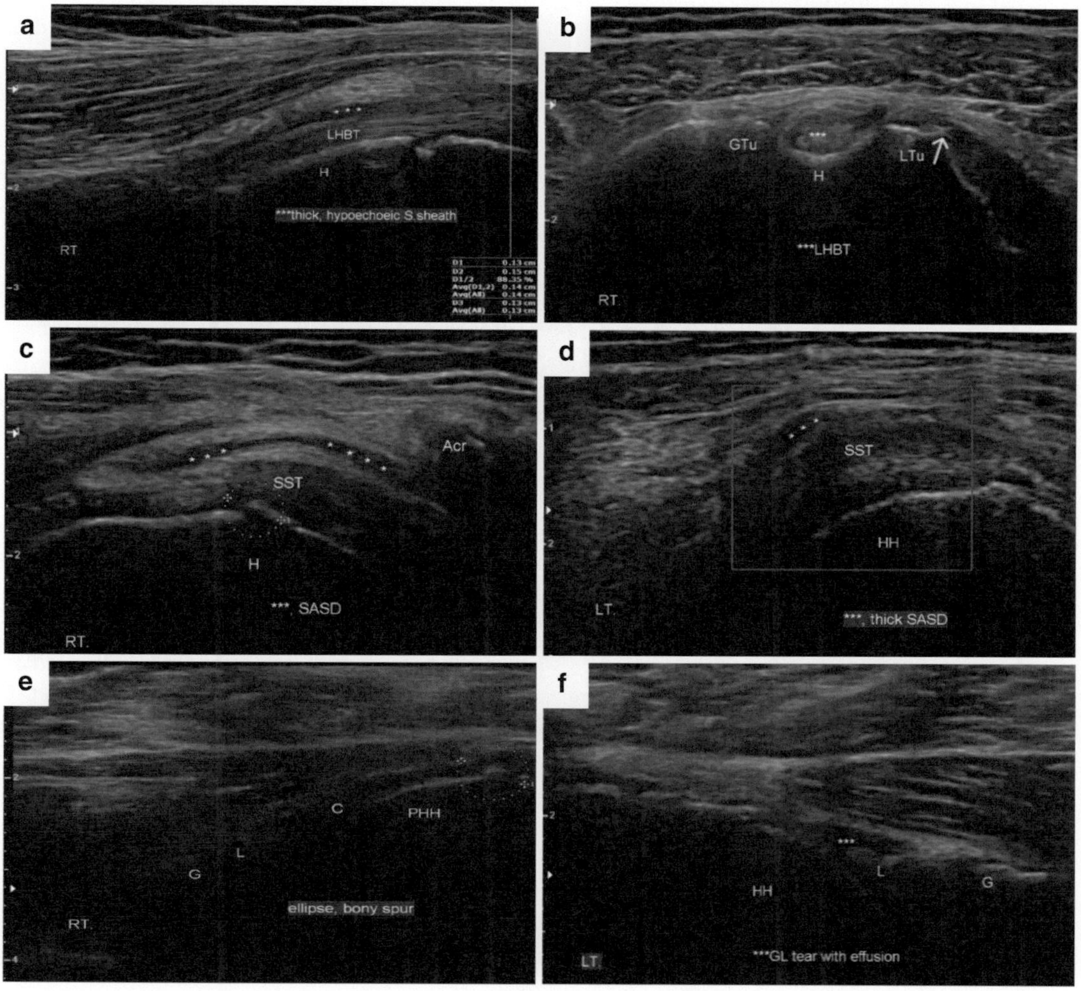

Fig. 7.7 Subacromial subdeltoid bursal thickening with glenoid labral tear. (**a**) Longitudinal scan of the anterior shoulder revealed thick and hypoechoic synovial sheath (asterisks) around the LHBT. (**b**) Short axis scan depicted the LHBT within the bicipital groove with cortical growth from the LTu (white arrow). (**c**, **d**) Oblique longitudinal scans of the lateral shoulder explored thick and hypoechoic SASD and cortical growth from the humeral head (**c**, ellipse). (**e**, **f**) Short axis scans of posterior shoulder at the GHJ exposed hypoechoic and torn GL that communicated between supraglenoid area and GHJ. *Acr* acromion, *ER* external rotation, *GTu* greater tuberosity, *GHJ* glenohumeral joint, HH humeral head, *GL/L* glenoid labrum, *LHBT* long head biceps tendon, *SST* supraspinatus, *SuT* subscapularis tendon, *SASD* subacromio subdeltoid bursa

observed to impinge upon the adjacent hypoechoic subscapularis tendon (SuT). The bilateral glenoid labrum was examined posteriorly (Fig. 7.7e–f), and a dynamic assessment revealed an anechoic gap within the posterior glenoid labrum on the left side (Fig. 7.7f), accompanied by a slightly compressible anechoic accumulation over the glenoid labrum connected to the joint cavity. Additionally, irregularities in the cortical surface of the humeral heads were noted (Fig. 7.7f), along with variations in articular cartilage thickness on either side.

Impressions Subacromial subdeltoid bursal thickening with glenoid labral tears.

Case Summary 8 A 36-year-old housewife reported experiencing pain and localized swelling in her left lateral ankle. She had sustained a lateral ankle sprain from a fall several months prior. The discomfort intensified with weight-bearing activities such as standing and walking but improved during periods of rest. Clinical assessment revealed tenderness localized to the area just below and in front of the lateral malleolus. Furthermore, the anterior drawer test was positive. Radiographic imaging of the ankle and foot did not reveal any signs of cortical disruption around the lateral malleolus. To gain additional information, an ultrasound was performed.

Ultrasound Findings The peroneal tendons, specifically the peroneus longus and peroneus brevis, presented a thickened and hypoechoic appearance; however, their structural integrity was preserved, with no signs of splitting or loss of tendon volume (Fig. 7.8a–b). There was an absence of increased Doppler activity in the vicinity of the tendons. The calcaneofibular ligament was intact beneath the tendons, whereas the anterior talofibular ligament (ATFL) was disrupted at its fibular attachment. Examination of the lateral malleolus (LM) revealed an anechoic gap between the hyperechoic fragment of the ATFL and the LM. The measured distance from the LM to the talus was 5.4 mm, which increased to 7.6 mm during dorsiflexion of the ankle joint (Fig. 7.8c–d). No fluid accumulation was detected in the talocrural joint recess. Further evaluation of the posterior heel area revealed a thickened and hypoechoic Achilles tendon that remained intact.

Impressions Peroneal tendinosis with anterior talofibular ligament tear.

Case Summary 9 A septuagenarian female reported right knee pain. There was no audible or palpable joint crepitus, and no sign of clinical joint effusion was detected. There was medial joint line tenderness, along with genu varus deformity. Her erythrocyte sedimentation rate was 84 mm/1 hr. X-ray of the knee revealed a reduction in the medial tibiofemoral joint space, marginal osteophytes, subchondral cysts, and sclerosis. An ultrasound of the knee was scheduled.

Ultrasound Findings Mild anechoic compressible collection in the anterior joint recess was revealed. The synovial membrane appeared thick and hypoechoic but was neither branched nor frond-like in appearance. In the suprapatellar area, prefemoral fat thickness was measured as 6.9 mm on the long axis. Antero-inferiorly, a poorly compressible anechoic mass with increased Doppler activity was revealed beneath the patellar tendon (Fig. 7.9a–c). Medially, there was a moderate joint line osteophyte. The medial meniscus was hypoechoic, torn, and extruded (4.8 mm from the medial joint line) (Fig. 7.9d). On the flexed knee, the mean medial femoral condylar cartilage thickness revealed 1.8 mm. Two compartmental anechoic compressible cystic collections with increased Doppler activity were observed around the SMT tendon (5.9e–f). No Baker's cyst was detected.

Impressions Deep infrapatellar cyst and semimembranosus tendon bursitis.

Case Summary 10 A 60-year-old farmer reported experiencing persistent pain in his left knee over the past 2 months. Additionally, the patient noted the presence of a painless, soft, cystic mass in the back of the knee without signifi-

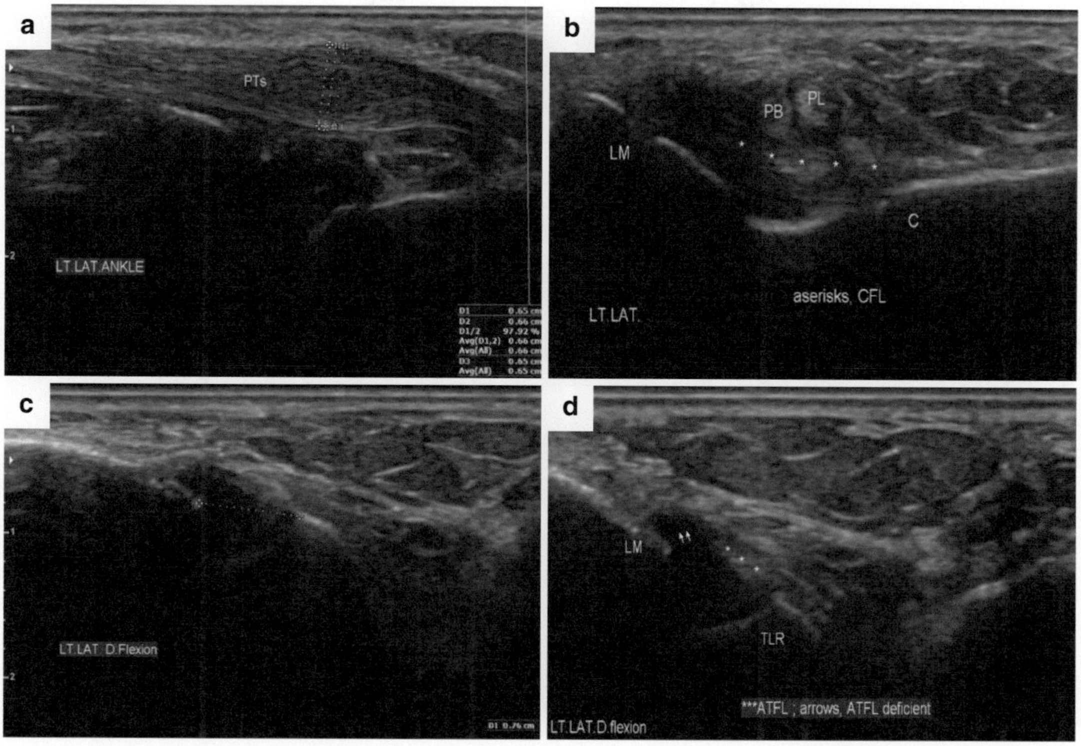

Fig. 7.8 Peroneal tendinosis with anterior talofibular ligament tear. (**a**) Lateral oblique longitudinal scan of the infra-malleolar foot revealed thick and hypoechoic PTs (PL, PB). (**b**) Short axis scan of lateral infra-malleolar area depicted intact, hypoechoic-hyperechoic CFL underneath the PL & PB (asterisks). (**c**, **d**) Anterior to the lateral malleolus, oblique longitudinal scan of the lateral foot measured talo-fibular distances (asterisks) 5.4 mm (**c**). and 7.6 mm (**d**) during neutral and ankle dorsiflexion, respectively. (**d**) ATFL appeared, thick, hypoechoic (asterisks), afibrillar, and lost integrity (arrows), more apparent on ankle dorsiflexion. *ATFL* anterior talofibular ligament, *CFL* calcaneofibular ligament, *C* calcaneus, *LM* lateral malleolus, *PB* peroneus brevis, *PL* peroneus longus, *PTs* peroneal tendons, *TLR* talus bone

cant limitations in the range of motion of the joint. Tenderness was demonstrated along the medial joint line, and there was a positive sign of clinical effusion. The valgus stress test for medial collateral ligament integrity was negative. He denied any recent falls or joint trauma and did not mention any other joint-related issues. An X-ray revealed no signs of joint space narrowing, marginal osteophytes, subchondral cysts, or sclerosis.

Ultrasound Findings The anterior joint recess exhibited distension characterized by anechoic and compressible fluid accumulation (Fig. 7.10a–b). A flexible, hyperechoic, and poorly compressible mass was observed traversing the anterior joint recess, displaying heightened Doppler activity. The synovial membrane was thick and hypoechoic and neither branched nor looked frond-like. The thickness of the prefemoral fat was measured as 1.03 cm in the short axis and 1.00 cm in the long axis (Fig. 7.10a–b). The medial meniscus (MM) was extruded by 4.0 mm, accompanied by a torn anechoic cleft extending from the medial region to the posterior region of the MM; however, no osteophytes were detected along the medial joint line. The medial femoral condylar (MFC) cartilage smoothness and thickness were maintained (Fig. 7.10b–d). The femoral condylar cartilage thicknesses were 1.8 mm, 2.3 mm, and 2.4 mm for the MFC, the intercondylar region, and the lateral femoral condylar areas, respectively. The medial collateral ligament appeared hypoechoic, and the thickness

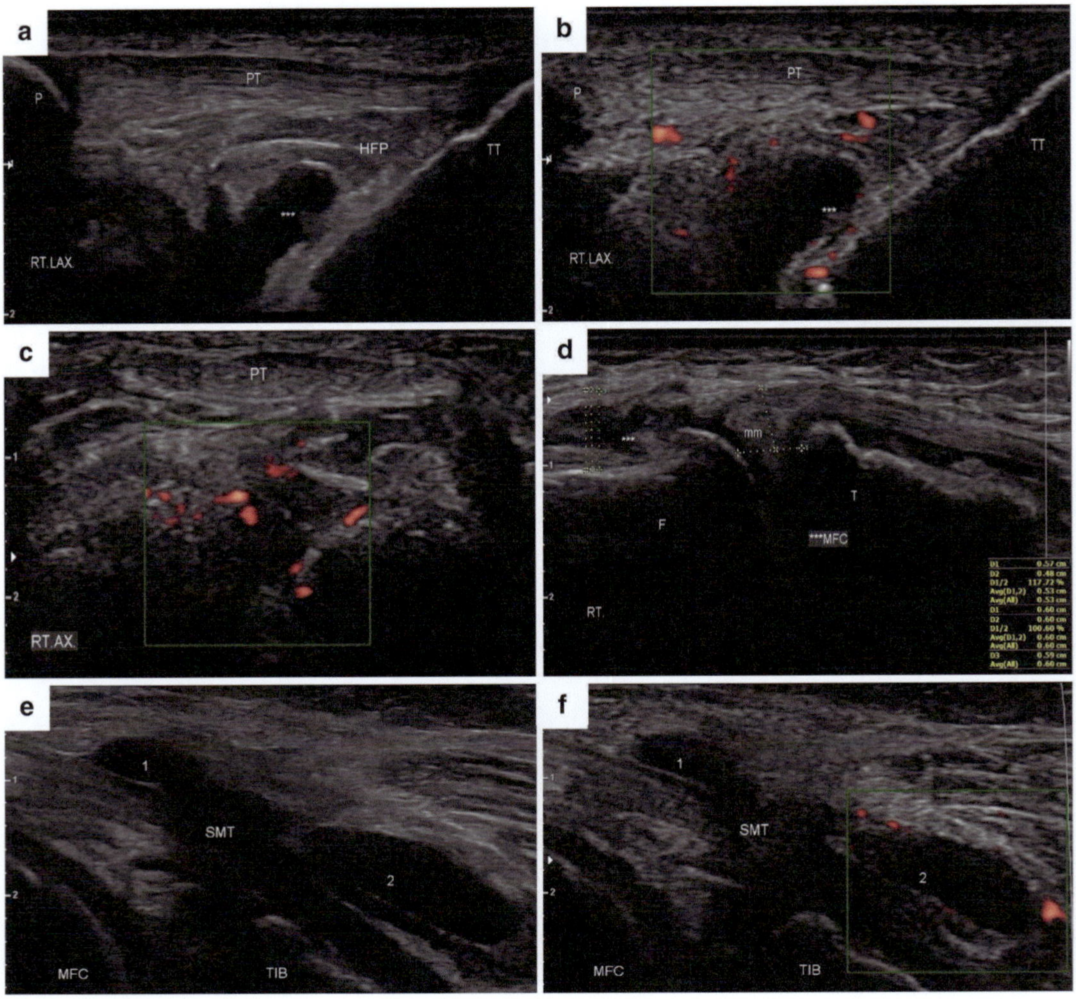

Fig. 7.9 Deep infrapatellar cyst and semimembranosus tendon bursitis. (**a, b**) Longitudinal scans of the infrapatellar knee revealed poorly compressible, anechoic mass (asterisks) behind the fibrillar PT and within the Hoffa's fat pad (**a**, HFP), (without (**a**) and with (**b**) increased Doppler signal. (**c**) Short axis scan of the infrapatellar knee depicted poorly compressible, anechoic cyst within the Hoffa's fat pad with increased Doppler activity. (**d**) Longitudinal scan of the medial knee explored joint line osteophyte and medial meniscal extrusion. (**e**, **f**) Posterior, longitudinal scan of medial knee demonstrated compressible, anechoic collection around the hypoechoic SMT. *F* femur, *HFP* Hoffa's fat pad, *MFC* medial femoral condyle, *mm* medial meniscus, *PT* patellar tendon, *SMT* semimembranosus tendon, *T* tibia, *TIB* tibia

was 6.9 mm. Additionally, a poorly compressible cystic mass was noted within Hoffa's fat pad (Fig. 7.10e), with no Doppler signal. Posteriorly, a superficial Baker's cyst was identified, characterized by anechoic and compressible accumulation, with septation and hyperechoic debris within (Fig. 7.10f–h). No hypoechoic-anechoic compressible collection was detected surrounding the semimembranosus tendon.

Impressions Medial meniscal tear, deep infrapatellar cyst, and Baker's cyst.

Case Summary 11 A 52-year-old male presented with persistent pain and swelling on the outer side of his right elbow, which had lasted for one year (Fig. 7.11a). The onset of his symptoms coincided with an incident where he lifted an 8-kilogram weight while working as an electri-

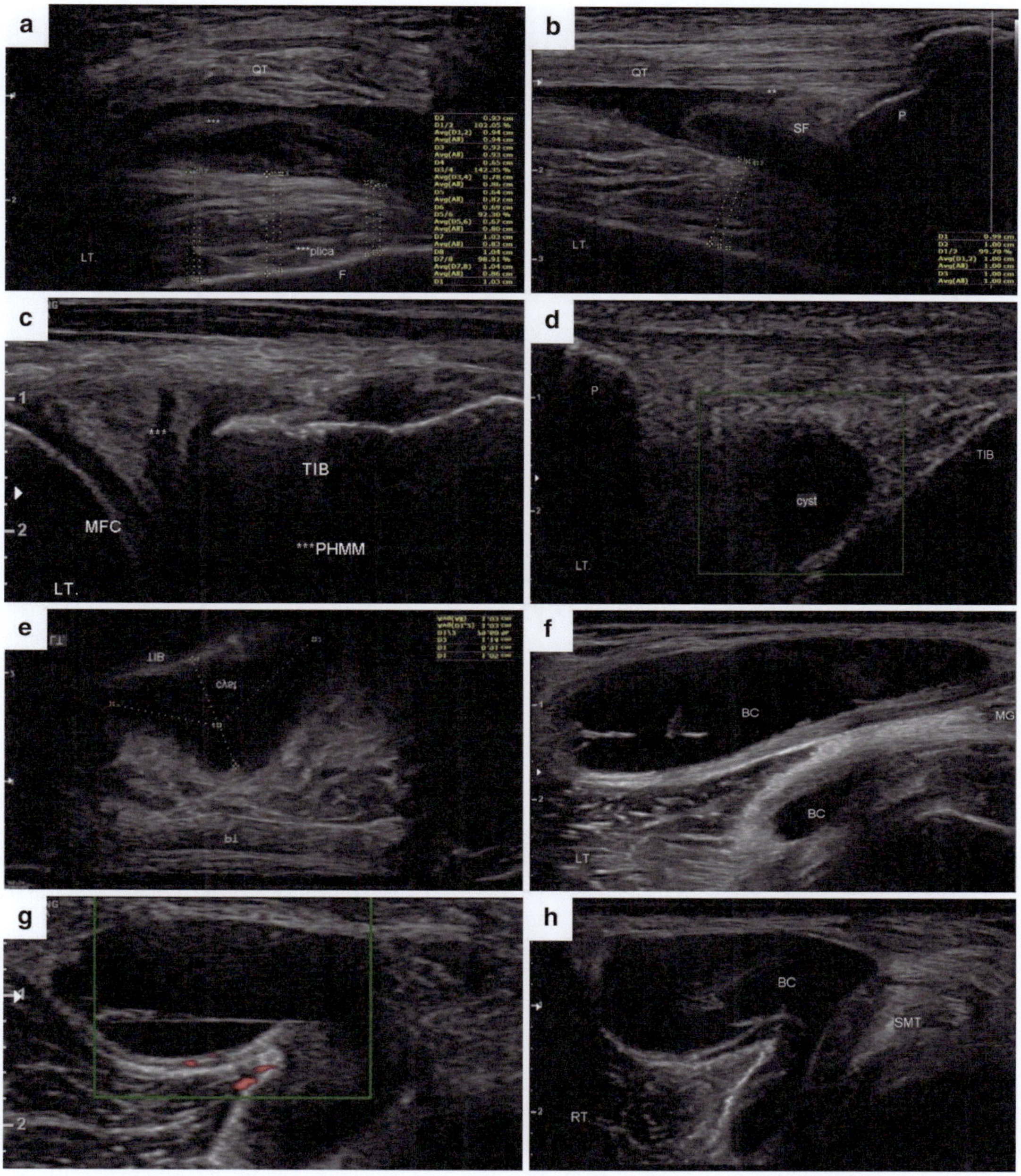

Fig. 7.10 Medial meniscal tear, deep infrapatellar cyst, and Baker's cyst. (**a**, **b**) Short and longitudinal axes scans of the suprapatellar knee revealed synovial plica (asterisks) with effusion (SF). (**c**) Posterior longitudinal scan of the medial knee depicted anechoic cleft extending from deep to peripheral part of posterior horn of MM. (**d**, **e**) Longitudinal and short axes scans localized poorly compressible, anechoic cyst within the Hoffa's fat pad, respectively. (**f–h**) Longitudinal and short axes scans of the posterior knee explored Beak-shaped Baker's cyst (**g, h**) with compressible, anechoic collection (**f-h**), and increased cyst wall Doppler activity (**g**). *F* femur, *MM* medial meniscus, *MFC* medial femoral condyle, *PT* patellar tendon, *SF* synovial fluid, *SMT* semimembranosus tendon, *TIB* tibia

cian overseas. Although he did not report any limitations in the elbow's range of motion, he experienced discomfort during movement of the joint. An X-ray of the lateral elbow revealed no signs of fractures in the distal humerus or the proximal radius and ulna. Upon physical exami-

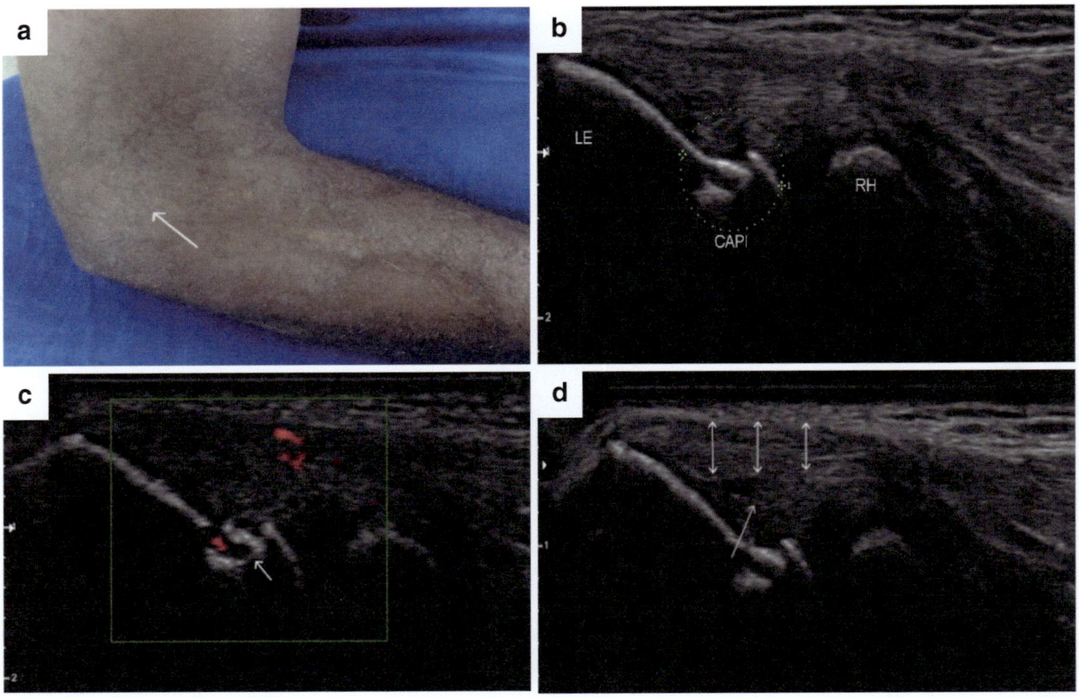

Fig. 7.11 Elbow radial collateral ligament tear with distal humeral fracture. (**a**) Focal swelling of the lateral elbow (white arrow). (**b, c**) Longitudinal scans of the lateral elbow revealed cortical discontinuity in the capitellum (**a**, ellipse, **b**, arrow) with increased Doppler activity (**c**, red spots) (**d**) Longitudinal scan of the lateral elbow depicted CET with loss of fibrillar pattern (double arrows) and hypoechoic, thick LCL (single arrow). *CAPI* capitellum, *CET* common extensor tendon, *LCL* lateral collateral ligament, *LE* lateral epicondyle, *RH* radial head

nation, there was noticeable swelling at the lateral epicondyle, and Maudsley's maneuver yielded a positive result. An ultrasound of the lateral elbow was recommended.

Ultrasound Findings The superficial fibrillar common extensor tendon, which typically appears hyperechoic, was noted to be hyperechoic-hypoechoic. Additionally, the radial collateral ligament (RCL) was thickened and hypoechoic, accompanied by increased Doppler activity (Fig. 7.11b–d). A cortical defect was identified on the distal humerus at the capitellum, which also exhibited increased Doppler activity (Fig. 7.11b–d).

Impression Radial collateral ligament tear with distal humeral fracture.

Case Summary 12 A 21-year-old electrician had been experiencing right shoulder pain and significant movement limitations for the last six weeks. This condition followed a proximal humerus fracture and a limp on the right arm resulting from exposure to high-voltage electricity a few weeks prior. The patient did not indicate any notable morning stiffness, headache, weight loss, or fever. While he could initiate shoulder abduction, all passive movements were restricted, and attempting to scratch his back aggravated pain. Furthermore, an examination of the right upper extremity's nervous system revealed normal elbow flexion and extension; an intact bicep, tricep, and supinator reflexes; and a floppy tricep muscle exhibiting decreased muscle tone.

An X-ray of the shoulder confirmed a fractured humeral head and separation of the humeral neck from the humeral head (Fig. 7.12a). An ultrasound of the shoulder was performed.

Ultrasound Findings The long head of the biceps tendon (LHBT) appeared fibrillar, with no evidence of peritendon effusion; an increase in

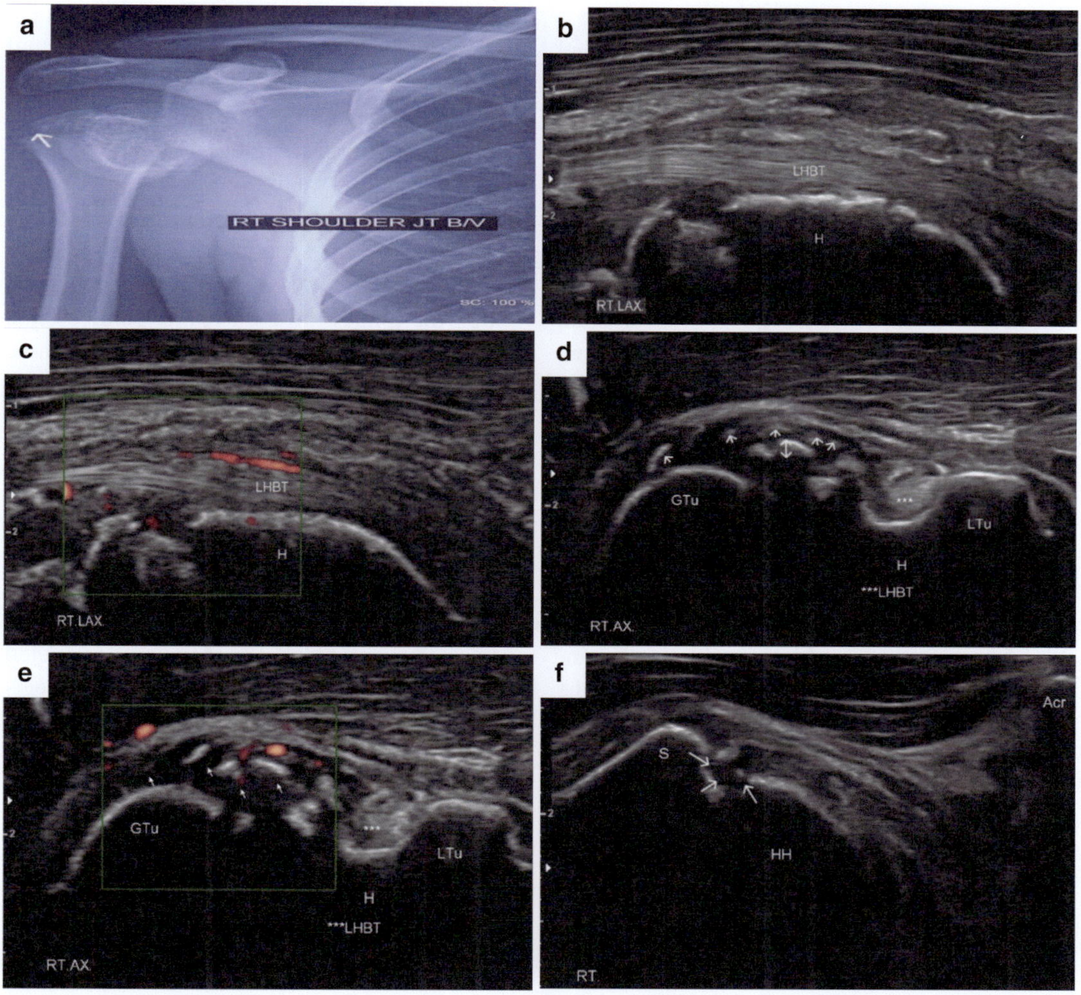

Fig. 7.12 Humeral head fracture with supraspinatus tendon tear. (**a**) X-ray revealing humeral head fracture (white arrow, cortical discontinuity). (**b**, **c**) Longitudinal scans of the anterior shoulder revealed fibrillar long head of the biceps tendon with increased Doppler activity (**c**) and cortical irregularity (**b**, **c**). (**d**, **e**) Short axis scans of the anterior shoulder at the bicipital groove depicted cortical discontinuity in the GTu with hyperechoic bone fragments (with posterior acoustic shadowing) within the SST. (**f**) Oblique longitudinal scan of the lateral shoulder revealed cortical defect in the HH and hypoechoic, torn SST. *GTu* greater tuberosity, *H* humerus, *HH* humeral head, *LTu* lesser tuberosity, *LHBT* long head of biceps tendon

Doppler activity was observed in the LHBT. The IA-LHBT was intact. A thick hypoechoic synovial sheath was clearly visible surrounding the LHBT (Fig. 7.12b–c). The transverse humeral ligament (THL) was noted to be thick, hypoechoic, and convex (Fig. 7.12d). Moreover, the supraspinatus tendon (SST) was noted to be hypoechoic and thick, with a loss of the fibrillar pattern and increased Doppler activity. Cortical integrity was distorted across the greater tuberosity (Fig. 7.12d–f). Hyperechoic noncompressible masses with posterior acoustic shadowing were observed within the SST with increased DA (Fig. 7.12d–e). Neither the subacromial subdeltoid nor the subcoacoid bursa exhibited bursal wall thickening or distension with compressible accumulation.

Impression The scan findings align with fractures of the humeral head, cortical defects in the greater tuberosity, supraspinatus tendon tears, and long head of bicep tendinosis.

Case Summary 13 A 66-year-old man with a medical history of ischemic heart disease and hypertension experienced an abrupt onset of intense pain in his right great toe. His current history of medication included olmesartan and low-dose aspirin. He had previously experienced a similar episode a few months prior, although he could not recall the exact date, which improved with pain relief medications. During these episodes, the patient reported being free of pain. There were no indications of renal dysfunction, recent foot injuries, intra-articular steroid treatments, or any surgical procedures in the affected area. An X-ray of the great toe indicated soft tissue swelling, and no cortical erosion was observed. Upon physical examination, the toe exhibited erythema, a shiny appearance, edema, and warmth, with severe tenderness preventing the physician from examining the joint further. While the serum uric acid and erythrocyte sedimentation rates were within normal limits, the C-reactive protein levels were elevated. Unfortunately, examination of the synovial fluid via polarized microscopy could not be conducted. Additional evaluation through ultrasound provided further insights.

Ultrasound Findings Synovial membrane was hypoechoic and thickened (Fig. 7.13a), and there was increased Doppler activity (Fig. 7.13b). Within the joint, a mild anechoic, compressible collection was noted. An irregular, hyperechoic deposit was noted on the metatarsal head cartilage, whereas hyperechoic tophi were observed within the thick synovium (Fig. 7.13c–d). No cortical defects were detected.

Impression Gouty arthritis.

Case Summary 14 A 55-year-old male presented with complaints of pain and restricted movement in his right shoulder, which had per-

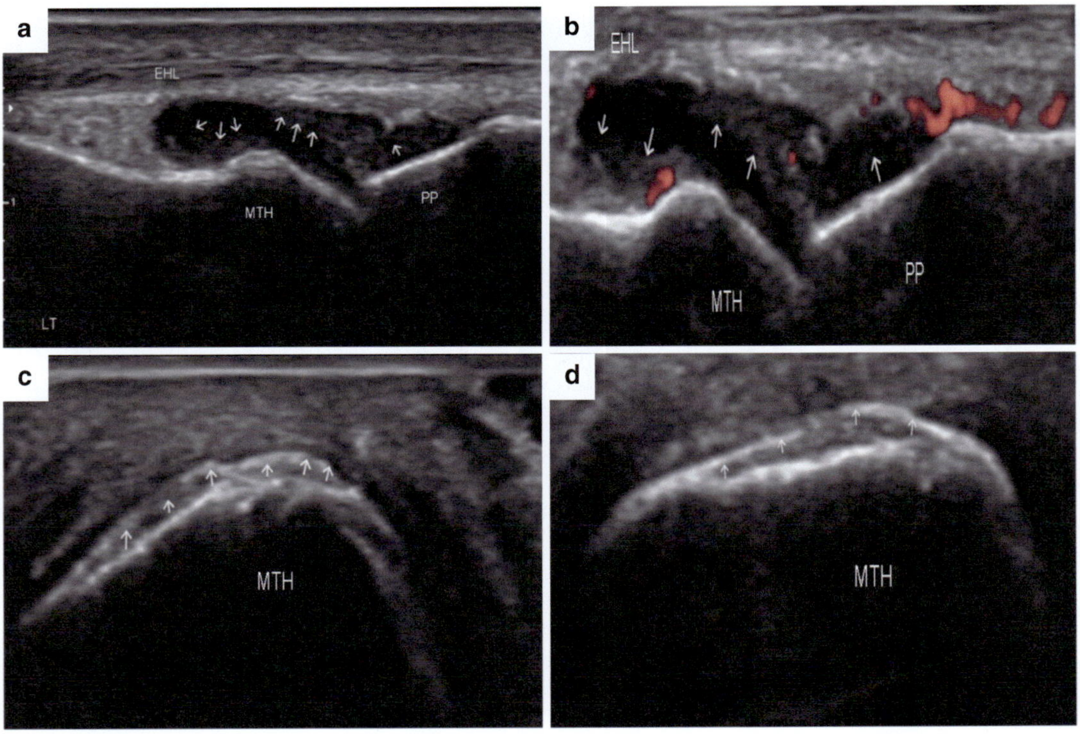

Fig. 7.13 Gouty arthritis. (**a, b**) Longitudinal scans of the anterior aspect of the first metatarsophalangeal joint revealed thick and hypoechoic synovial membrane (white arrows) with increased Doppler signals (red spots) (**b**). (**c, d**) Short axis scans of the first MTH depicted hyperechoic, rough double contour sign over the anechoic cartilage (white arrows). *EHL* extensor hallucis longus, *MTH* metatarsal head, *PP* proximal phalanx

sisted for three months. Upon clinical assessment, he exhibited discomfort during shoulder movements, with a positive result for the painful arc sign. Additionally, both Hawkin's test and Apley's scratch test yielded positive results. External rotation was painful when the shoulder was in the abducted position. Importantly, there were no signs of significant morning stiffness, headache, weight loss, or fever. The patient denied any recent falls and reported no history of diabetes mellitus, hypertension, or ischemic heart disease.

Ultrasound Findings The long head of the biceps tendon (LHBT) exhibited a fibrillar appearance, with signs of peritendon effusion and increased Doppler activity (Fig. 7.14a–d). The intra-articular LHBT was intact. A

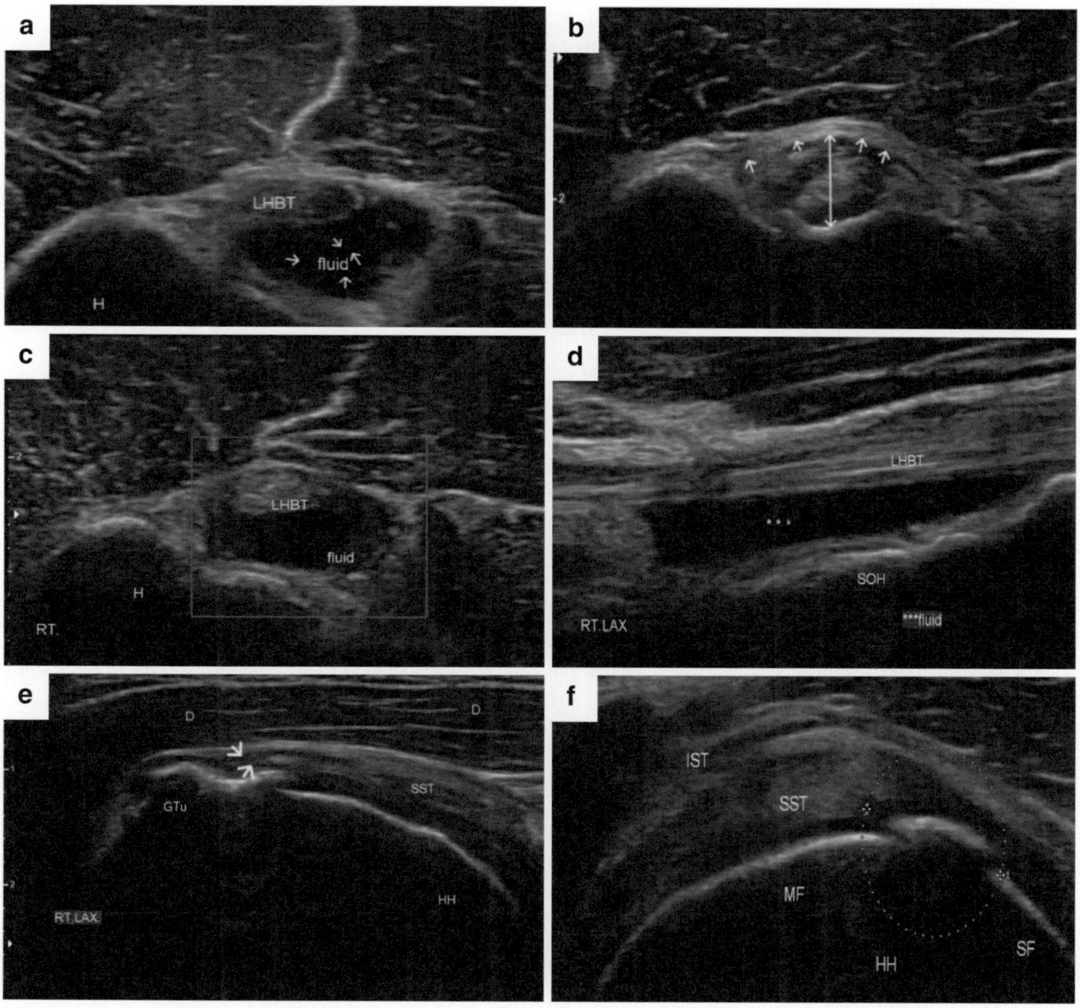

Fig. 7.14 Supraspinatus tendon tear with long head biceps tenosynovitis. (**a**–**c**) Short axis scans of the anterior shoulder at the bicipital groove revealed anechoic, compressible collection (**a**, **c**) around the LHBT with increased Doppler activity (**c**) and convex THL (**b**) (double arrow). (**d**) Longitudinal scans of the anterior shoulder at the bicipital groove depicted anechoic-hypoechoic compressible collection (asterisks) behind the fibrillar LHBT. (**e**) Longitudinal scan revealed full-thickness SST tear at GTu. (**f**) Longitudinal scan of the SST explored anechoic defect in the echogenic HH cortex with hypoechoic SST. *GTu* greater tuberosity, *IST* infraspinatus tendon, *LHBT* long head of biceps tendon, *MF* medial facet, *SST* supraspinatus tendon, *SF* superior facet, *SOH* shaft of humerus, *THL* transverse humeral ligament

hypoechoic, thick synovial sheath surrounding the LHBT was noted. The transverse humeral ligament appeared hyperechoic and displayed a convex shape. At the footprint of the greater tuberosity, a full-thickness tear of the supraspinatus tendon (SST) was present, characterized by a loss of cortical irregularity (Fig. 7.14e), with the SST appearing hypoechoic and torn in its midsection as well (Fig. 7.14f). Dynamic examination revealed that abduction and external rotation were limited. Both the subacromial and subdeltoid bursa, as well as the subcoracoid bursa, showed no signs of bursal wall thickening or distension with compressible collection. The posterosuperior glenoid labrum was intact, exhibited a triangular hyperechoic texture, and showed no evidence of tearing or extrusion during dynamic assessment. There was no indication of glenohumeral joint effusion.

Impression Supraspinatus tendon tear with long head bicep tenosynovitis.

Case Summary 15 A 30-year-old woman presented with pain and swelling in her right middle toe (Fig. 7.15a), with reduced mobility over the last 18 months. She noted that the discomfort began following a blunt injury to the toe, which was sustained from a fall off her bed. Upon physical examination, significant swelling and limited range of motion, particularly at the proximal interphalangeal joint, were limited. X-ray imaging revealed narrowing of the joint space and the presence of osteophytes (Fig. 7.15b). The ultrasound findings are detailed below.

Ultrasound Findings Reduced proximal interphalangeal joint space with a hypoechoic and thick synovial capsule was revealed (Fig. 7.15c). Increased Doppler activity (Fig. 7.15c) was revealed over the thick and extensor digitorum tendon (Fig. 7.15d). The joint line osteophyte was prominent.

Impression Extensor digitorum tenosynovitis.

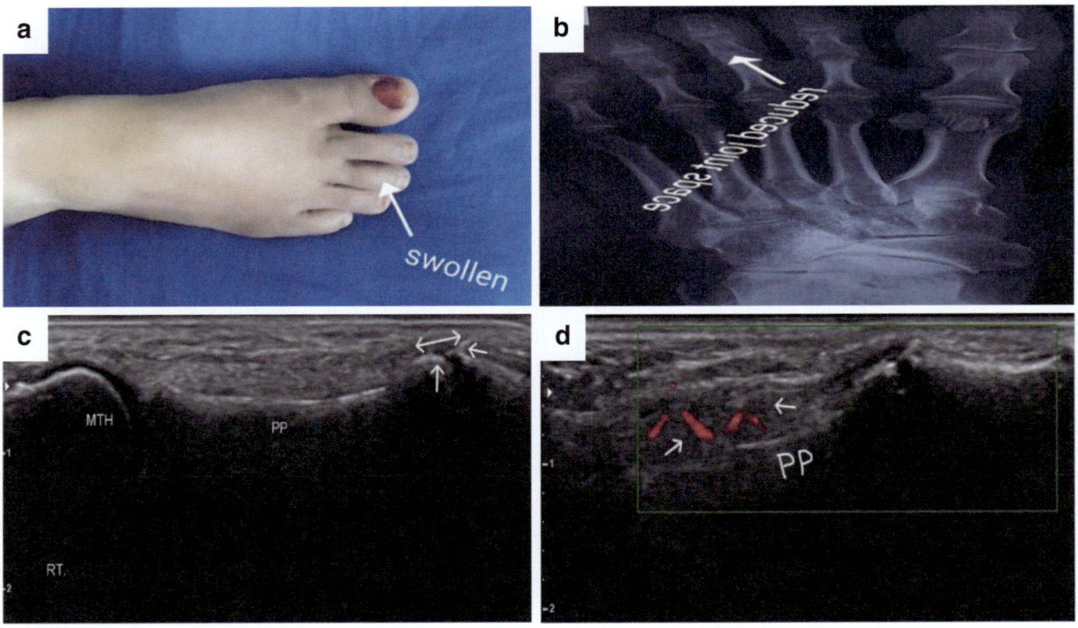

Fig. 7.15 Extensor digitorum tenosynovitis of toe. (**a**) Swollen middle toe. (**b**) Radiology revealed reduced joint space width, cortical erosion, and osteophyte. (**c**) Longitudinal scan of the digit revealed osteophytes in proximal interphalangeal joint (single arrows) and synovial thickening (double arrows). (**d**) Long axis scan explored hypoechoic and thick extensor digitorum tendon (arrows) with increased Doppler signal (red dots). *MTH* metatarsal head, *PP* proximal phalanx, *RT* right

Case Summary 16 The patient suffered from persistent pain and deformity in the left knee joint, which significantly impaired physical function for a prolonged duration. X-ray examinations revealed narrowed medial tibio-femoral joint spaces accompanied by subchondral cysts, sclerosis, and osteophytes (Fig. 7.16a).

Ultrasound Findings Mild anechoic compressible collection was noted in the anterior joint recess. The prefemoral fat thickness was 5.5 mm along the long axis and 7.7 mm along the short axis. There were no visible noncompressible, hyperechoic, pliable masses traversing the joint recess. The synovial membrane appeared normal, showing no signs of thickening, branching, or frond-like appearance. Severe osteophytes were noted along the medial joint line, and the medial meniscus was torn and 1.05 cm medially extruded (Fig. 7.16b). The cartilage thickness of the medial femoral condyle decreased, with a mean thickness of 1.0 mm *(a positive chondral print sign);*

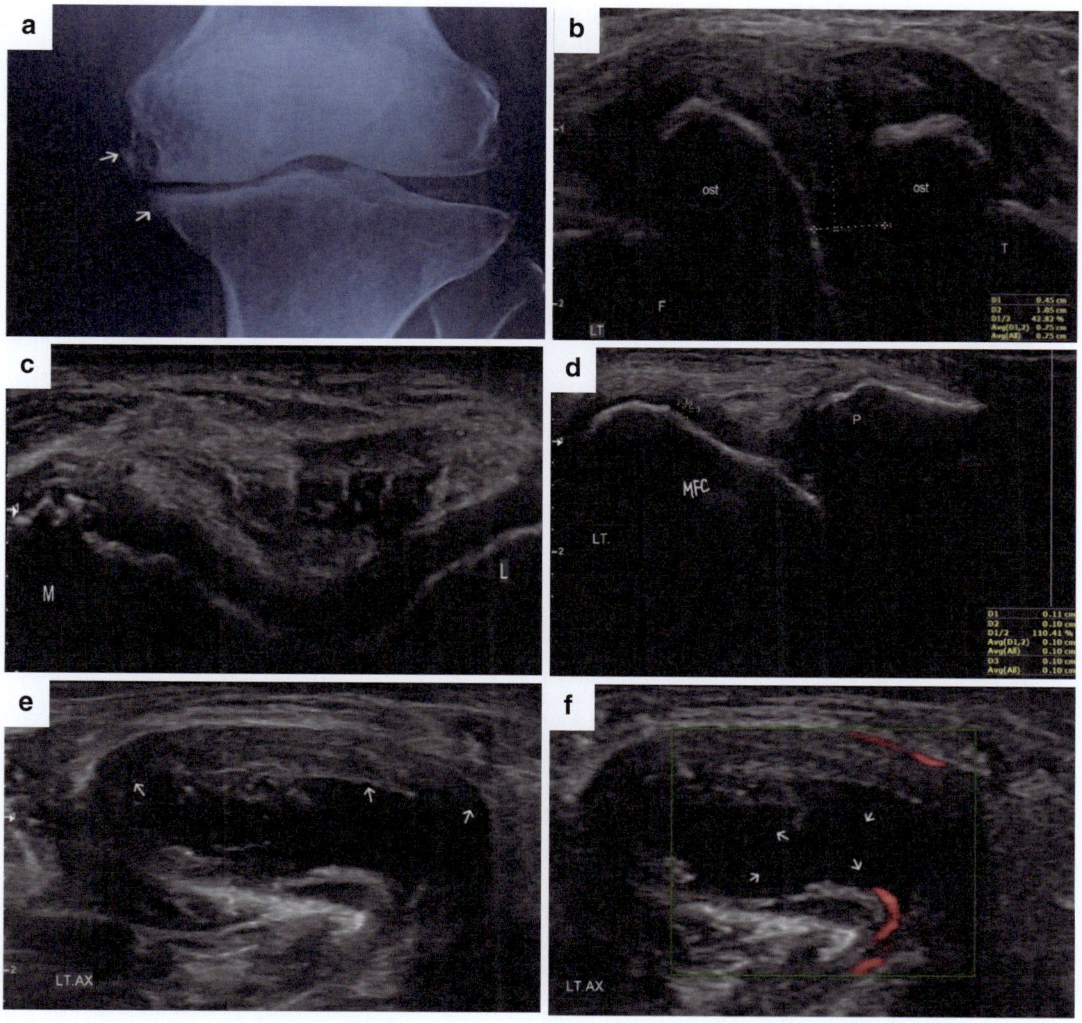

Fig. 7.16 Baker's cyst in knee osteoarthritis. (**a**) X-ray knee revealed medial joint line osteophyte. (**b**) Longitudinal scan of the medial knee depicted tibio-femoral joint line osteophytes and MME. (**c**, **d**) Transverse scan of the suprapatellar knee (**c**) and short axis scan of the MFC (**d**) demonstrated reduced cartilage sharpness and thickness. (**e**, **f**) Short axis scans of posterior knee demonstrated a beak-shaped Baker's cyst with anechoic, compressible collection, increased cyst wall thickness (white arrows) and Doppler signals (red spots). *L* lateral, *LT* left, *MFC* medial femoral condyle, *F* femur, *Ost* osteophyte, *P* patella, *M* medial, *MME* medial meniscal extrusion

however, the cartilage thickness remained intact in the intercondylar and lateral femoral condylar regions (Fig. 7.16c–d). Additionally, a large anechoic and compressible Baker's cyst was documented posteriorly, with no increased Doppler activity detected in its wall. No hypoechoic-anechoic compressible collection surrounding the semimembranosus tendon was noted (Fig. 7.16e–f).

Impression Baker's cyst in knee osteoarthritis.

Case Summary 17 A 52-year-old homemaker reported experiencing pain localized in the medial aspect of her left knee joint. This discomfort intensified during routine activities that required knee flexion, such as kneeling for prayers, using the toilet, and ascending stairs. She did not report any notable morning stiffness. Her medical history was unremarkable for any joint injuries, recent falls, or surgical interventions. There was no other joint pain, and her thyroid function was normal. Upon physical examination, there were no signs of joint effusion, and anterior–posterior drawer tests were negative. However, tenderness was noted along the medial joint line. X-ray examination of the knee revealed a medial femoral osteophyte, significant narrowing of the medial tibio-femoral joint space, and subchondral sclerosis, along with increased radioopacity on the medial side of the knee (Fig. 7.17a).

Ultrasound Findings The anterior joint recess was not distended with anechoic compressible collection, and there was no synovial thickening or branching. A noncompressible, hyperechoic, pliable mass was not identified. The prefemoral

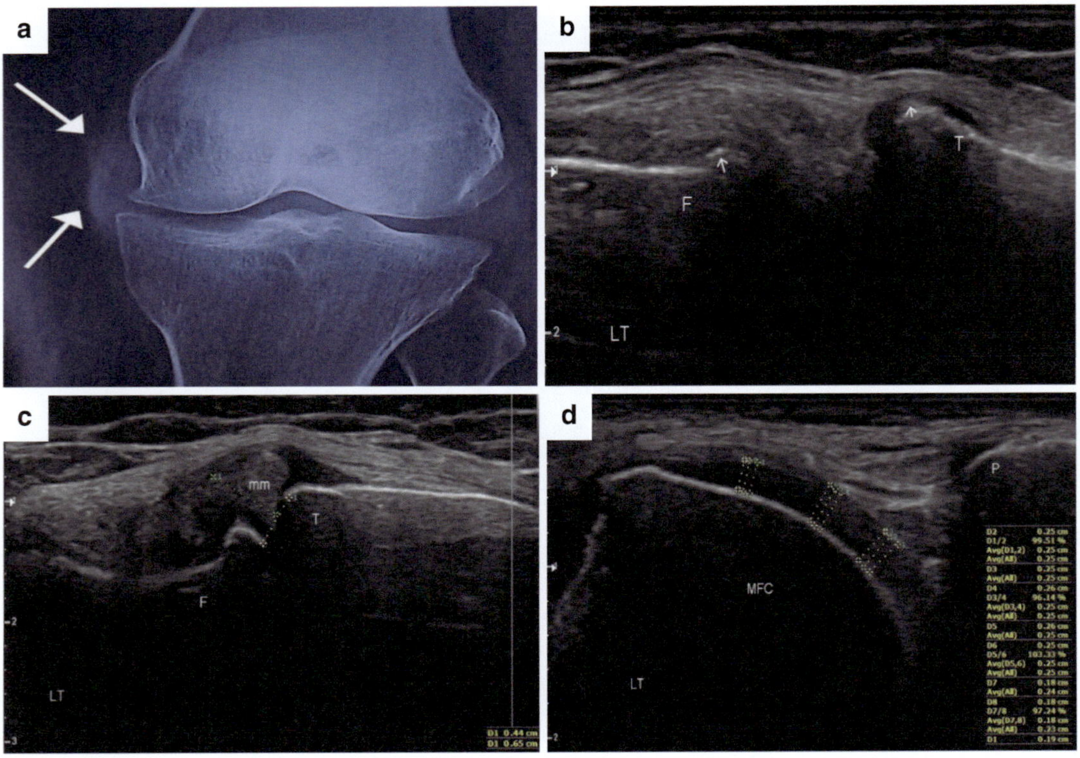

Fig. 7.17 Medial meniscal extrusion in knee osteoarthritis. (**a**) X-ray knee revealed reduction of the medial joint space width with mild femoral osteophyte. (**b**) Longitudinal scan of the medial knee depicted mild joint line osteophyte. (**c**) Longitudinal scan of medial knee explored severe grade MME. (**d**) Short axis scan of the MFC demonstrated echogenic cartilage but thickness preserved. *F* femur, *LT* left, *MME* medial meniscal extrusion, *mm* medial meniscus, *MFC* medial femoral condyle, *P* patella, *T* tibia

fat thickness was recorded as 4.1 mm in the long axis and 3.6 mm in the short axis. Notably, a mild osteophyte was observed along the medial joint line (Fig. 7.17b), and the medial meniscus was torn and extruded by 6.5 mm from the joint line, which in turn pushed the medial collateral ligament (Fig. 7.17c). There was no evidence of an anechoic, noncompressible cystic mass within the extruded medial meniscus. The thickness of the femoral condylar cartilage was intact, although it appeared echogenic (Fig. 7.17d). Posteriorly, there was no documentation of a superficial Baker's cyst or a hypoechoic-anechoic compressible collection surrounding the semimembranosus tendon.

Impression Medial meniscal extrusion in knee osteoarthritis.

Case Summary 18 A 70-year-old patient presented with persistent pain and swelling in the left posterior heel. Upon examination, tenderness was noted at the insertion of the Achilles tendon, although the tendon itself was found to be intact, as confirmed by the Thompson maneuver. The patient reported no history of trauma to the rearfoot and had no prior medical conditions, such as diabetes mellitus, ischemic heart disease, dyslipidemia, or hypertension. Additionally, there were no signs of joint pain or swelling. An X-ray of the foot revealed soft tissue swelling. Further evaluation of posterior heel pain via ultrasound was performed.

Ultrasound Findings The Achilles tendon (AT) exhibited a thickened and hypoechoic appearance, accompanied by disruption of its fibrillar architecture (Fig. 7.18a–b). Additionally, a linear hyperechoic mass, which was noncompressible, was identified within the AT; however, the integrity of the AT was preserved, as confirmed through dynamic assessment. At the site where the tendon is attached to the posteroinferior calcaneus, hyperechoic, noncompressible bony growth was observed, which displayed posterior acoustic shadowing and was continuous with the

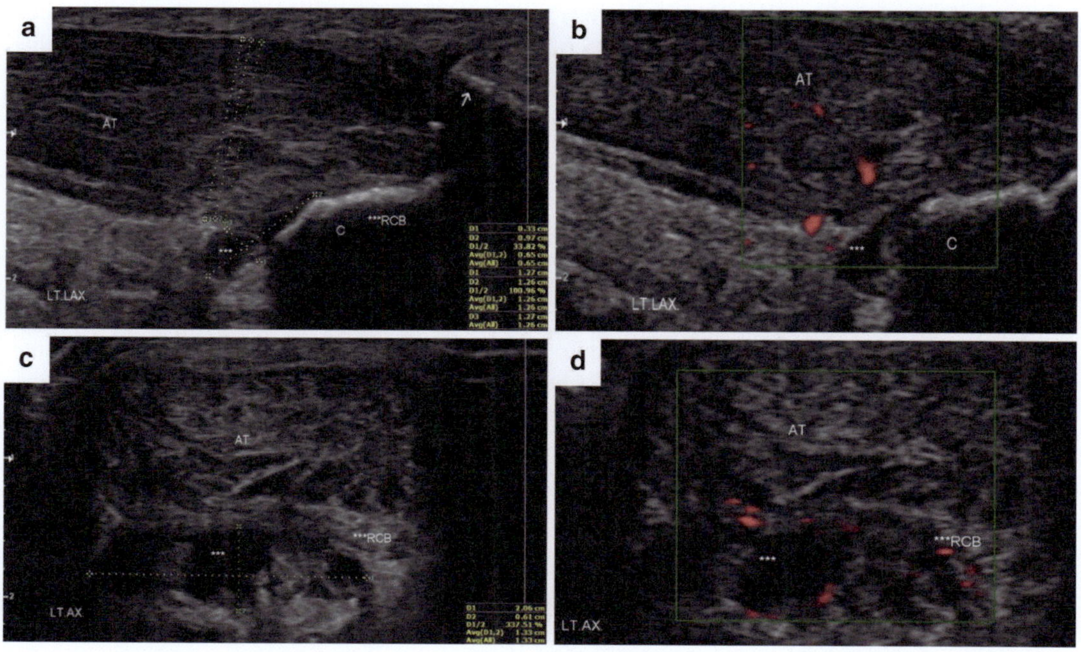

Fig. 7.18 Achilles tendinopathy with retrocalcaneal bursitis. (**a, b**) Longitudinal scans of the posterior heel revealed thick and hypoechoic Achilles tendon with loss of fibrillar pattern, increased Doppler signal (**b**), anechoic, compressible collection noted in the RCB (**a**, **b**, asterisks), and hyperechoic calcaneal growth (**a**, arrow). (**c, d**) Short axis scans explored anechoic, compressible collection in the RCB with increased bursal wall Doppler activity (**d**). *AX*, short axis, *AT* Achilles tendon, *C* calcaneus, *RCB* retro-calcaneal bursa, *LT LAX* left long axis

calcaneus (Fig. 7.18a). Furthermore, the retrocalcaneal bursa (RCB) was noted to be distended with anechoic and compressible fluid collection (Fig. 7.18c–d). There was also an increase in Doppler activity detected in both the AT and RCB.

Impression Achilles tendinopathy with retrocalcaneal bursitis.

Case Summary 19 A 45-year-old woman with a background of obesity and hypothyroidism presented with discomfort and swelling in her left posterolateral ankle. During the clinical assessment, tenderness was documented not only in the posterior heel but also around the lateral ankle area. Furthermore, a solid, swollen mass that was not tender and exhibited a positive slip sign was detected in the posterolateral region of the ankle. The range of motion of the ankle remained within normal limits. Further evaluation under ultrasound was performed.

Ultrasound Findings The subcutaneous fatty layer revealed areas of hypoechoic areolar fatty tissue interspersed with an interrupted hyperechoic septum (Fig. 7.19a–b). The Achilles tendon appeared hypoechoic, lost its fibrillar pattern, and demonstrated signs of thickening of hypoechoic paratenon, with no notable increase in Doppler activity (Fig. 7.19c–d). A hyperechoic, noncompressible mass with posterior acoustic shadowing was observed continuous with the posterior calcaneus. Dynamic scanning confirmed the integrity of the Achilles tendon. The retrocalcaneal bursa was not distended, with anechoic, compressible accumulation. Later, the peroneal tendons appeared thick and hypoechoic, along with a disruption in their fibrillar pattern (Fig. 7.19e–f). An intact hypoechoic peroneal retinaculum was observed around the peroneal tendons (Fig. 7.19e–f).

Impression Achilles tendon and peroneal tendon tendinopathy with lipoma.

Case Summary 20 A 55-year-old man reported experiencing pain and swelling in his right posterior heel for the last two months. These issues affected his ability to perform daily tasks, especially when he stood erect or walked for a long time. He denied any recent injuries or problems with his footwear. The other joints appeared normal, with no complaints regarding the patient's neck or lower back. Upon clinical examination, there was noticeable swelling and tenderness in the posterior heel, with soft tissue overlying the hard bony calcaneus. The movements of both the ankle and subtalar joints were within normal limits. An X-ray of the left foot revealed a prominent calcaneal spur along with soft tissue swelling in the posterior heel and lower leg (Fig. 7.20a).

Ultrasound Findings The Achilles tendon was thick and hypoechoic with disruption of its fibrillar architecture (Fig. 7.20b). Deeper tendon fibers displayed signs of discontinuity, accompanied by an increased Doppler signal (Fig. 7.20b–c). Hyperechoic bony protrusion was observed, which caused posterior acoustic shadowing and was continuous with the posterosuperior calcaneal spur (Fig. 7.20b–c). A noncompressible, hyperechoic mass was also detected within the tendon (Fig. 7.20d).

Impression Hugland syndrome.

Case Summary 21 A patient with knee osteoarthritis presented with bilateral knee pain, swelling, and limited range of motion, which affected his physical function for a long period of time. The pain exacerbated with activity, and there was no significant morning stiffness. X-ray results revealed reduced medial tibio-femoral joint spaces with subchondral cysts, sclerosis, and osteophyte formation (Fig. 7.21a).

Ultrasound Findings Anechoic compressible accumulation was not observed in the anterior joint recess. The synovial membrane was not thickened; it was neither branched nor had a

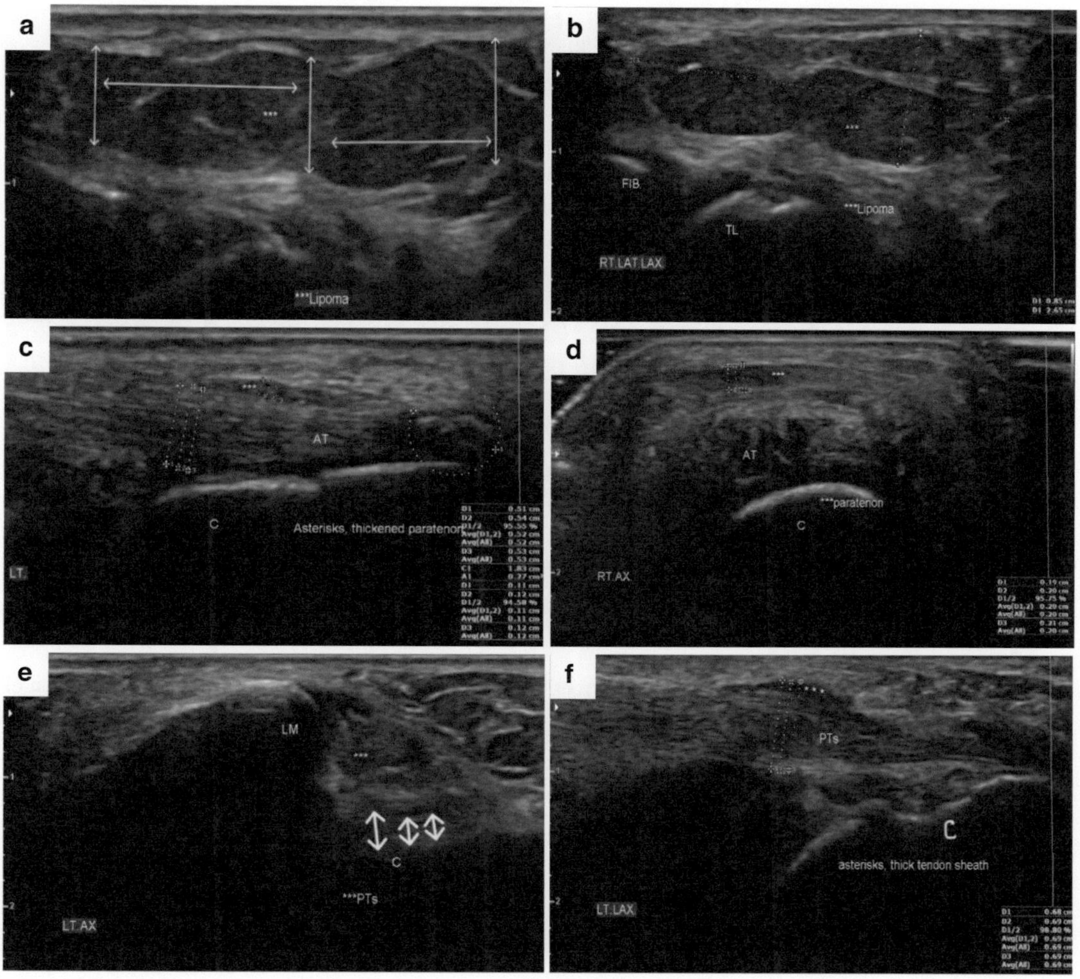

Fig. 7.19 Achilles and peroneal tendinopathy with lipoma. (**a**, **b**) Oblique longitudinal scans of the lateral ankle revealed a noncompressible, hypoechoic subcutaneous mass (asterisks and double arrows). (**c**, **d**) Longitudinal scans of the posterior heel demonstrated afibrillar Achilles tendon (**c**), covered with a thick hypoechoic paratenon (asterisks) (**d**) (**e**, **f**) Short axis and longitudinal scans of the peroneal tendons (PTs) (asterisks) at the LM appeared hypoechoic,) and exhibited a loss of fibrillar pattern (**e**) with thick and hypoechoic sheath (**f**) (asterisks) intact calcaneofibular ligament (double arrows) explored beneath the PTs (**e**). *AT* Achilles tendon, *C* calcaneus, *LM* lateral malleolus, *PTs* peroneal tendons

frond-like appearance. There was no evidence of noncompressible, hyperechoic, pliable masses in either anterior joint recess. Mild to moderate osteophytes and medial meniscus extrusion (5.6 mm) in the right knee were noted medially (Fig. 7.21b). Bilaterally, the medial femoral condylar (MFC) cartilage appeared echogenic with a reduction in thickness (positive chondral print sign) (Fig. 7.21c, e), and the MFC thicknesses were 1.2 mm and 1.1 mm on the right (Fig. 7.20d) and left (Fig. 7.21f) knees, respectively. Posteriorly, no superficial Baker's cyst or semimembranosus tendon bursal cyst was visualized.

Impression Reduced cartilage thickness in patients with knee osteoarthritis.

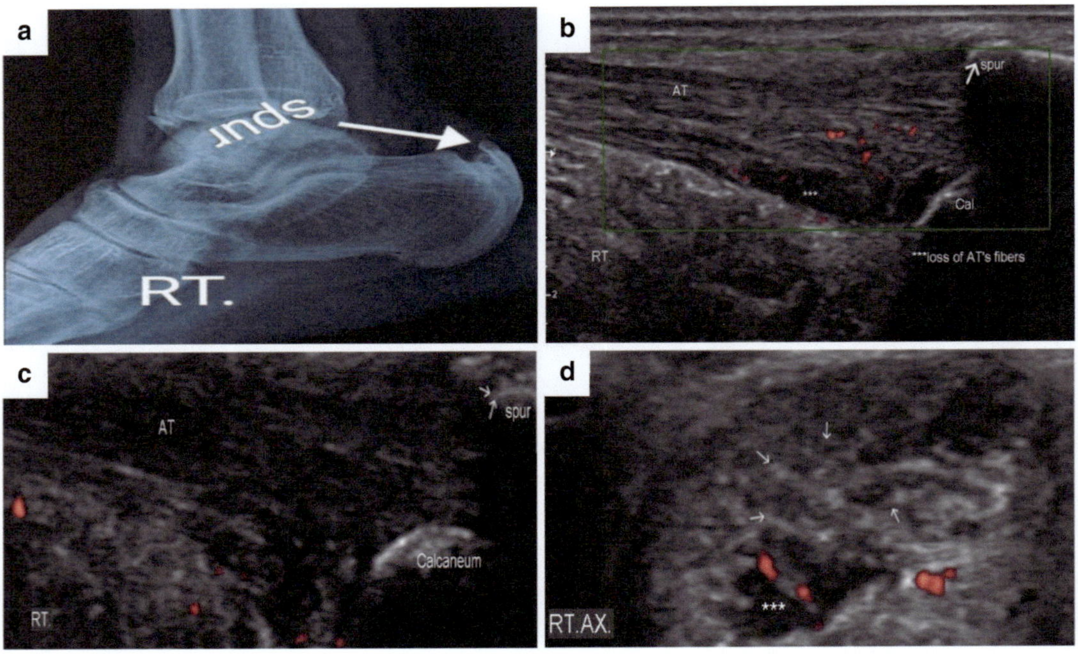

Fig. 7.20 Hugland syndome. (**a**) X-ray ankle/foot revealed posterior calcaneal spur (arrow). (**b**, **c**) Longitudinal scans of the posterior heel demonstrated thick and hypoechoic Achilles tendon with loss of fibrillar pattern, increased Doppler signals (red spots), and calcaneal spur (**b**, **c**) (arrows). (**d**) Short axis scan of the posterior calcaneus depicted hyperechoic lesions (arrows) within the hyperechoic-hypoechoic Achilles tendon with increased Doppler signals (red spots). *AT* Achilles tendon, *Cal* calcaneus, *RT* right

Case Summary 22 An elderly individual, aged 65 years, presented with complaints of a swollen and painful right ankle joint, along with a limited range of motion for a few days. The patient denied any other joint problems. There was no significant morning stiffness associated with these symptoms. Physical examination revealed that the joint was swollen and that the joint line was tender. No tenderness was elicited over the malleolus. X-ray findings indicated soft tissue swelling. Despite treatment with naproxen sodium (500 mg twice per day for 5 days) and oral steroids, the patient's symptoms did not improve. There were elevated serum inflammatory biomarkers. He was also seropositive for an anti-cyclic citrullinated peptide antibody. An ultrasound of the ankle was performed.

Ultrasound Findings A mild, compressible, anechoic collection was noted within the talocrural joint, accompanied by a thick synovial membrane displaying heightened Doppler activity (Fig. 7.22a–c). Moreover, an interface sign was observed over the talar dome (Fig. 7.22c). Ultrasound-guided aspiration (Fig. 7.22d) of the cloudy, hazy fluid yielded was subjected to cytology, staining, and culture analysis. The culture findings revealed the presence of gram-positive cocci in the clusters, suggesting the initiation of antibacterial therapy.

Impression Septic arthritis in the ankle.

Case Summary 23 A 70-year-old woman who was generally in good health presented with issues related to her right shoulder, specifically pain and a noticeable decrease in her range of motion that had persisted for several months. She experienced limitations in shoulder abduction, rotation, and extension, making activities challenging, especially activities requiring shoulder abduction. She did not report a painful arc during shoulder abduction. An intra-articular steroid injection was administered, but it did not provide

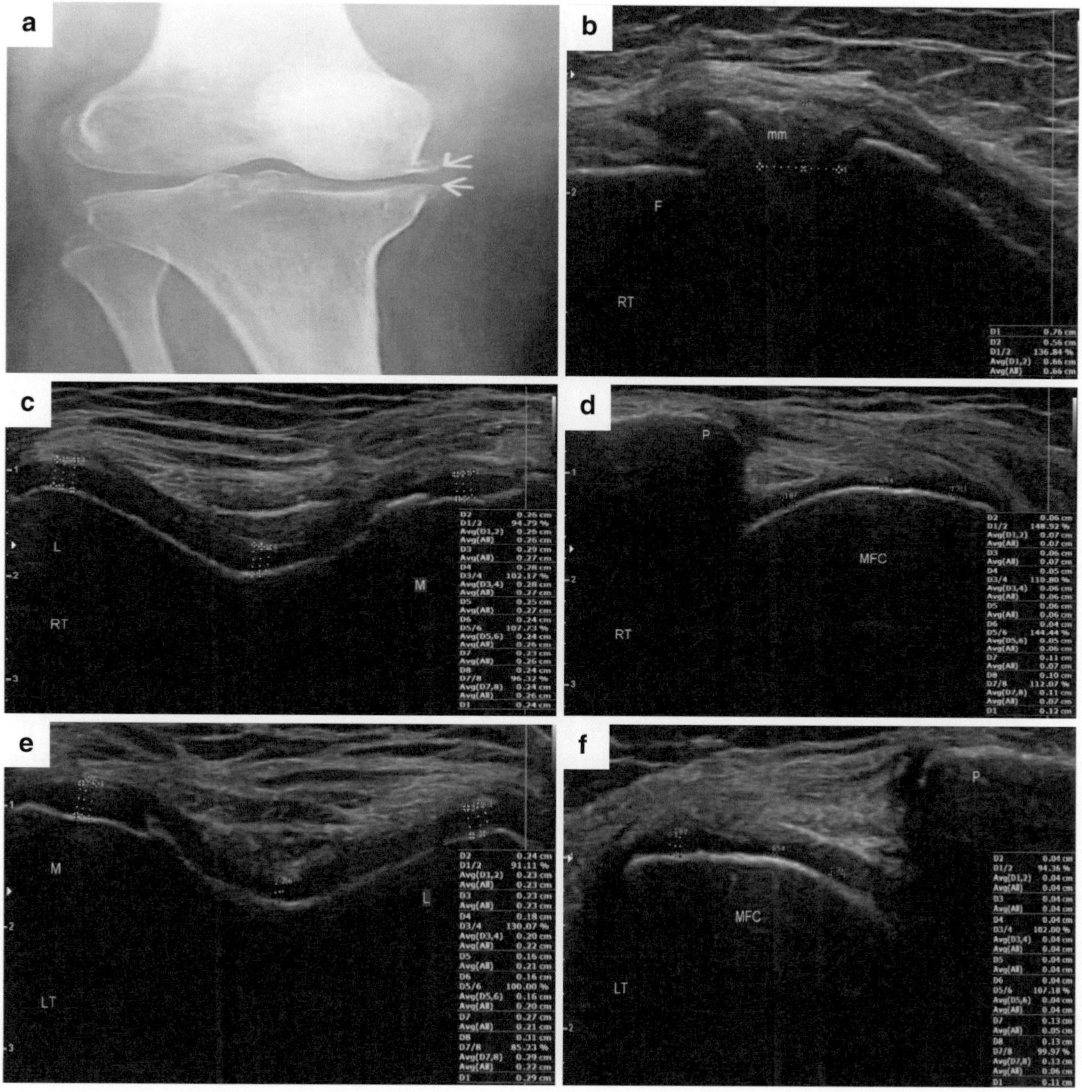

Fig. 7.21 Cartilage thickness changes in knee osteoarthritis. (**a**) X-ray right knee showing medial joint line osteophytes (single arrows). (**b–f**) Medial longitudinal, transverse suprapatellar, and short axes scans of the MFC revealed medial meniscal extrusion (**b**), joint line osteophytes (**b**), and reduced femoral condylar cartilage thickness (**c-f**) in both knees. (**c**, **e**) Transverse suprapatellar scans of the flexed knees demonstrated reduced femoral condylar cartilage thickness and sharpness (**d**, **f**) Short axis scans of the MFC of both knees explored the reduced cartilage sharpness and thickness. *F* femur, *L* lateral, *LT* left, *M* medial, *MFC* medial femoral condyle, *mm* medial meniscus, *P* patella, *RT* right

substantial relief from her discomfort. Further evaluation under ultrasound was performed.

Ultrasound Findings The transverse humeral ligament was hyperechoic and displayed a convex shape. The bicipital tendon appeared fibrillar, maintaining its integrity, whereas compressible anechoic fluid collection was present behind the long head of the bicipital tendon, accompanied by heightened Doppler activity. The subacromial-subdeltoid bursa (SASD) was found to be distended with compressible anechoic fluid

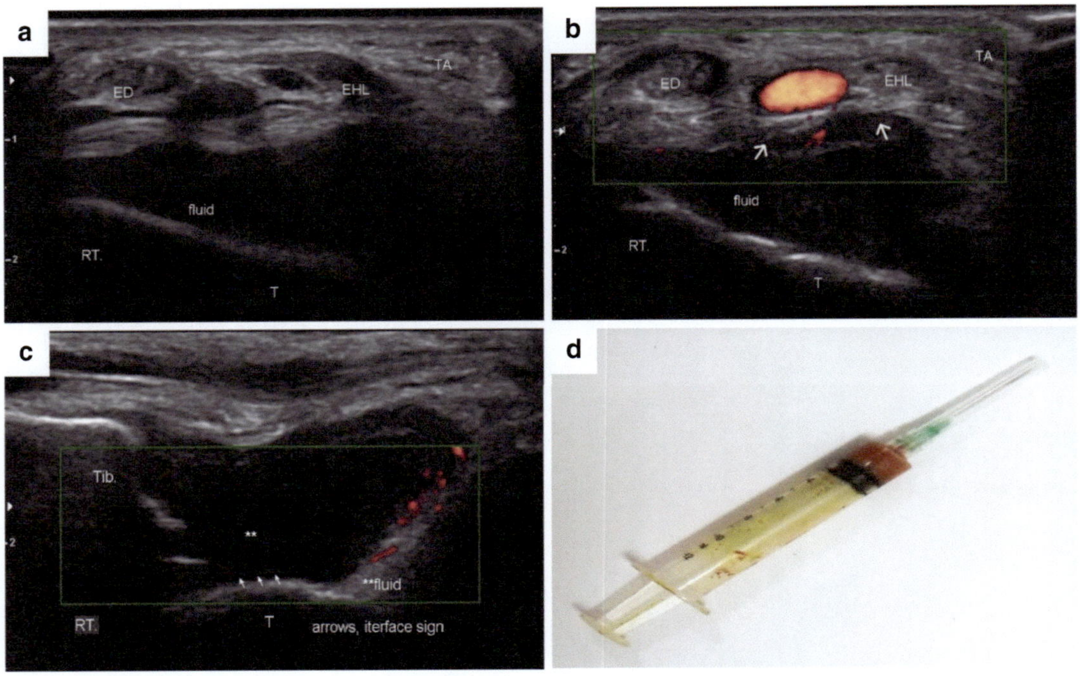

Fig. 7.22 Ankle septic arthritis. (**a**, **b**) Short axis scans of the anterior ankle revealed compressible and anechoic collection in the talocrural joint with increased synovial membrane thickness (**b**, arrows). (**c**) Longitudinal scan of the anterior ankle explored compressible collection in the joint with increased synovial Doppler signal (red spots). (**d**) Cloudy, opaque-green fluid aspirated from the joint cavity. *ED* extensor digitorum, *EHL* extensor hallucis longus, *TA* tibialis anterior, *Tib/T* tibia, *RT* right

accumulation, spreading over the anterolateral aspect of the shoulder (Fig. 7.23a–c). The SASD bursa was aspirated and treated with a steroid and lidocaine injection (Fig. 7.23d). An intralesional steroid injection was also given around the bicipital tendon (Fig. 7.23d).

Impression Subacromial subdeltoid bursitis.

Case Summary 24 A 43-year-old sales executive employed at a pharmaceutical company faced recurring pain and swelling in his right big toe. He noted that these painful episodes had been occurring more frequently over the last few years, particularly after undergoing a cardiac procedure. The discomfort made walking difficult for him. He had diabetes mellitus and no recent injury to the foot. His current medication history included bisoprolol, low-dose aspirin, atorvastatin, amlodipine, febuxostat (40 mg/day), and olmesartan. An X-ray of his ankle and foot revealed soft tissue swelling. The laboratory results revealed normal serum uric acid and creatinine levels.

Ultrasound Findings The synovial membrane in the first metatarsophalangeal joint exhibited thickening (Fig. 7.24a) and elevated Doppler signals (Fig. 7.24b). A double contour sign was identified over the metatarsal head (Fig. 7.24c–d).

Impression Gouty arthritis.

Case Summary 25 A woman in her middle age presented with discomfort at the base of her right middle finger (Fig. 7.25a). She also described a tingling feeling in both her middle and ring fingers. Tenderness was noted at the ring finger's base. She had no prior diagnosis of diabetes mellitus, and her thyroid function was normal. The

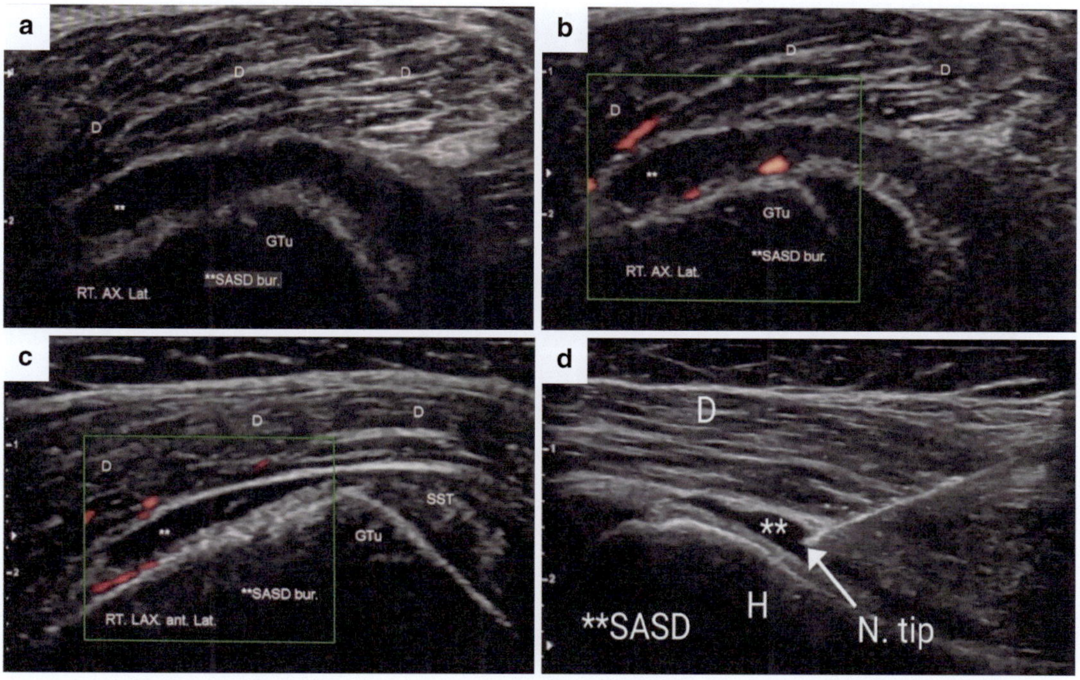

Fig. 7.23 Subacromial subdeltoid bursitis. (**a-c**) Short and longitudinal scans of thel lateral shoulder t s revealed compressible and anechoic collection in the SASD bursa with increased bursal wall Doppler activity (**b, c**). (**d**) Needle tip (N tip) inserted into the bursa using in-plane ultrasound technique for aspiration and steroid injection. *AX* short axis, *D* deltoid, *GTu* greater tuberosity, *H* humerus, *LTu* lesser tuberosity, *LAX* long axis, *N tip* needle tip, *SASD* subacromial subdeltoid bursa

clinical assessment suggested the possibility of a trigger finger; however, to exclude other potential diagnoses, an ultrasound was arranged.

Ultrasound Findings An anechoic-hypoechoic noncompressible mass with well-defined margins and posterior acoustic enhancement, although no sign of internal vascularity was observed at the ring finger base (Fig. 7.25b–d). A long-axis view revealed the fibrillar tendon with an anechoic, poorly compressible cystic mass obstructing the fibrillar tendon (Fig. 7.25d). The A1 pulley was not thickened, nor was any tenosynovial thickening or fluid accumulation revealed.

Impressions 1. Ganglion cyst. DD: 1. Pulley cyst; 2. Giant cell tumor of the flexor sheath.

Case Summary 26 A 42-year-old male complained of pain localized in the right anterior thigh, which significantly hindered his mobility and daily activities. During the clinical assessment, firm and tender soft tissue was noted in the middle thigh. The patient disclosed that he had experienced an injury to his thigh caused by a cow's horn. X-ray imaging revealed soft tissue swelling. The preliminary diagnosis indicated a quadriceps muscle tear. Further assessment of the anterior thigh was performed with ultrasound, with the findings outlined below.

Ultrasound Findings Axial and longitudinal scanning of the anterior thigh muscles, namely, the rectus femoris (RF), vastus lateralis (VL), medialis (VM), and intermedius (VI), revealed increased thickness and *hypoechogenicity* (Fig. 7.26a–f). The proximal region of the RF and VL muscle fibers presented evidence of tearing accompanied by an increase in Doppler signals (Fig. 7.26c–e). Additionally, hyperechoic non-

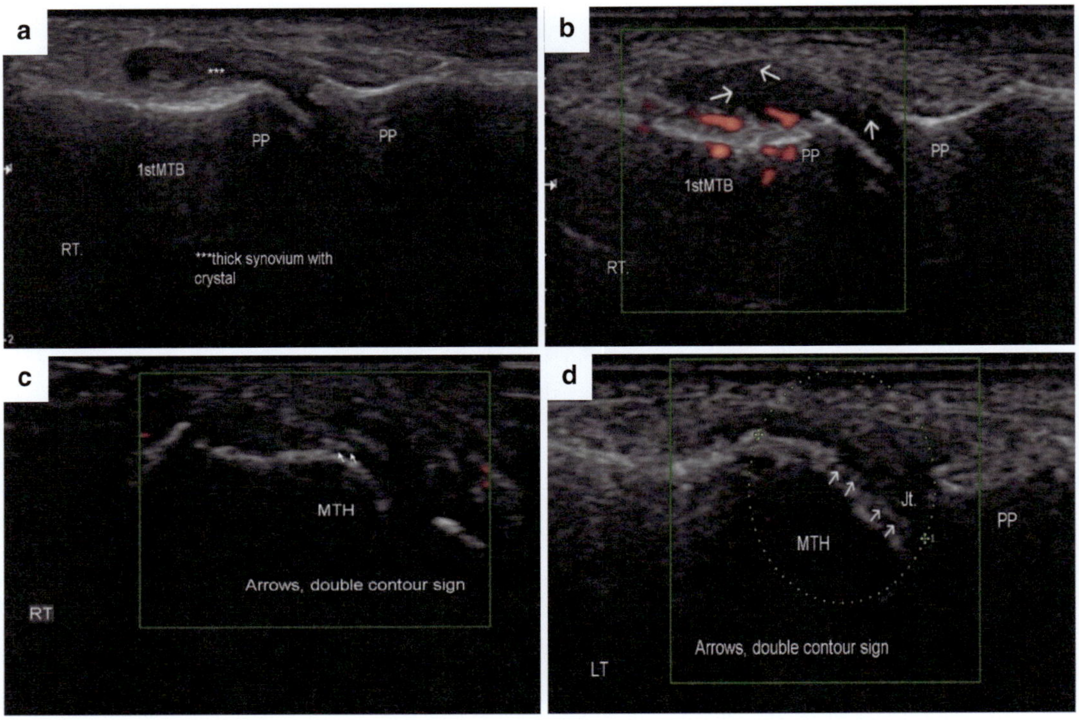

Fig. 7.24 Gouty arthritis. (**a, b**) Longitudinal scans of the anterior aspect of the first metatarsophalangeal joint revealed thick and hypoechoic synovial membrane (asterisks and arrows) with increased Doppler activity (**b**, red spots). (**c, d**) Short and longitudinal axes scans of the MTH, respectively explored Double contour sign over the MTH cartilage (white arrows). *MTH* metatarsal head, *MTB* metatarsal bone, *PP* proximal phalanx

compressible masses exhibiting posterior acoustic shadowing were observed within the anterior thigh muscles (Fig. 7.26a–b, d, f).

Impression Quadricep muscle tear with myositis ossificans.

Case Summary 27 A 29-year-old Bangladeshi expatriate employed as a chef presented with symptoms of pain and swelling in the right lateral elbow, exacerbated by repetitive use during daily activities over the course of 1 month. Physical examination revealed tenderness in the lateral elbow region, which was more prominent below the lateral epicondyle. Maudsley's maneuver was eventful. The range of motion of the elbow was not restricted.

Ultrasound Findings The assessment of the lateral elbow revealed that the superficial common extensor tendon of the forearm was echogenic-hypoechoic (Fig. 7.27a). In contrast, the radial collateral ligament (RCL) was noted to be thickened (mean 4.6 mm) and showed signs of partial tearing (anechoic cleft with hypoechoic changes) (Fig. 7.27b–d). Valgus stress testing did not indicate any gap within the RCL. There were no cortical defects identified on the distal humerus.

Impression Radial collateral ligament tear.

Case Summary 28 An 85-year-old male reported experiencing pain and weakness in his right shoulder for several years, which was accompanied by restricted movements and difficulties in performing daily activities. He denied any recent injuries to the shoulder and did not report any neck pain that radiated to the ipsilateral upper extremity. Upon examination, the shoulder girdle appeared atrophied. The Hawkins

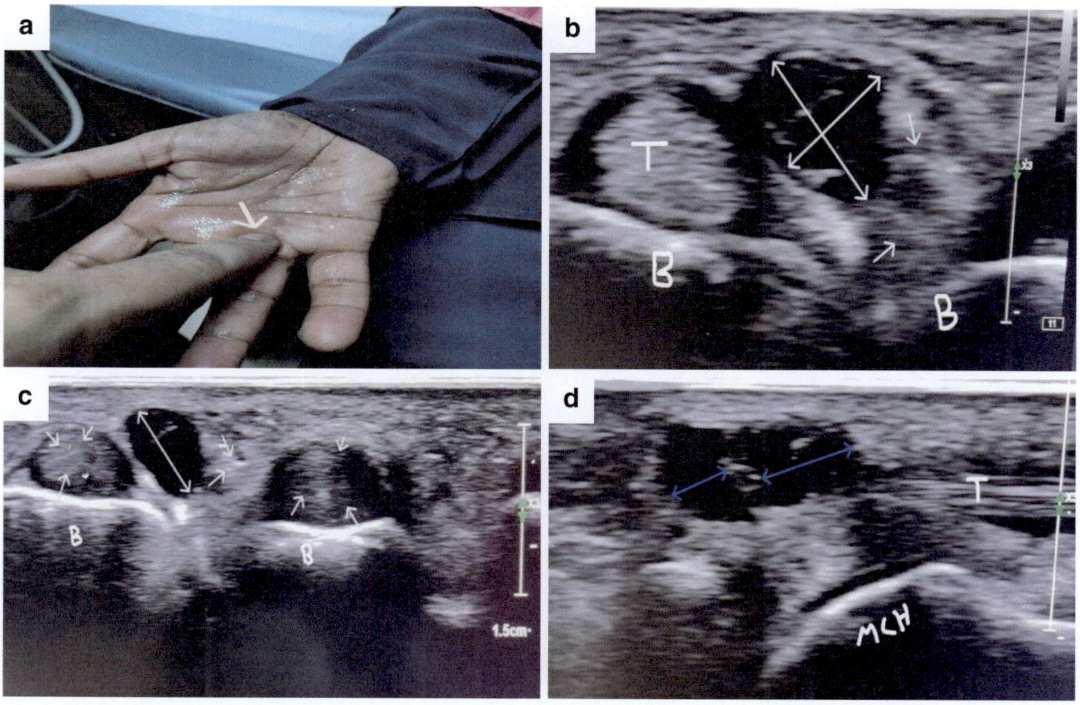

Fig. 7.25 A ganglion cyst mimics trigger finger. (**a**) Area of focal pain and swelling (arrow). (**b**, **c**) Short axis scans at the distal palmar crease of the ring finger revealed an anechoic-hypoechoic, poorly compressible cyst (double arrows) adjacent to the hyperechoic-hypoechoic flexor tendon (**c**, white arrows). (**d**) Longitudinal scan over the respective finger explored the cystic mass (double arrows) obscuring the fibrillar tendon (T). *B* bone, *MCH* metacarpal head, *T* tendon

maneuver was negative, and both external and internal rotations were unrestricted in both the abduction and neutral positions of the shoulder. Notably, the patient did not experience significant morning stiffness, headache, weight loss, or fever. His medical history of diabetes mellitus, hypertension, or cardiovascular conditions was uneventful. An X-ray of the shoulder revealed increased radiopaque changes in the greater tuberosity.

Ultrasound Findings The long head of the biceps tendon (LHBT) displayed a hypoechoic characteristic with a disrupted fibrillar architecture. A thick, hypoechoic synovial sheath enveloped the LHBT. The intra-articular LHBT was intact. Peritendon anechoic compressible accumulation was not observed. The synovial capsule was noted to be thick and hypoechoic. In the modified Middleton shoulder position, the supraspinatus tendon (SST) was found to have a full-thickness tear on both short- and long-axis imaging, with the adjacent deltoid muscle encroaching over the humeral head (HH) (Fig. 7.28a–b). The subscapularis tendon exhibited a loss of its fibrillar pattern, appearing thick and hypoechoic, whereas the infraspinatus tendon was echogenic. Cartilage thickness over the humeral head appeared diminished and exhibited a rough echotexture (Fig. 7.28c). The posterosuperior glenoid labrum (GL) appeared hypoechoic (Fig. 7.28d).

Impression Supraspinatus tendon tear with deltoid herniation.

Case Summary 29 A 42-year-old overweight woman complained of discomfort in her left

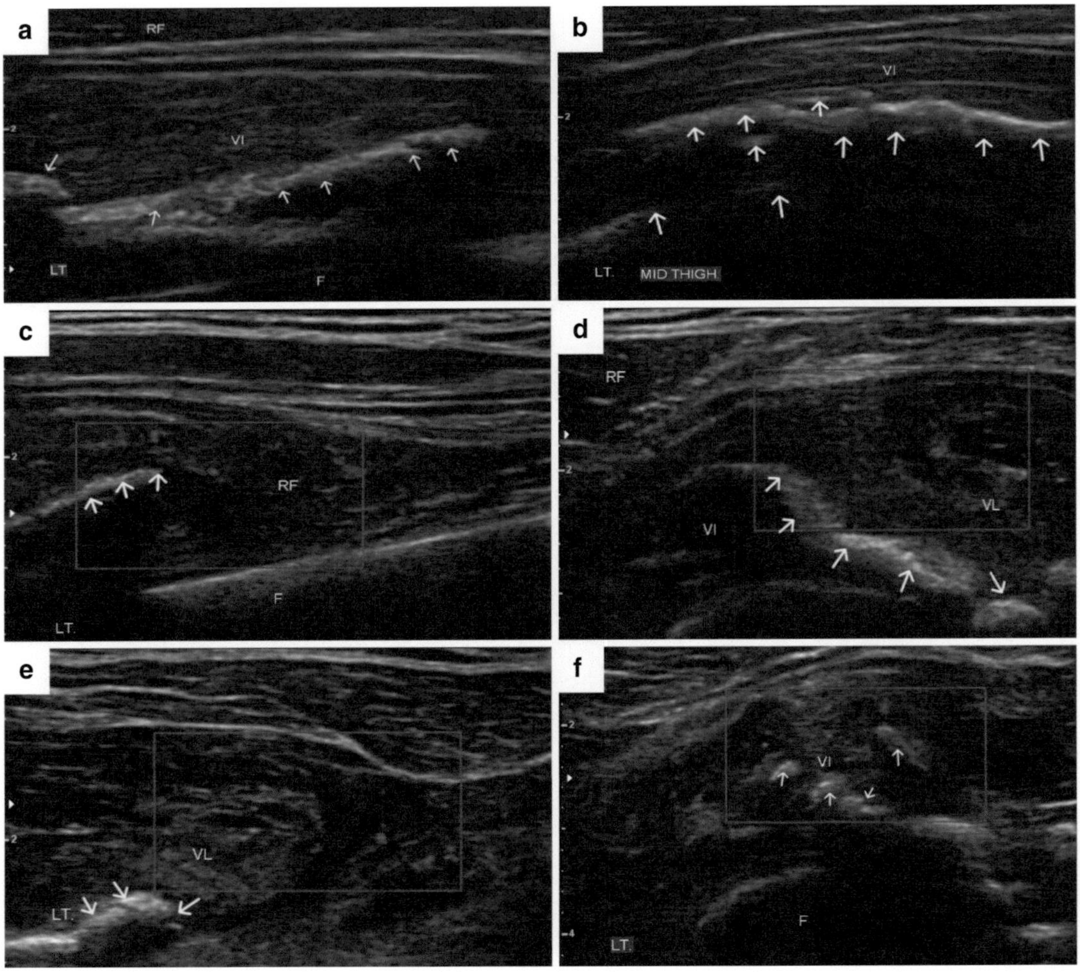

Fig. 7.26 Quadricep muscle tear with myositis ossificans. (**a–f**) Longitudinal and short axes scans of the anterior thigh revealed VI, VL, and RF muscles thick and hypoechoic with hyperechoic lesions with posterior acoustic shadowing (white arrows). (**c–e**) Sustained tears were depicted in VL and VI muscles. *F* femur, *RF* rectus femoris muscle, *VI* vastus intermedius muscle, *VL* vastus lateralis muscle, *VM* vastus medialis muscle

knee, particularly during activity and movement. Although there was no visible swelling in the joint and the examination for fluid accumulation yielded normal results, she did exhibit some muscle atrophy in the quadriceps area. However, the joint range of motion was not limited. Further examination via ultrasound was performed.

Ultrasound Findings The anterior joint recess showed no signs of distension from anechoic, compressible fluid collections, nor was there any presence of a noncompressible, hyperechoic, pliable mass within the joint cavity. The synovial membrane did not branch or appear frond-like. The prefemoral fat thickness was recorded as 5.2 mm along the long axis and 4.9 mm along the short axis. Medially, no medial joint line osteophytes were noted; the medial meniscus appeared hypoechoic but remained intact, showing no signs of tearing or extrusion. Sonopalpation elicited medial knee pain. The medial collateral ligament was intact. The medial femoral condylar cartilage appeared echogenic, with a mean thickness of 2.1 mm (Fig. 7.29a).

In addition to the patella, a poorly compressible, smooth-walled septate mass was identified beneath the patellar tendon within Hoffa's fat pad, extending laterally toward the lateral joint line (Fig. 529b). The lateral meniscus was torn, accompanied by anechoic, compressible fluid

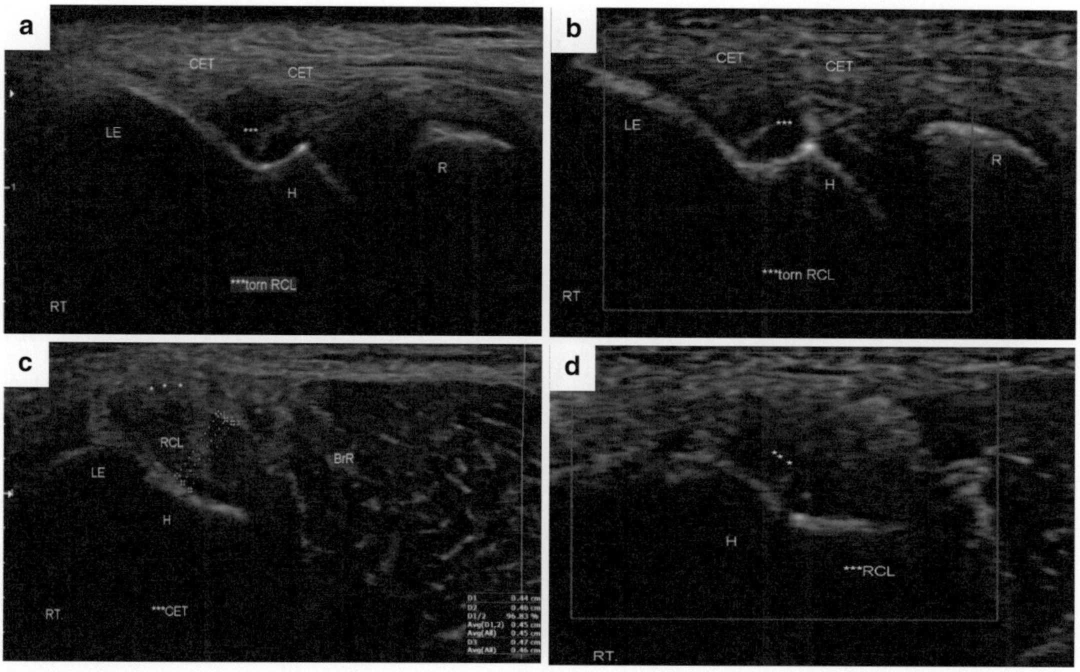

Fig. 7.27 Elbow radial collateral ligament tear. (**a**, **b**) Longitudinal scans of the lateral elbow revealed thick, hypoechoic, and torn RCL assessed on dynamic assessment (asterisks). (**c**, **d**) Short axis scans of the lateral elbow unveiled thick, hypoechoic, and torn RCL assessed dynamically (asterisks). *BrR* brachioradialis muscle, *CET* common extensor tendon, *H* humerus, *LE* lateral epicondyle, *RCL* radial collateral ligament, *R* radial head

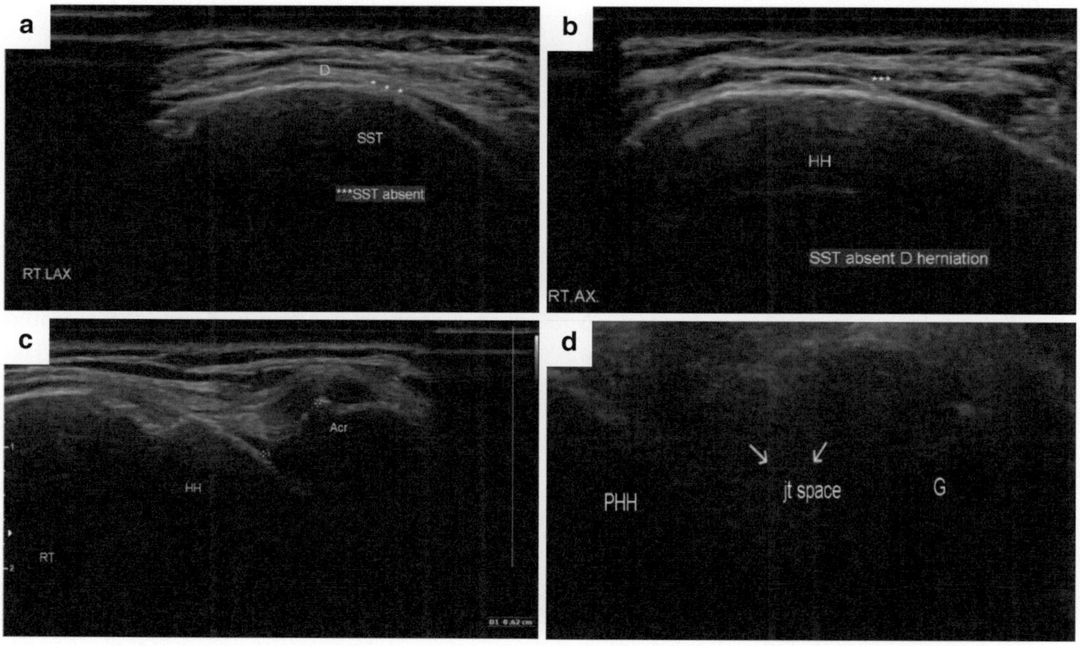

Fig. 7.28 Supraspinatus tendon tear with deltoid herniation. (**a**, **b**) Longitudinal scans of lateral shoulder revealed SST absent over the humeral head (asterisks), and the deltoid approached to the HH. (**c**) The distance between HH and Acr measured 0.65 cm. (**d**) Short axis scan of posterior shoulder at the GHJ depicted the glenoid labrum hypoechoic (white arrows). *Acr* acromion, *D* deltoid, *G* glenoid, *GHJ* glenohumeral joint, *HH* humeral head, *PHH* posterior humeral head, *SST* supraspinatus tendon

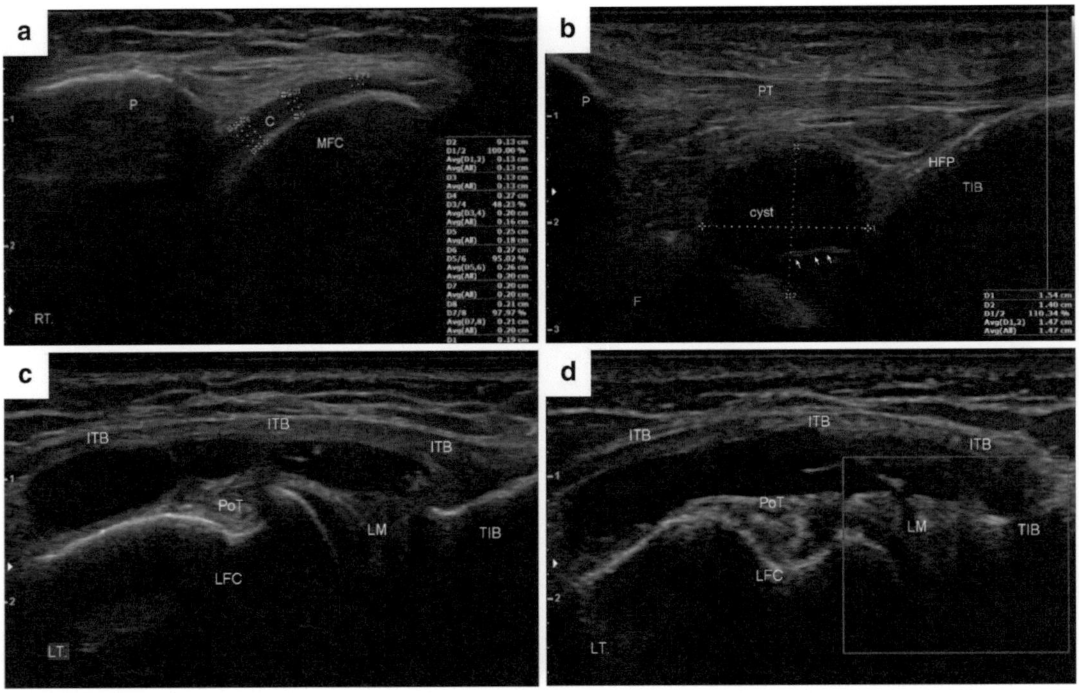

Fig. 7.29 Lateral meniscal tear with parameniscal and deep infrapatellar cysts. (**a**) Short axis scan of the MFC revealed cartilage thickness preserved. (**b**) Anterior, longitudinal scan of infra-patellar knee revealed anechoic, poorly compressible cystic lesion beneath the PT and within the Hoffa's fat pad (HFP). (**c**–**d**) Laterally, longitudinal scan revealed an anechoic, compressible mass underneath the ITB communicating with the joint cavity through the torn LM. *ITB* iliotibial band tendon, *HFP* Hoffa's fat pad, *LM* lateral meniscus, *LFC* lateral femoral condyle, *MFC* medial femoral condyle, *PT* patellar tendon, *PoT* popliteal tendon, *TIB* tibia

accumulation beneath the lateral collateral ligament and iliotibial band complex, which leaked through the lateral meniscus (Fig. 7.29c–d). Notably, no increased Doppler activity was detected in the cyst wall (Fig. 7.29d). Baker's cyst or bursal swelling around the semimembranosus tendon was not documented.

Impression Lateral meniscal tear with a parameniscal and deep infra-patellar cyst.

Case Summary 30 A 23-year-old individual presented with persistent low back and hip pain accompanied by notable morning stiffness, which has been linked to axial spondyloarthropathy. Upon physical examination, both Patrick's and Gaenslen's tests yielded positive results. X-ray assessment of the hip revealed no distinct abnormalities. An ultrasound of the hip joint was conducted.

Ultrasound Findings During the examination of the anterior hip, notable thickening of the joint recess was observed, although there was no corresponding increase in Doppler activity. The recess had an average thickness of 6.8 mm, and no compressible collection was found within it (Fig. 7.30a–b). The femoral head maintained its normal contour; however, the cartilage appeared echogenic, and the thickness was reduced. The anterior labrum remained hyperechoic and was appropriately aligned throughout the dynamic assessment (Fig. 7.30a–b).

Impression Hip synovial hypertrophy.

Case Summary 31 A 55-year-old Bangladeshi man reported experiencing tingling and numbness in the radial aspect of his left hand, with exacerbation of symptoms at night, during daily activities, and in cold weather. The symptoms

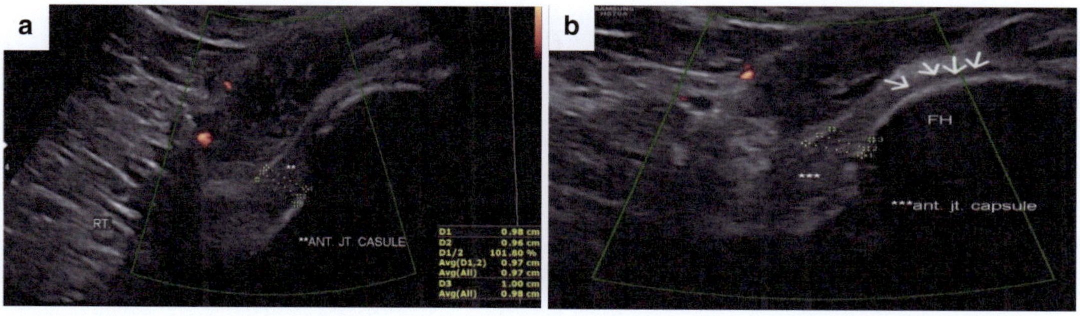

Fig. 7.30 Hip synovial hypertrophy in ankylosing spondylitis. (**a**, **b**) Longitudinal, oblique anterior hip scans revealed the thick and hypoechoic synovial membrane without Doppler activity. (**b**) Femoral head cartilage appeared hyperechoic with loss of cartilage thickness (white arrows). *FH* femoral head

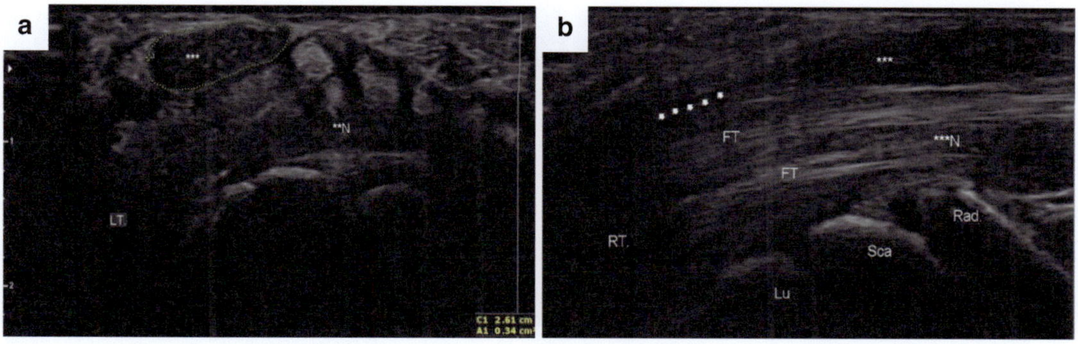

Fig. 7.31 Carpal tunnel syndrome. (**a**) Short axis scan of the volar wrist revealed an increased cross-sectional area of the hypoechoic median nerve (asterisks). (**b**) Longitudinal scan of the volar wrist explored thick and hypoechoic flexor retinaculum (arrows) compressed the median nerve at the tunnel with dilatation of the proximal nerve (asterisks). *FT* flexor tendon, *Lu* lunate, *Rad* radius, *RT* right, *Sca* scaphoid

had been ongoing for months and involved three and a half fingers along the radial distribution. Notably, there was no wasting of the thenar eminence. The patient had no diabetes mellitus, and his thyroid function was normal. Past medical history was unremarkable for significant trauma. The patient's clinical picture was consistent with left carpal tunnel syndrome. Further evaluation under ultrasound was performed.

Ultrasound Findings The flexor tendons located on the volar side of the wrist, including the flexor digitorum superficialis, flexor digitorum profundus, and flexor pollicis longus, exhibit normal echotexture and thickness. The median nerve was noted to be transversely elongated, measuring a total cross-sectional area of 2.61 cm^2 at the proximal carpal tunnel (Fig. 7.31a). Proximal to compression (Fig. 7.31b), the nerve appeared dilated with loss of the fascicular pattern. Moreover, the epineurium appeared hypoechoic.

Impression Severe carpal tunnel syndrome.

Case Summary 32 A woman aged 50 years presented with the complaint of tingling in the radial aspect of both hands, which worsened at night, during daily activities, and in cold weather. The symptoms have been ongoing for months and involve the radial three and a half fingers. Clinical examination revealed positive Tinel's and Phalen's signs and reversed Phalen's signs, with no evidence of wasting the thenar eminence. The patient had no history of diabetes mellitus, and her thyroid function was normal. There was no significant past trauma around the wrists or proximal forearm. The clinical picture is suggestive of bilateral carpal tunnel syndrome. Further examination via ultrasound was performed.

Ultrasound Findings The flexor tendons located at the volar aspect of both wrists, specifically the flexor digitorum superficialis, flexor digitorum profundus, and flexor pollicis longus, were observed to have normal echogenicity and thickness during both static and dynamic scanning. The median nerve was found to be transversely elongated on both sides, with a total cross-sectional area of 1.66 cm^2 in the right hand (Fig. 7.32a–b) and 1.77 cm^2 in the left hand (Fig. 7.32c–d) at the proximal carpal tunnel.

Impression Bilateral severe carpal tunnel syndrome.

Case Summary 33 A 32-year-old man presented with bilateral hip joint pain with impaired daily activities. Clinical assessment revealed bilateral positive Patrick's tests. X-ray findings indicated the absence of osteophytes, and the femoral head contour was maintained. The patient reported experiencing back pain with significant morning stiffness. Axial spondyloarthritis was the diagnosis. Further examination of the hips via ultrasound was performed.

Ultrasound Findings The anterior joint capsule was thickened; thickness revealed more than 5 mm bilaterally (right—9.4 mm, left—10.5 mm); no increased Doppler activity was noted (Fig. 7.33a–b). The contour of the left femoral head was maintained (Fig. 7.33b); however, it was deformed on the right side (Fig. 7.33a). There was no compressible collection in the joint cavity. The anterior labrum was hyperechoic, and no defects were revealed on dynamic maneuvers.

Impression Bilateral hip synovial hypertrophy.

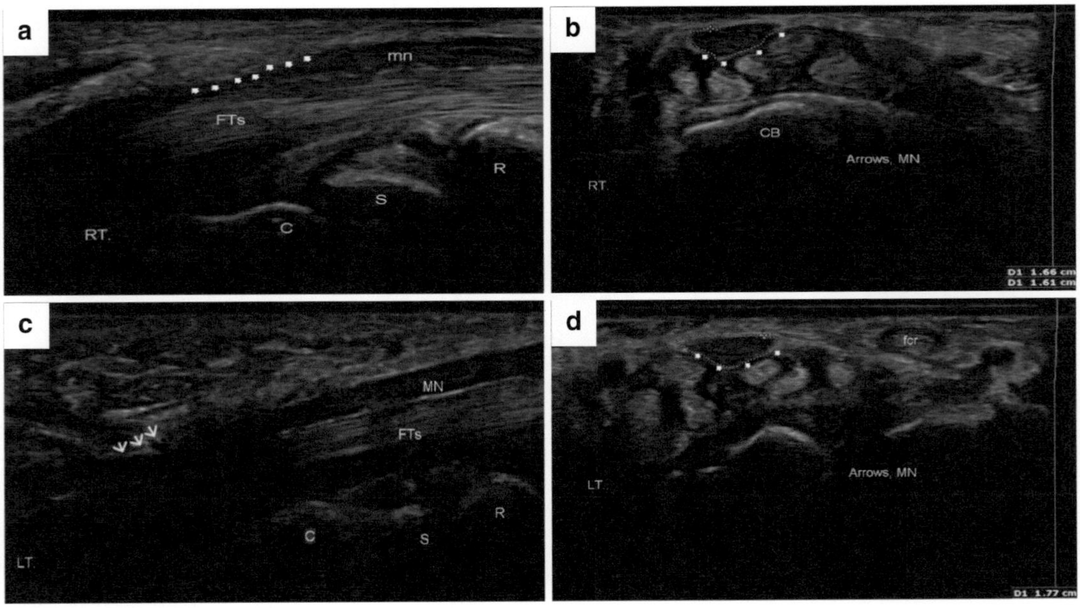

Fig. 7.32 Bilateral carpal tunnel syndrome. (**a**) Longitudinal scan of the right volar wrist revealed the constricted MN at the tunnel (thick arrows) with a proximal dilated nerve segment. (**b**) Short axis scan of the right volar wrist unveiled an increased cross-sectional area of the MN. (**c**) Longitudinal scan of the left volar wrist depicted a thick and hypoechoic flexor retinaculum compressed the MN at the tunnel (arrows). (**d**) Short axis scan of the left volar wrist demonstrated an increased cross-sectional area of the MN (in dots) at the carpal tunnel. *C* capitellum, *CB* carpal bone, *FTs* flexor tendons, *MN* median nerve, *LT* left, *RT* right, *S* scaphoid

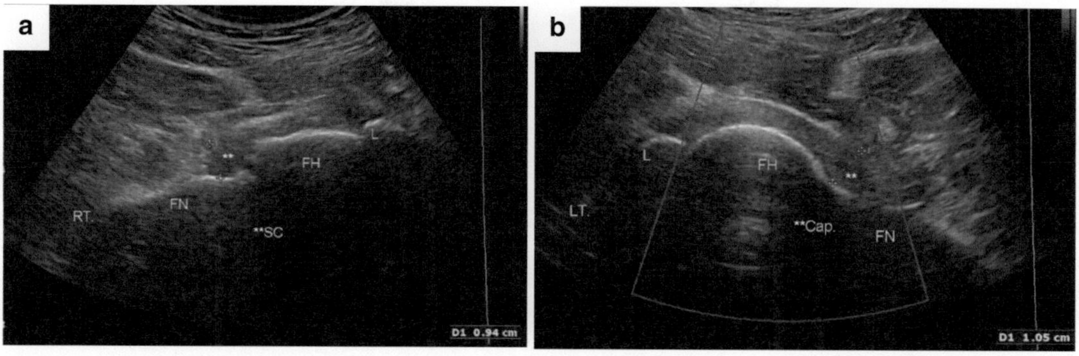

Fig. 7.33 Bilateral hip synovial hypertrophy in ankylosing spondylitis. (**a**) Oblique, longitudinal scan of the right anterior hip revealed thick and hypoechoic synovial membrane(asterisks), with deformed femoral head. (**b**) Oblique longitudinal scan of the left anterior hip revealed thick and hypoechoic synovial membrane (asterisks) with normal femoral head contour. *Cap/SC* synovial capsule, *FH* femoral head, *FN* femoral neck, *L* labrum, *LT* left, *RT* right

Case Summary 34 A 30-year-old female patient presented with complaints of pain and swelling in her right dorsal wrist, which had persisted for several months. Her medical history included rheumatoid arthritis and hypothyroidism. During the clinical examination, a soft, cystic mass was observed on the ulnar aspect of the dorsal wrist. This finding was indicative of a ganglion cyst, and further examination via ultrasound was performed.

Ultrasound Findings Scanning of the sixth dorsal wrist compartment revealed a fibrillar extensor carpi ulnaris (ECU) tendon covered with a thick and hypoechoic synovial sheath (Fig. 7.34a–d). Increased Doppler activity was noted in the ECU tendon sheath (Fig. 7.34b, d).

Impression Extensor carpi ulnaris tenosynovitis.

Case Summary 35 A 30-year-old male presented with swelling in the right knee joint that had persisted for several years. He also reported experiencing low back pain accompanied by significant stiffness in the morning. During the physical examination, the right knee joint was swollen, exhibiting a restricted range of motion, which was similarly noted in the hip joints. The synovial membrane in the knee appeared thickened, and a positive cross-fluctuation test indicated severe effusion within the knee joint. X-ray of the pelvis and hip revealed signs of hip joint space narrowing, subchondral sclerosis, and marginal bony growth (Fig. A). The sacroiliac joint revealed ankylosis. On the basis of these findings, a clinical diagnosis of ankylosing spondylitis was established, prompting further evaluation of the right knee joint through ultrasound.

Ultrasound Findings The anterior recess exhibited distension due to compressible anechoic fluid collection. The synovial membrane was noted to be thickened and hypoechoic and exhibited a villous appearance (Fig. 7.35b–c), with no significant Doppler activity detected. Cartilage thickness measurements over the medial femoral condyle indicated a thickening of 2.7 mm. Both the intercondylar and lateral femoral condylar cartilage displayed hyperechoic characteristics and a loss of smoothness, which was particularly pronounced in the lateral femoral condyle. Additionally, a cystic mass containing a poorly compressible anechoic collection was observed beneath the lateral head of the gastrocnemius muscle (Fig. 7.35d).

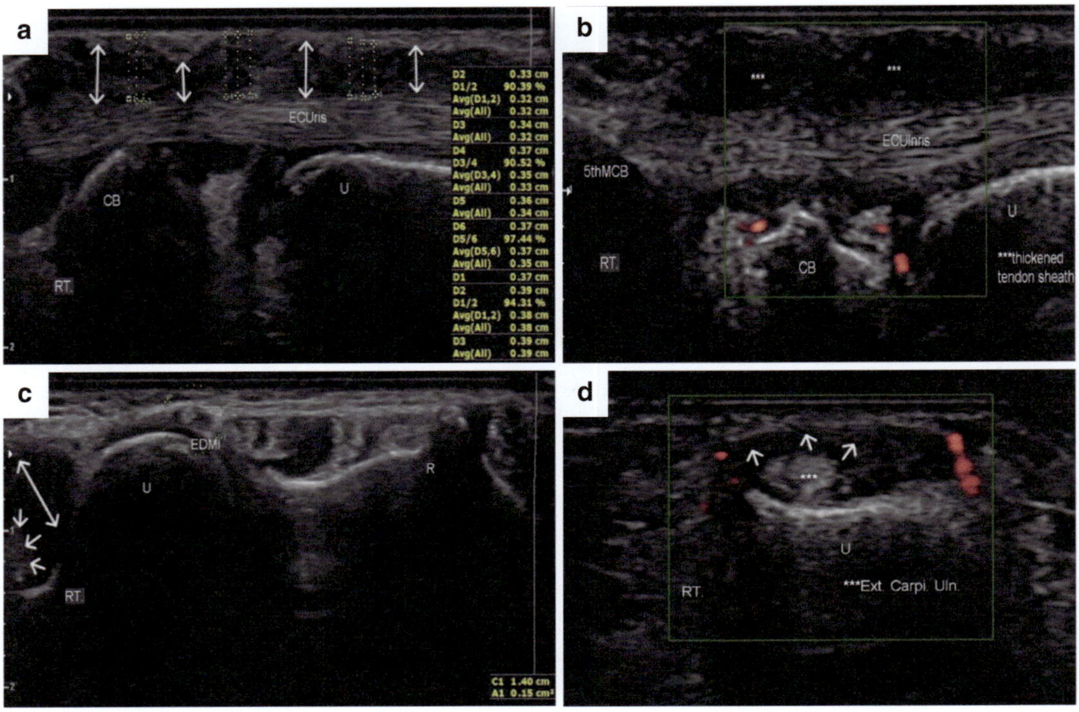

Fig. 7.34 Extensor carpi ulnaris tenosynovitis. (**a**, **b**) Longitudinal scans of the sixth dorsal wrist compartment revealed the fibrillar ECUris tendon surrounded by thick and hypoechoic tenosynovial sheath (adouble arrows, **b**, asterisks). (**c**) Short axis scan of the sixth compartment depicted a hyperechoic-hypoechoic tendon (arrows) surrounded by a thick, hypoechoic synovial sheath (double arrow). (**d**) Short axis scan explored a thick hypoechoic synovial sheath (arrows) with increased Doppler activity (red dots) enveloping the hyperechoic (ECUris) tendon (asterisks). *CB* carpal bone, *EDMi* extensor digiti minimi, *ECUris* extensor carpi ulnaris, *RT* right, *U* ulna

Impression Lipoma arborescence with ganglion cyst in knee synovitis in ankylosing spondylitis.

Case Summary 36 A 43-year-old male lumberjack presented with acute, intense pain in his left shoulder joint, accompanied by restricted range of motion for the previous three days. There were no reports of morning stiffness, headache, weight loss, or fever. The patient denied any recent falls; however, she had a medical history of diabetes mellitus, hypertension, and ischemic heart disease. Upon examination, painful movements of the shoulder were severely limited in all directions (limited circumduction). Apley's scratch test and the Hawkins maneuver were negative. Further investigation under ultrasound was performed.

Ultrasound Findings The long head bicep tendon (LHBT) exhibited a fibrillar structure, and the intra-articular portion of the LHBT was intact (Fig. 7.36a). The synovial sheath appeared thickened, accompanied by increased Doppler activity (Fig. 7.36a). Mild anechoic and compressible accumulation was noted around the LHBT (Fig. 7.36a). Anteriorly, the deep deltoid fibers over the LHBT displayed a loss of their fibrillar pattern, evolving into complex sonographic characteristics that varied from hypoechoic to hyperechoic with heightened Doppler activity. The transverse humeral ligament was noted to be hypoechoic and convex, also demonstrating significant Doppler activity, with the LHBT positioned within the bicipital groove. Additionally, the supraspinatus tendon (SST) was thickened and hypoechoic, with a tear present in the bursal-SST region.

The subcoracoid bursa (Fig. 7.36b, c) and the subacromial-subdeltoid (SASD) bursa (Fig. 7.36a, d–f) were thick and hypoechoic. An

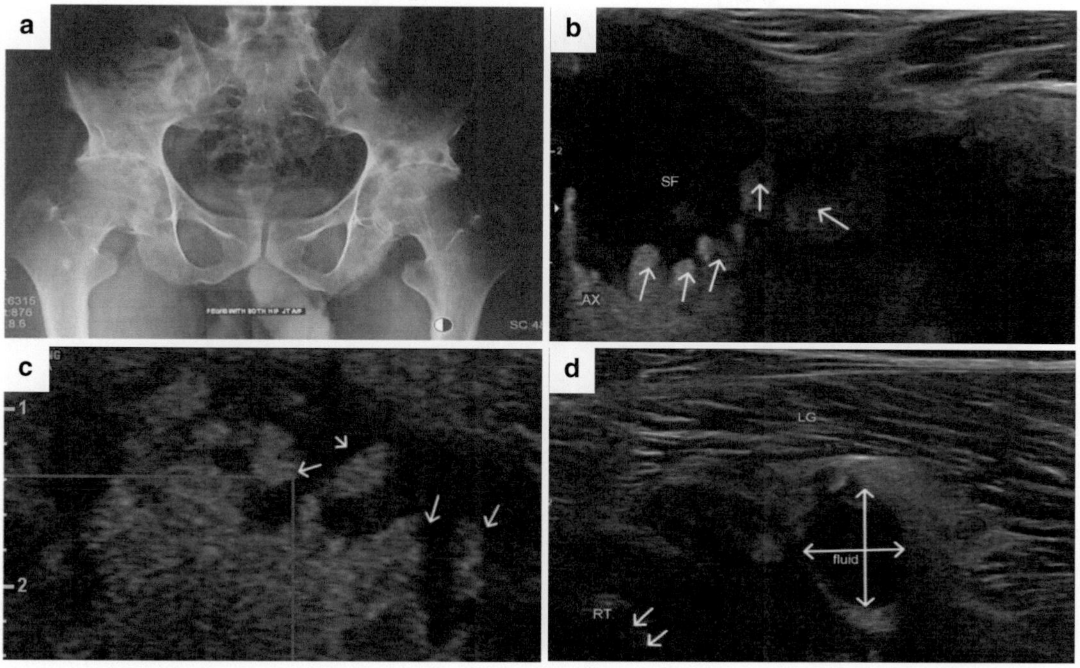

Fig. 7.35 Lipoma arborescence with ganglion cyst in knee synovitis in ankylosing spondylitis. (**a**) X-ray revealing bilateral hip joint ankylosis. (**b**, **c**) Transverse scans of the suprapatellar knee joint explored villous synovium (white arrows) with anechoic, compressible synovial fluid (SF), no increased Doppler signal depicted in the synovium. (**d**) Poorly compressible anechoic mass explored deep to the lateral gastrocnemius (LG) muscle. *AX* short axis, *LG* lateral gastrocnemius, *RT* right, *SF* synovial fluid

echogenic and thick SASD extended over the LHBT (Fig. 7.36a). Mild anechoic compressible collection was noted within the SASD bursa (Fig. 7.36f). The subscapularis tendon appeared echogenic and intact. The cartilage of the humeral head was hypoechoic, yet the contour of the humeral head was maintained. Upon dynamic scanning, the posterosuperior glenoid labrum was confirmed to be intact, and no glenohumeral joint effusion was observed.

Impressions Subacromial subdeltoid and subcoracoid bursitis.

Case Summary 37 A 68-year-old male presented with discomfort, swelling, and a sensation of tightness in his left leg, which he attributed to a feeling of crushing while fishing with a net in the village pond. Clinical evaluation revealed tenderness and tightness in the calf muscle, accompanied by localized warmth. An X-ray indicated soft tissue swelling in the leg, prompting an initial diagnosis of calf muscle injury. Further imaging under ultrasound was performed.

Ultrasound Findings Examination of the posterior aspect of the left leg revealed an incomplete tear in the medial head of the gastrocnemius muscle (MHG) (Fig. 7.37a–b). Anechoic compressible accumulation was noted, extending from the proximal region of the MHG to the midsection, with dimensions of 3.68 cm by 1.34 cm in the cross-sectional area, accompanied by several Doppler spots (Fig. 7.37a–c). Both dynamic and static imaging techniques were used to verify the integrity of the Achilles tendon. The lateral head of the gastrocnemius muscle was found to be intact (Fig. 7.37d).

Impression Medial head of the gastrocnemius muscle tear.

Case Summary 38 A 40-year-old male patient presented with pain and swelling in his right

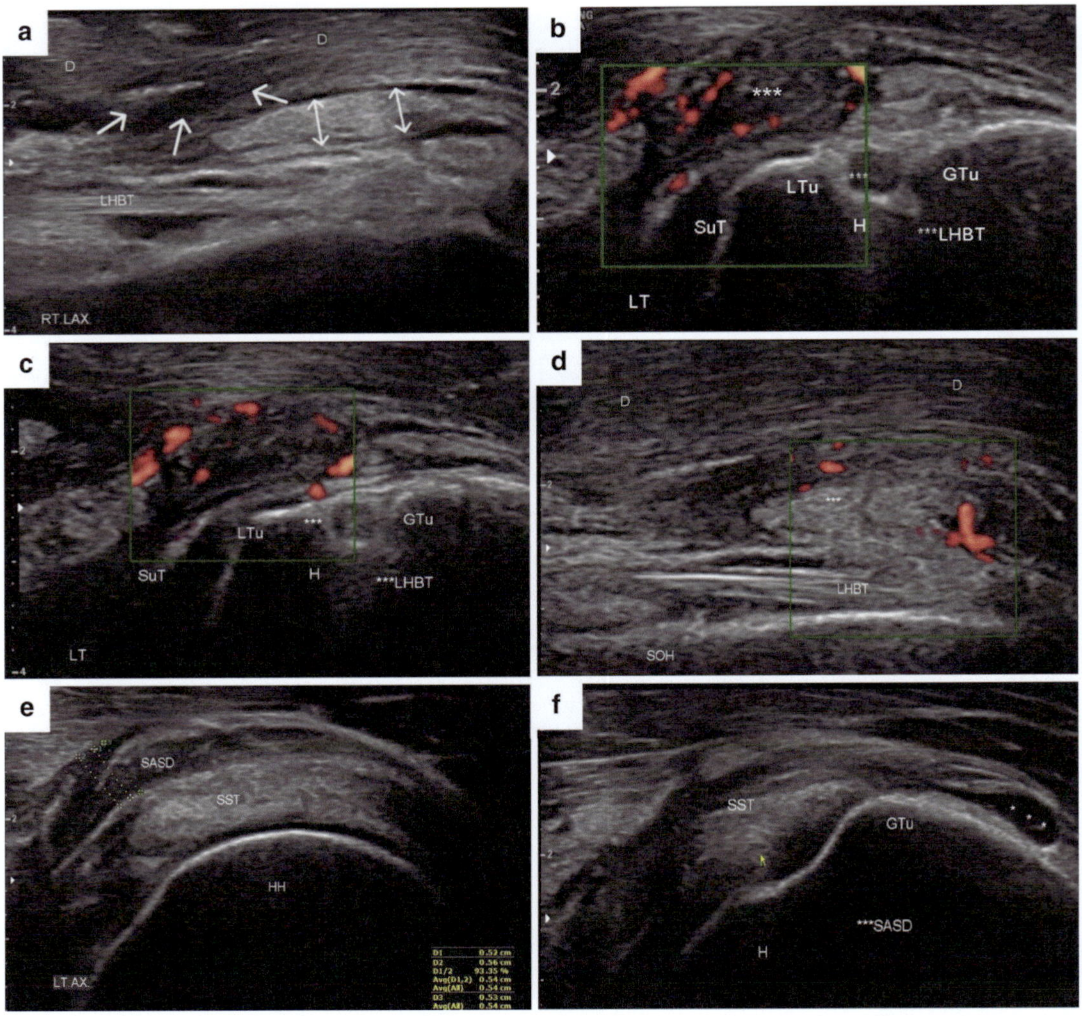

Fig. 7.36 Subacromial subdeltoid and subcoracoid bursitis. (**a**) Longitudinal scan of the anterior shoulder at the bicipital groove revealed hypoechoic and torn deeper deltoid fibers with thick, echogenic SASD bursa (double arrows). (**b**, **c**) Short axis scans of the anterior shoulder at the bicipital groove depictede the thick and hypoechoic SASD (**b**, asterisks) and hypoechoic subcoracoid bursa (**c**) in relation to LTu with increased Doppler signals (**b**, red dots). (**d**) Longitudinal scan of the anterior shoulder at the bicipital groove explored the thickened and echogenic SASD (asterisks) with increased Doppler signal (red dots). (**a**, **e**, **f**) Longitudinal (**a**) and short axis scans (**e**, **f**), respectively unveiled thick and hypoechoic SASD bursa with mild compressible collection (asterisks) (**f**). *GTu* greater tuberosity, *H* humerus, *HH* humeral head, *LTu* lesser tuberosity, *SuT* subscapularis tendon, *LHBT* long head of biceps tendon, *SASD* subacromial subdeltoid bursa, *SOH* shaft of humerus

elbow that had persisted for 4–5 days. Upon clinical examination, there was an increase in local temperature and tenderness noted on the antero-postero-lateral aspect of the elbow, whereas Maudsley's maneuver yielded negative results, and the range of motion in the joint remained intact. Although the X-ray findings were normal, indicating only soft tissue swelling, the clinical symptoms raised concerns for cellulitis. Further assessment via ultrasound was performed.

Ultrasound Findings The flexor muscles in the forearm demonstrated normal echogenicity and thickness (Fig. 7.38a). There were no indications of thickening at the origin of the common exten-

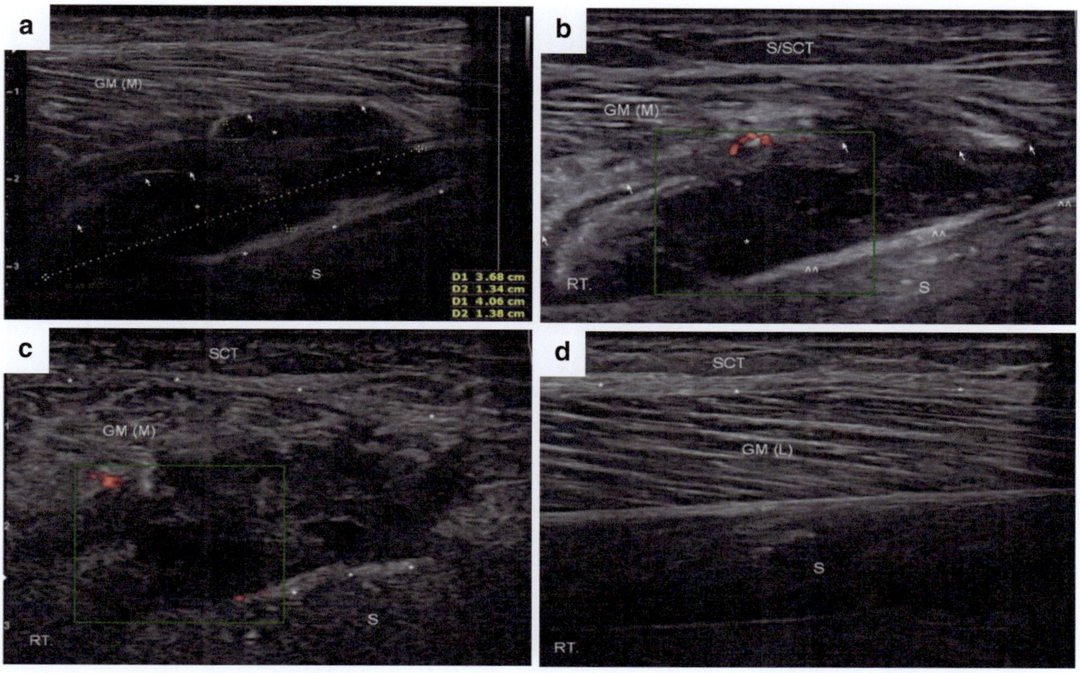

Fig. 7.37 Medial head of the gastrocnemius muscle tear. (**a–c**) Longitudinal scans of the posterior, proximal leg revealed the torn medial head of the gastrocnemius muscle with compressible collection (**a-c**) and increased Doppler signals (**b**, **c**) (red spots). (**d**) Longitudinal scan of the posterior and proximal lateral leg revealed fibrillar lateral gastrocnemius muscle. *GM(L)* lateral gastrocnemius, *GM* medial gastrocnemius, *S* soleus, *SCT* subcutaneous fat

sor tendons located at the right lateral epicondyle. Moreover, the anterior radiocapitellar, trochleoulnar, and posterior joint recesses were all normal, with no accumulation observed in any of the joint recesses assessed. Nonetheless, there was a notable increase in the thickness of the subcutaneous tissue, accompanied by the presence of hypoechoic lobules interspersed with hyperechoic linear bands (cobblestone appearance) (Fig. 7.38b–c). Additionally, an increase in Doppler spots was detected on the antero-postero-lateral regions of the elbow (Fig. 7.38d–f). The olecranon fossa and bursa were both assessed to be normal, with no abnormalities identified during the evaluation.

Impression Elbow cellulitis.

Case Summary 39 A 50-year-old expatriate from Bangladesh presented with complaints of pain and swelling on the lateral aspect of his right elbow, which had persisted for approximately 5—6 months. He could not recall any recent trauma to the region. Elbow full range of motion was maintained. He had diabetes mellitus. Radiographic imaging revealed no fractures in the elbow bones. The patient received treatment with intralesional steroid injection. Upon physical examination, significant swelling was observed on the outer elbow, accompanied by tenderness in that area and a positive Maudsley test result. The tennis elbow was diagnosed, and further evaluation of the region was performed via ultrasound.

Ultrasound Findings Ultrasound examination of the lateral elbow revealed a noncompressible, hyperechoic mass traced over the lateral epicondyle (Fig. 7.39a). The superficial common extensor tendon (CET) appeared hyperechoic–

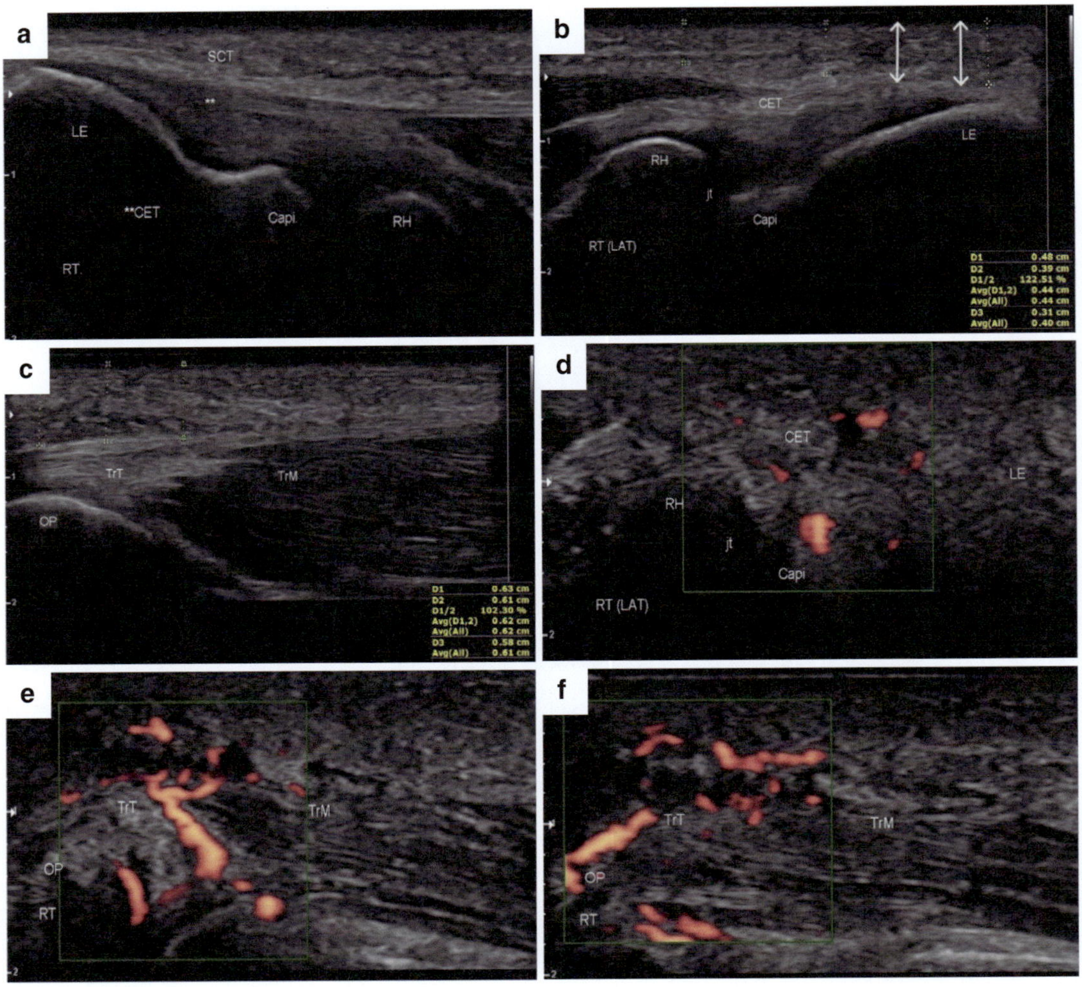

Fig. 7.38 Elbow cellulitis. (**a**) Longitudinal scan of the right lateral elbow. (**b**) Longitudinal scans of the lateral elbow showed SCT fat thick and hypoechoic (double arrows). (**c**) Longitudinal scan of the posterior elbow depicted hypoechoic and afibrillar TrT. (**d–f**) Longitudinal scans of lateral (**d**) and posterior flexed elbow (**e**, **f**) explored increased Doppler activity at CET and TrT, respectively. *CET* common extensor tendon, *Cap* capitellum, *RH* radial head, *TrM* triceps muscle, *TrT* triceps tendon

hyperechoic, and the fibrillar echotexture was distorted (Fig. 7.39a–b). Underneath the CET, a partial tear characterized by an anechoic cleft was identified in the radial collateral ligament (RCL) (Fig. 7.39b–d). No increase in Doppler activity was noted. When varus stress was applied to the elbow, which was partially flexed, and the forearm was supinated, an anechoic gap was observed in the RCL. No cortical defects were detected on the distal humerus at the capitellum.

Impression Radial collateral ligament tear.

Case Summary 40 A 60-year-old man presented with right shoulder pain and limited mobility, which hindered his ability to perform everyday tasks such as scratching his back. He had experienced a fall a year prior with an outstretched hand. Importantly, he had no history of diabetes mellitus, hypertension, dyslipidemia, or heart disease, and he did not report any significant morning stiffness, headache, weight loss, or

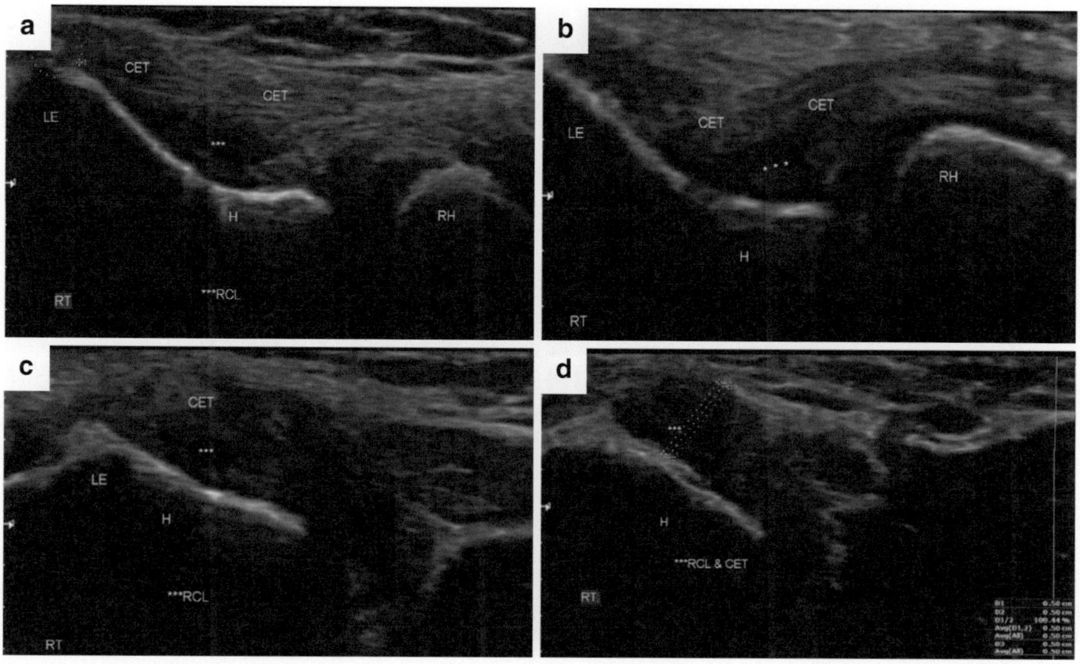

Fig. 7.39 Elbow radial collateral ligament tear. (**a, b**) Longitudinal scans of the lateral elbow revealed CET hyperechoic to hypoechoic with loss of fibrillar pattern (**b**), RCL appeared hypoechoic and torn (**a, b**) (asterisks). (**c, d**) Short axis scans of the lateral elbow at the lateral epicondyle depicted thick and hypoechoic RCL with intrasubstance tear (**b, d**) (asterisks). *CET* common extensor tendon, *LE* lateral epicondyle, *RCL* radial collateral ligament, *RH* radial head, *RT* right

fever. Upon physical examination, the Hawkins and shoulder drop arm tests yielded positive results, and a painful arc test could not be performed. The right shoulder girdle resulted in more muscle wasting than did the left shoulder girdle. Radiographic assessments revealed radio-opacity and cortical irregularities at the greater tuberosity, along with changes in the humeral head contour. Further evaluation under ultrasound was performed.

Ultrasound Findings The long head of the biceps tendon (LHBT) appeared hypoechoic with loss of the fibrillar pattern, yet there was no evidence of peritendinous effusion or heightened Doppler activity. The LHBT remained intact and continuous distally at the myotendinous junction. A thick and hypoechoic synovial sheath enveloped the LHBT (Fig. 7.40a–b). The transverse humeral ligament appeared thick, hypoechoic, and convex in shape (Fig. 7.40a–b).

The supraspinatus tendon (SST) also appeared thick and hypoechoic, with a reduction in tendon thickness in the middle (Fig. 7.40c). An incomplete full-thickness tear of the SST was identified at the greater tuberosity (Fig. 7.40d–e). The subscapularis tendon increased in thickness and appeared hypoechoic, accompanied by an intrasubstance hyperechoic mass (Fig. 7.40f). The subacromial-subdeltoid bursa was neither thickened nor distended, with anechoic, compressible accumulation.

Both abduction and external rotation (ER) movements are limited, with the ER being particularly restricted in both the shoulder abduction and neutral positions. The humeral head cartilage thickness was maintained. The posterosuperior glenoid labrum was triangular and hyperechoic, showing no tears during dynamic assessment. There was no effusion within the glenohumeral joint.

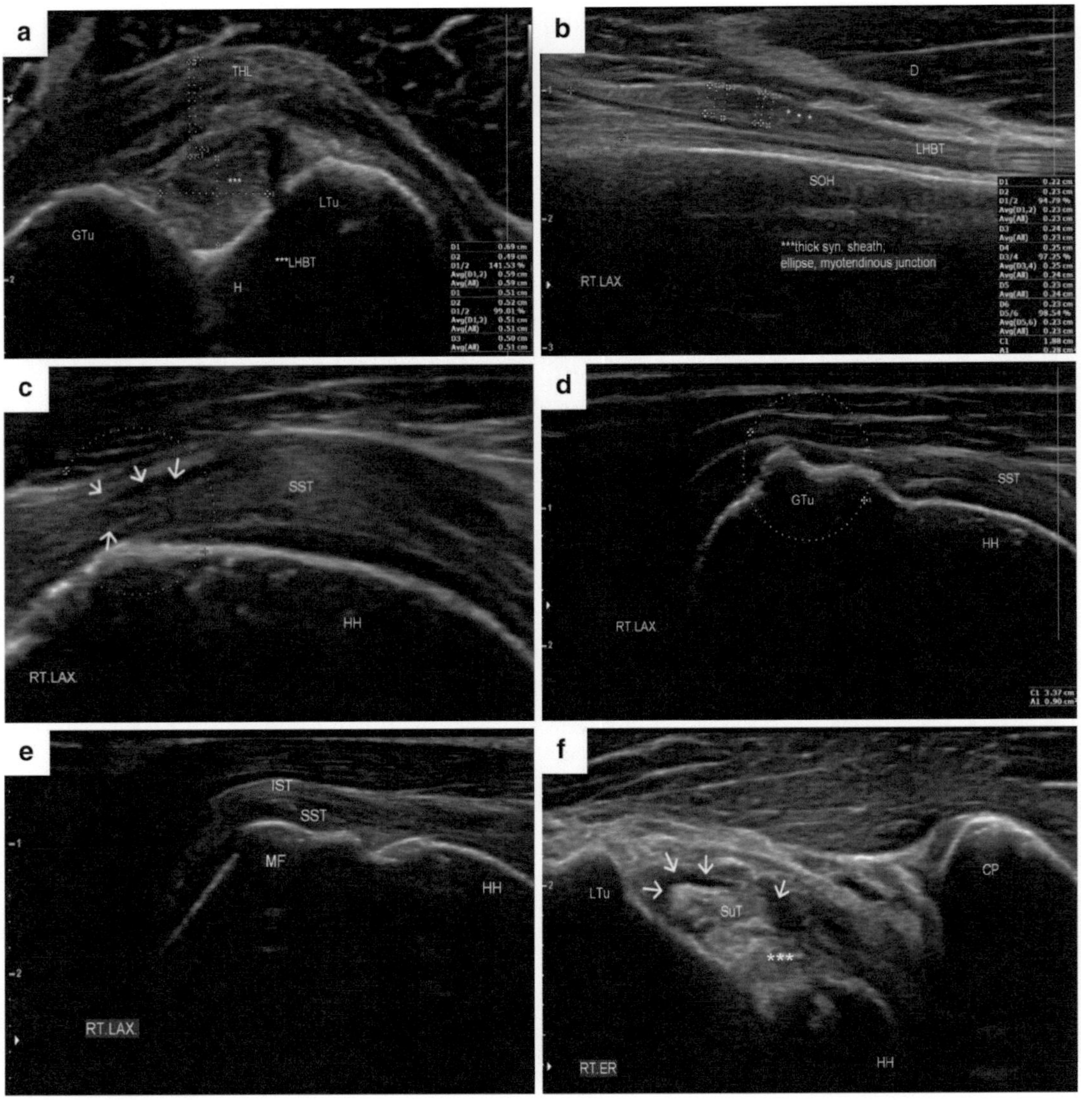

Fig. 7.40 Rotator cuff tear. (**a**, **b**) Short(**a**) and longitudinal axes (**b**) scans of the anterior shoulder revealed LHBT in the bicipital groove with thick, hypoechoic, and convex THL (**a**) and thick tenosynovial sheath anterior to the LHBT (**b**, asterisks). (**c**–**e**) Longitudinal scans of the lateral shoulder depicted an incomplete mid-portion SST tear (**c**) (white arrows) and a complete SST tear (**d**, **e**) at the GTu insertion (**d**, ellipse) with cortical defect (**d**, **e**). (**f**) Short axis scan of the anterior, externally rotated shoulder at the coracoid process level explored torn SuT with an anechoic split (white arrows), echogenic retracted SuT (asterisks) tendon revealed vicinity. *AX* short axis, *ER* external rotation, *GTu* greater tuberosity, *H* humerus, *IST* infraspinatus tendon, *LAX* long axis, *LTu* lesser tuberosity, *LHBT* long head of the biceps tendon, *SuT* subscapularis tendon, *SST* supraspinatus tendon, *SOH* shaft of the humerus

Impression Rotator cuff tear.

Case Summary 41 A 30-year-old male presented with pain in the right lateral ankle. He had experienced an ankle eversion injury 4 years prior. Upon examination, focal tenderness was noted in the retro-malleolar region, accompanied by an audible and palpable click. Lateral ankle ultrasound revealed the following findings.

Ultrasound Findings A longitudinal anechoic split at the lowest part of the peroneus brevis (PB) (deep to the peroneus longus) dividing it into two parts (Fig. 7.41a) was noted. The PB

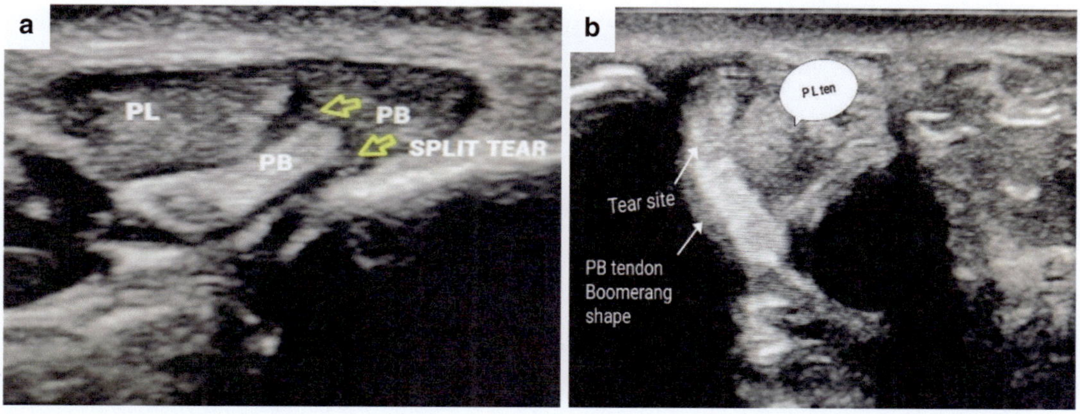

Fig. 7.41 Peroneus brevis split tear. (**a**) Short axis scan of the lateral ankle (infra-malleolar) depicted PB divided into two fragments with an anechoic cleft between them (yellow arrows). (**b**) Short axis scan revealed C-shaped (white arrows) PB creating a potential gap to trap PL vicinity. *PB* peroneus brevis, *PL* peroneus longus

becomes flat and "C"-shaped, encircling the peroneus longus (PL) tendon, giving the shape of a *"boomerang"* (Fig. 7.41b). Dynamic examination (on flexion and extension of the foot)—The PL tendon insinuates inside the tear area, with the superficial torn segments of the PB subluxating over the prominence of the lateral malleolus, producing a click.

Impression Peroneus brevis split tear.

Case Summary 42 A 65-year-old female patient presented with persistent pain and severe restriction of movement in her left knee joint, leading to impaired physical function over a period of several months. Despite the absence of clinical joint effusion, there was noticeable crepitus during movement and significant wasting of the anterior thigh muscle. A palpable, mobile mass was noted in the suprapatellar recess. An X-ray revealed grade IV knee osteoarthritis with increased radiopacity in the suprapatellar area (Fig. 7.42a). Further examination of the joint was performed via ultrasound.

Ultrasound Findings A large, hyperechoic, noncompressible lesion exhibiting posterior acoustic shadowing was observed in the anterior joint recess (Fig. 7.42b–d). This mass was mobile during knee flexion and dynamic scanning, accompanied by low-grade Doppler activity. The synovial membrane appeared thick and hypoechoic but not branched or frond-like in appearance (Fig. 7.42b–c). Severe-grade osteophytes were noted medially, yet the medial meniscus remained intact and was not extruded. In the lateral aspect, measurement of femoral cartilage thickness was hindered by a loose body obstructing the area (Fig. 7.42e). On the flexed knee, echogenic cartilage with nonuniform thickness was revealed (Fig. 7.42f). Posteriorly, anechoic compressible superficial Baker's cyst or hypoanechoic compressible fluid collection surrounding the semimembranosus tendon has not been documented.

Impression Synovial chondromatosis with synovial hypertrophy in knee osteoarthritis.

Case Summary 43 A 27-year-old female presented with discomfort localized to her left distal forearm, adjacent to the wrist joint, for the past few months, aggravated particularly during daily chores such as cooking, chopping vegetables, gripping objects tightly, lifting weights, doing laundry, washing her hands, and manipulating jars and door locks. There was no wrist joint swelling. Her medical history was unremarkable for diabetes mellitus, hypothyroidism, rheumatoid arthritis, or any recent trauma or childbirth. Maximum tenderness was noted over the distal radius vicinity to the styloid process. The Finkelstein test was positive. Additionally, a painless, soft, cystic mass with a smooth edge that did not adhere to the

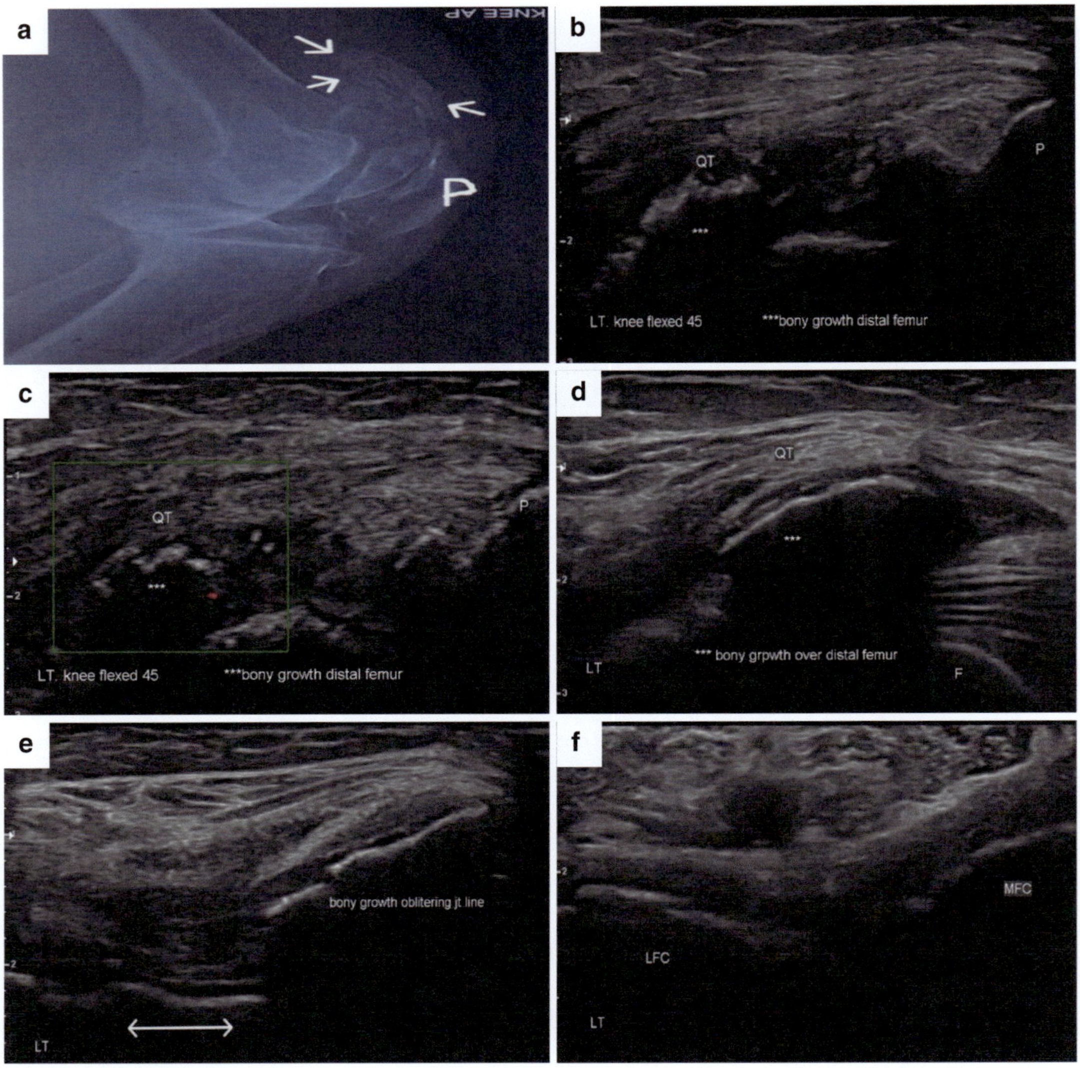

Fig. 7.42 Synovial chondromatosis with synovial hypertrophy in knee osteoarthritis. (**a**). X-ray revealed a radiopaque mass in the suprapatellar and prepatellar areas (white arrows). (**b**, **c**) Longitudinal scans of the suprapatellar knee revealed hyperechoic loose bodies with posterior acoustic shadowing (asterisks) impacted in the anterior joint recess. (**d**) Short axis scan of the suprapatellar flexed knee depicted hyperechoic mass (double arrows) with posterior acoustic shadowing obscured over the femoral condyle. (**e**, **f**) Transverse scans of the suprapatellar flexed knee explored reduced femoral condylar cartilage thickness. *LFC* lateral femoral condyle, *MFC* medial femoral condyle, *P* patella, *QT* quadriceps tendon

overlying skin, soft tissue, or underlying bone was revealed. The cyst became more pronounced with wrist flexion. Further examination via ultrasound was performed.

Ultrasound Findings Examination of the first dorsal wrist compartment revealed the absence of a hypoechoic and thickened synovial sheath surrounding the abductor pollicis longus (APL) and extensor pollicis brevis (EPB) tendons. Within this compartment, three tendons were identified, comprising one EPB and two APLs (Fig. 7.43a–b). Notably, the EPB was delineated from the APL by a hypoechoic fibrous septum (Fig. 7.43b), and the tendons displayed fibrillar echotexture. The tendons were not thickened. Furthermore, a poorly compressible, anechoic mass (Fig. 7.43c–d) was detected beneath the

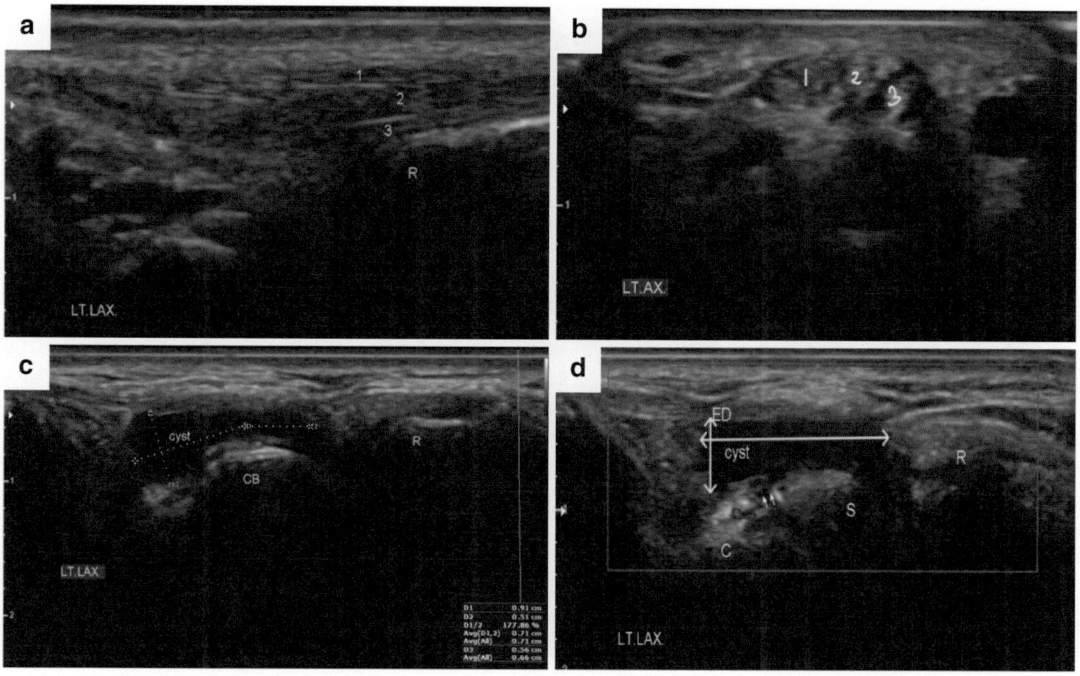

Fig. 7.43 Dorsal wrist ganglion cyst and de Quervain's tenosynovitis. (**a**, **b**) Longitudinal (**a**) and short axis (**b**) scans, respectively of the first dorsal wrist compartment revealed three extensor tendons (**b**, 1-APL, 2-accessory APL, 3-EPB). (**c**, **d**) Longitudinal scans of the dorsal wrist explored an anechoic, poorly compressible cystic mass (**c**, **d**) between carpal bones and distal radius (**d**, double arrows). *APL* abductor pollicis longus, *C/CB* carpal bone, *EPB* extensor pollicis brevis, *ED* extensor digitorum, *R* radius, *S* scaphoid

extensor digitorum tendon, which exhibited no heightened Doppler activity in its wall. This cyst measured 1.42 × 0.56 cm in the longitudinal dimension and was positioned distal to the joint line.

Impressions Dorsal wrist ganglion cyst and de Quervain's tenosynovitis.

Case Summary 44 A 55-year-old woman presented with primary concern of ongoing pain and swelling in her right ankle that had persisted for several months. She reported that the discomfort worsened with standing and walking during her daily activities but improved with rest. History of any recent or previous ankle injuries was insignificant; no history of joint pain elsewhere was reported. Her medical history was negative for diabetes mellitus, hypothyroidism, or chronic inflammatory arthritis. She also noted experiencing mild pain on the outer side of her ankle. Upon physical examination, tenderness was revealed at the anterior talocrural joint; both anterior and posterior drawer tests yielded negative results. X-ray imaging of the ankle revealed no significant soft tissue or bony abnormalities. Further evaluation of the ankle under ultrasound provided additional insights.

Ultrasound Findings Anteriorly, a decrease in cartilage thickness was observed on the talar dome, particularly on the medial side. Cartilage thickness was lower on the talar dome and greater on the medial aspect (Fig. 7.44a). In the inframalleolar region, the peroneal tendons appeared thick and hypoechoic (Fig. 7.44b). A hyperechoic bony growth originating from the lateral calcaneus pushed the peroneal tendons laterally (Fig. 7.44c–d), although the integrity of the tendons remained intact. Both the anterior talofibular ligament and the calcaneofibular ligament were found to be intact, as confirmed by both static and dynamic scanning.

Impression Osteoarthritis of the talocrural joint with peroneal tendinosis.

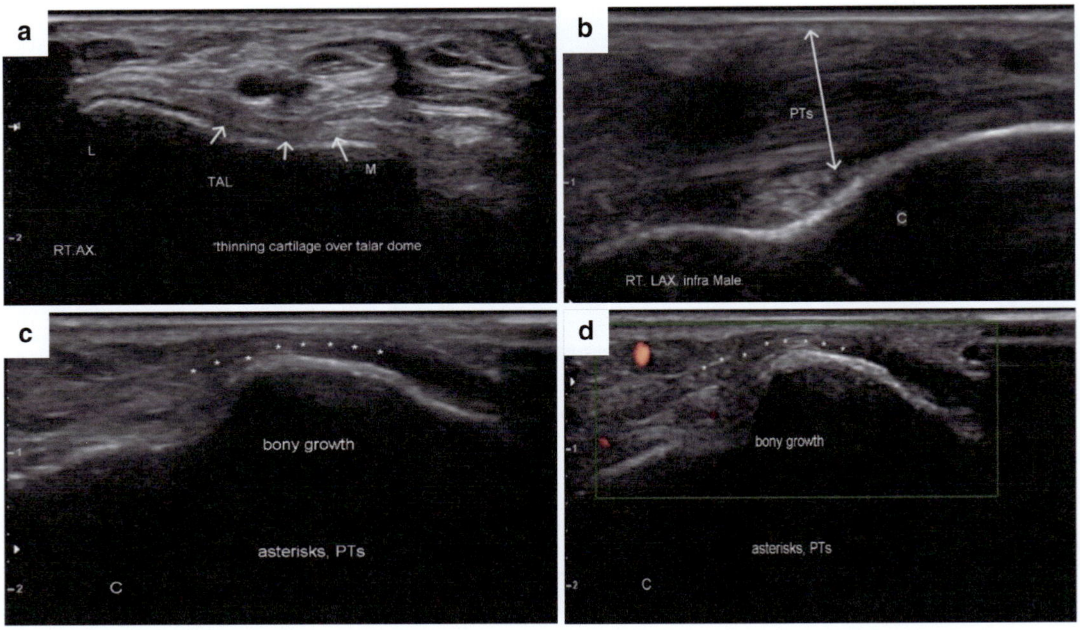

Fig. 7.44 Osteoarthritis of the talocrural joint with peroneal tendinosis. (**a**) Short axis scan of the anterior ankle revealed reduced articular cartilage thickness over the talar dome (white arrows). (**b**) Lateral oblique longitudinal scan of the ankle (inferior to lateral malleolus) unveiled thick, hypoechoic, and afibrillar PTs. (**c**, **d**) Longitudinal scans over the lateral ankle depicted hypoechoic PTs pushed by the calcaneal (bony) growth. *AX* axial, *C* calcaneus, *LAX* long axis, *L* lateral, *M* medial, *PTs* peroneal tendons, *TAL* talar, *RT* right

Case Summary 45 A 24-year-old woman presented with complaints of pain in her right dorsal hand and wrist, which interfered with her daily activities. She also noted experiencing tingling in the volar fingers, especially the first three, primarily at night. The patient recounted a fall that occurred a month earlier, which resulted in an injury to the dorso-radial area of her wrist and hand, causing persistent discomfort during her everyday tasks. Clinical examination revealed wrist joint line and distal dorsal forearm tenderness. The patient experienced pain when resisting finger extension and when attempting to abduct the wrist toward the ulnar side. Grade III tenderness was identified in the dorsal wrist region, and an attempt to perform Phalen's maneuver was thwarted by the patient's pain. Further examination via ultrasound was performed.

Ultrasound Findings In the sixth dorsal compartment, a hypoechoic-anechoic, poorly compressible, and thick synovial sheath enveloped the fibrillar extensor carpi ulnaris tendon (Fig. 7.45a–b). Localized tenderness was elicited during sonopalpation. Further scanning of the fourth dorsal compartment of the wrist revealed a thick hypoechoic synovial sheath enveloping the extensor digitorum and extensor indicis tendons, with no signs of heightened Doppler activity (Fig. 7.45c). The scanning process was extended to the volar side of the wrist, where an enlarged cross-sectional area of the median nerve was identified and measured 15.2 mm^2 (Fig. 7.45d). Longitudinal scanning revealed a thickened flexor retinaculum compressing the median nerve, with the epineurium appearing hyperechoic and no evidence of nerve bifurcation.

Impressions Extensor digitorum and extensor carpi ulnaris tenosynovitis with severe carpal tunnel syndrome.

Case Summary 46 A 55-year-old male reported experiencing tingling and sharp pain in the elbow,

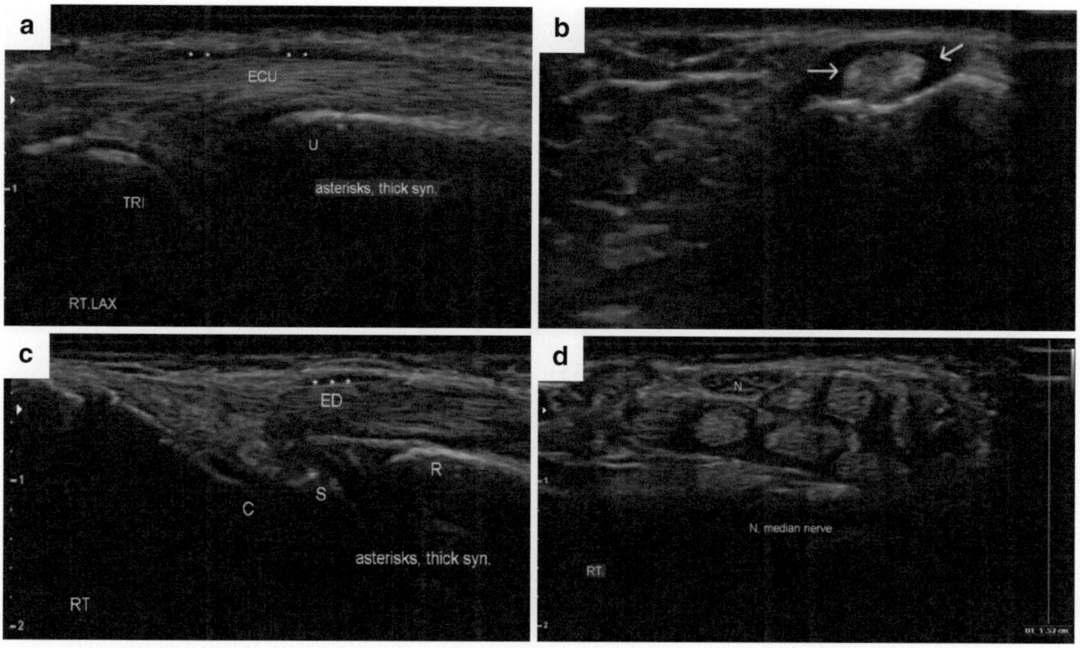

Fig. 7.45 Extensor carpi ulnaris and extensor digitorum tenosynovitis with carpal tunnel syndrome. (**a**, **b**) Longitudinal (**a**, asterisks) and short axis (**b**, arrows) scans, respectively over the dorsal wrist revealed thick and hypoechoic tenosynovial sheath around the fibrillar ECU tendon. (**c**) Longitudinal scan over the dorsal wrist depicted thick and hypoechoic tenosynovial sheath around the fibrillar ED tendon (asterisks). (**d**)Short axis scan of the volar wrist at the carpal tunnel explored increased cross-sectional area of the median nerve. *ECU* extensor carpi ulnaris, *ED* extensor digitorum, *N* median nerve, *R* radius, *S* scaphoid, *U* ulna

which radiated along the inner side of the forearm and was distributed down the fourth and fifth fingers for the past three months. Tinel's sign was positive at the cubital tunnel. Further scrutiny under ultrasound was performed.

Ultrasound Findings An anechoic and poorly compressible cystic mass in the distal cubital tunnel, which was located just lateral to the ulnar nerve (Fig. 7.46a–b). This cyst was noted to exert pressure on the nerve (Fig. 7.46b), causing it to flatten, and no Doppler signal was noted. The cyst neither communicated with the elbow joint (Fig. 7.46c) nor extended to the cubital tunnel (Fig. 7.46d). Ultrasound-guided cyst aspiration was carried out, followed by intralesional steroid injection (Fig. 7.46b).

Impression Epineural cyst of the ulnar nerve.

Case Summary 47 A middle-aged individual from Bangladesh presented with right foot drop and noticeable leg muscle wasting, especially on the outer side. Initially, he reported vague tingling sensations that remained clueless until lateral knee ultrasound was conducted. The knee joint was not swollen, and the range of motion of the joint was not restricted. Moreover, the left leg was more wasted than its right leg was. Ankle dorsiflexion and eversion were compromised. Common peroneal nerve compressive neuropathy was the provisional diagnosis. Ultrasound examination of the lateral knee was performed.

Ultrasound Findings A circumscribed, anechoic-hypoechoic, poorly compressible cystic lesion measuring 1.81 cm × 1.50 cm (Fig. 7.47a–b), noncommunicating with the joint cavity and compressing the common peroneal nerve vicinity, was noted at the fibular neck (Fib. 5.47b). The cystic lesion revealed posterior acoustic enhancement (Fig. 7.47a–b). Doppler activity was not noted in the cyst wall.

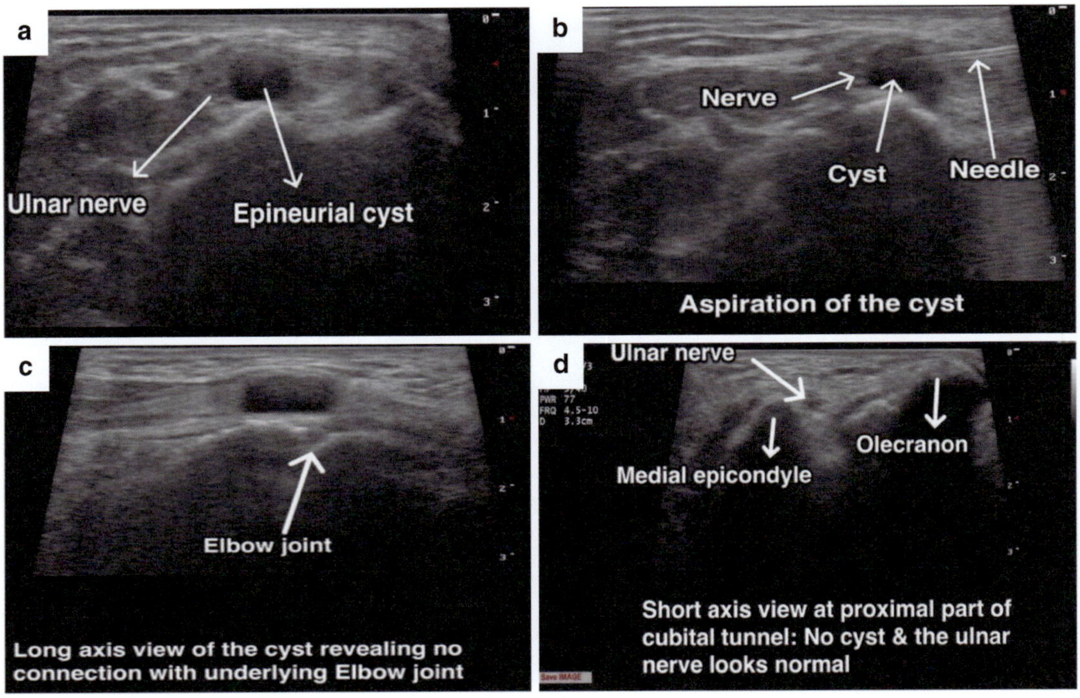

Fig. 7.46 Epineural cyst of the ulnar nerve. (**a**) Short axis scan of the medial elbow at medial epicondyle revealed noncompressible anechoic cyst (arrow) close to the nerve (arrow). (**b**) Short axis scan of the medial elbow depicted ultrasound-guided in-plane cyst aspiration (white arrows, needle trajectory). (**c**) Longitudinal scan of the medial elbow explored no connection between the cyst and the joint cavity. (**d**) The cyst did not extend to the proximal cubital tunnel as demonstrated on short axis scanning of the medial elbow

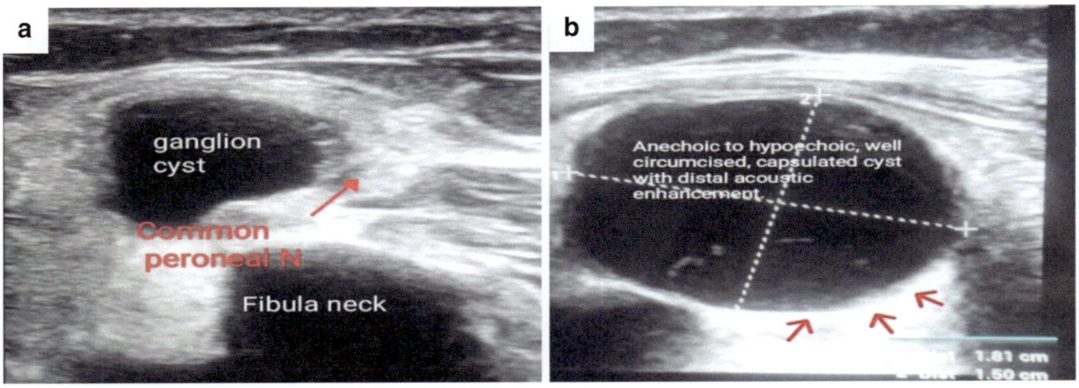

Fig. 7.47 Ganglion cyst compressing the common peroneal nerve at the fibular neck. (**a**) Short axis scan at the fibular neck revealed an anechoic, poorly compressible cystic mass compressing the adjacent common peroneal nerve (red arrow). (**b**) Short axis scan of the cyst explored the posterior acoustic enhancement artifact (red arrows). *Common peroneal N* common peroneal nerve

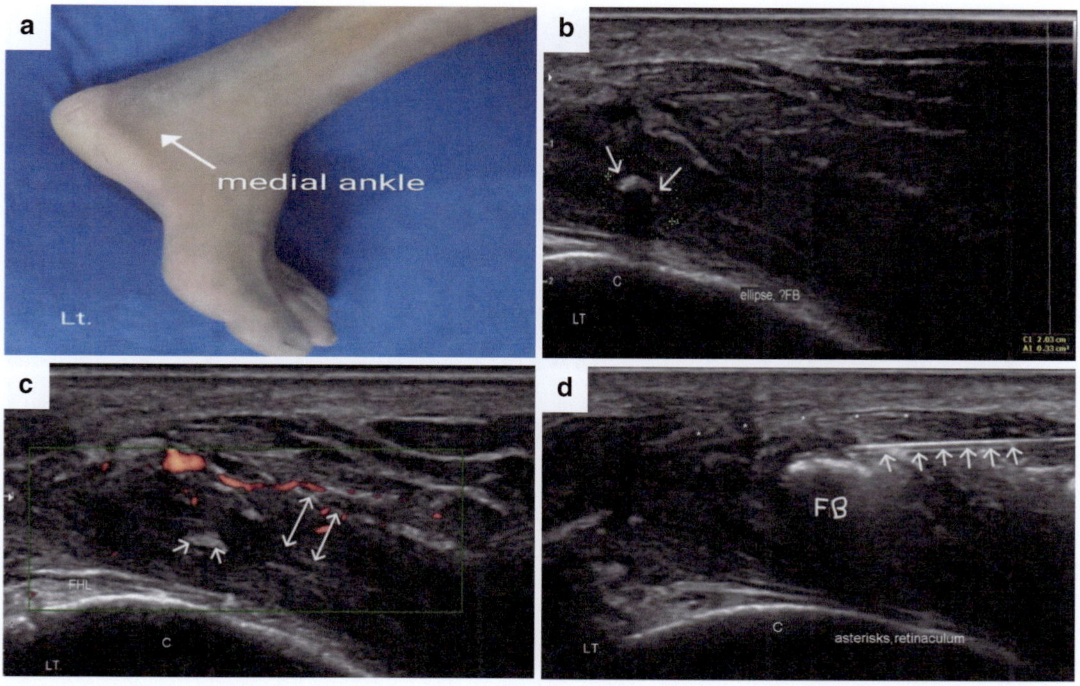

Fig. 7.48 Foreign body in the medial ankle compartment with flexor tenosynovitis. (**a**) Focal swelling of the medial ankle. (**b–d**) Longitudinal scans of the medial ankle revealed a hyperechoic, noncompressible mass (ellipse) with the posterior acoustic shadowing (white arrows) (**b–d**) and afibrillar flexor tendons with increased Doppler signal (**c**). (**c**) The tibial nerve appeared thick and hypoechoic with loss of the fascicular pattern (double arrows). (**d**) Longitudinal scan revealed needle trajectory (white arrows) during in-plane ultrasound injection in the medial ankle compartment. *C* calcaneus, *FB* foreign body, *FHL* flexor hallucis longus, *Lt* left

Impressions Ganglion cyst compressing the common peroneal nerve at the fibular neck.

Case Summary 48 A 65-year-old male presented with a chief complaint of pain and swelling, accompanied by numbness in the medial ankle, heel, and sole, which persisted for approximately six weeks (Fig. 7.48a). The patient recalled having a bamboo piece lodged in his left foot, which he managed to remove; however, he was unsure if any remnants were left behind. Upon physical examination, the medial ankle was visibly swollen, and a positive Tinel's sign was detected. An X-ray of the ankle indicated soft tissue swelling, prompting further investigation. Ultrasound scanning of the medial ankle was performed.

Ultrasound Findings The medial ankle compartment exhibited enlargement with outward bulging of the flexor retinaculum. A hyperechoic mass with posterior acoustic shadowing was revealed (Fig. 7.48b–d). The tibialis posterior, flexor halluces longus, and flexor digitorum tendons appeared hypoechoic with loss of the fibrillar pattern; nevertheless, they remained intact as assessed dynamically, and there was increased Doppler activity. The posterior tibial nerve appeared enlarged, with a cross-sectional area of 3.36 cm. The tibial nerve lost its fascicular pattern. The posterior tibial artery demonstrated intact flow.

Impression Foreign body in the medial ankle with flexor tenosynovitis.

Case Summary 49 A patient reported the complaint of medial knee pain with limping and compromised daily activities, including walking, standing from sitting, and bending the knee for a few days. Physical examination revealed no joint line tenderness, and maximum focal tenderness

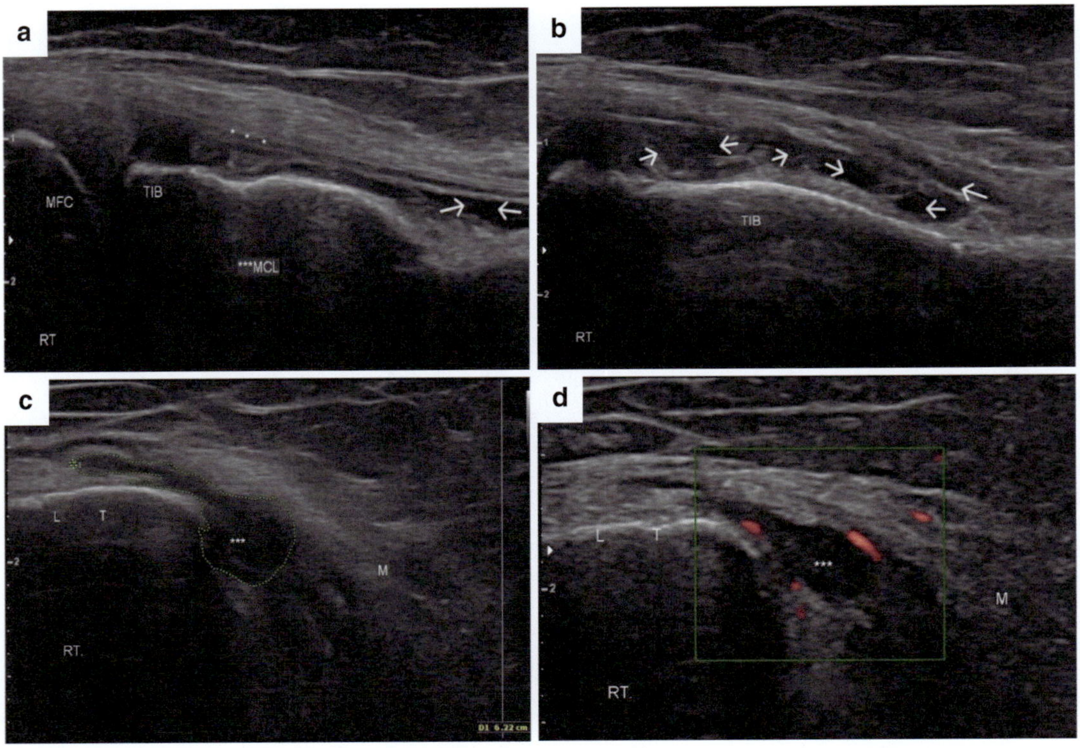

Fig. 7.49 Anserine bursitis. (**a**, **b**) Longitudinal scans over the proximal medial tibia revealed hypoechoic-anechoic compressible collection in the hypoechoic anserine bursa (white arrows). (**c**, **d**) Short axis scans of the proximal medial tibia depicted increased cross-sectional area of the bursa (**c**) with increased Doppler activity (**d**) in the bursal wall (asterisks). *L* lateral, *MFC* medial femoral condyle, *M* medial, *RT* right, *T* tibia, *TIB* tibia

was elicited in the proximal medial tibia just below the medial joint line. There was no sign of clinical effusion in the anterior joint recess. X-ray revealed a medial joint line osteophyte. He had no other joint complaints. Further examination of the medial knee via ultrasound was performed.

Ultrasound Findings Medially, attachment of the fibrillar pes anserina tendon to the proximal medial tibia was revealed. Anechoic compressible collection was noted around the tendon (Fig. 7.49a–c), with an increased Doppler signal (Fig. 7.49d).

Impression Anserine bursitis.

Case Summary 50 A 50-year-old female presented with a chief complaint of persistent pain in her right shoulder during movement over the course of several months. The patient denied experiencing any significant morning stiffness, headache, weight loss, or fever. She reported a recent fall but had no known history of diabetes mellitus, hypertension, or ischemic heart disease. Upon examination, the patient exhibited painful movements in the affected shoulder, with a positive painful arc and Hawkin's maneuver. Apley's scratch test was negative. External rotation elicited pain when the shoulder was in abduction or neutral positions. X-ray revealed cortical erosion over the greater tuberosity (Fig. 7.50a). Further assessment under ultrasound was performed (Fig. 7.50b–h).

Ultrasound Findings The long head of the biceps tendon (LHBT) exhibited a fibrillar pattern with associated peri-tendon effusion, while there was no notable increase in Doppler activity. The intra-articular LHBT remained intact. The synovial sheath surrounding the LHBT appeared thick. In contrast, the supraspinatus tendon (SST) was thickened (Fig. 7.50c), with the SST foot-

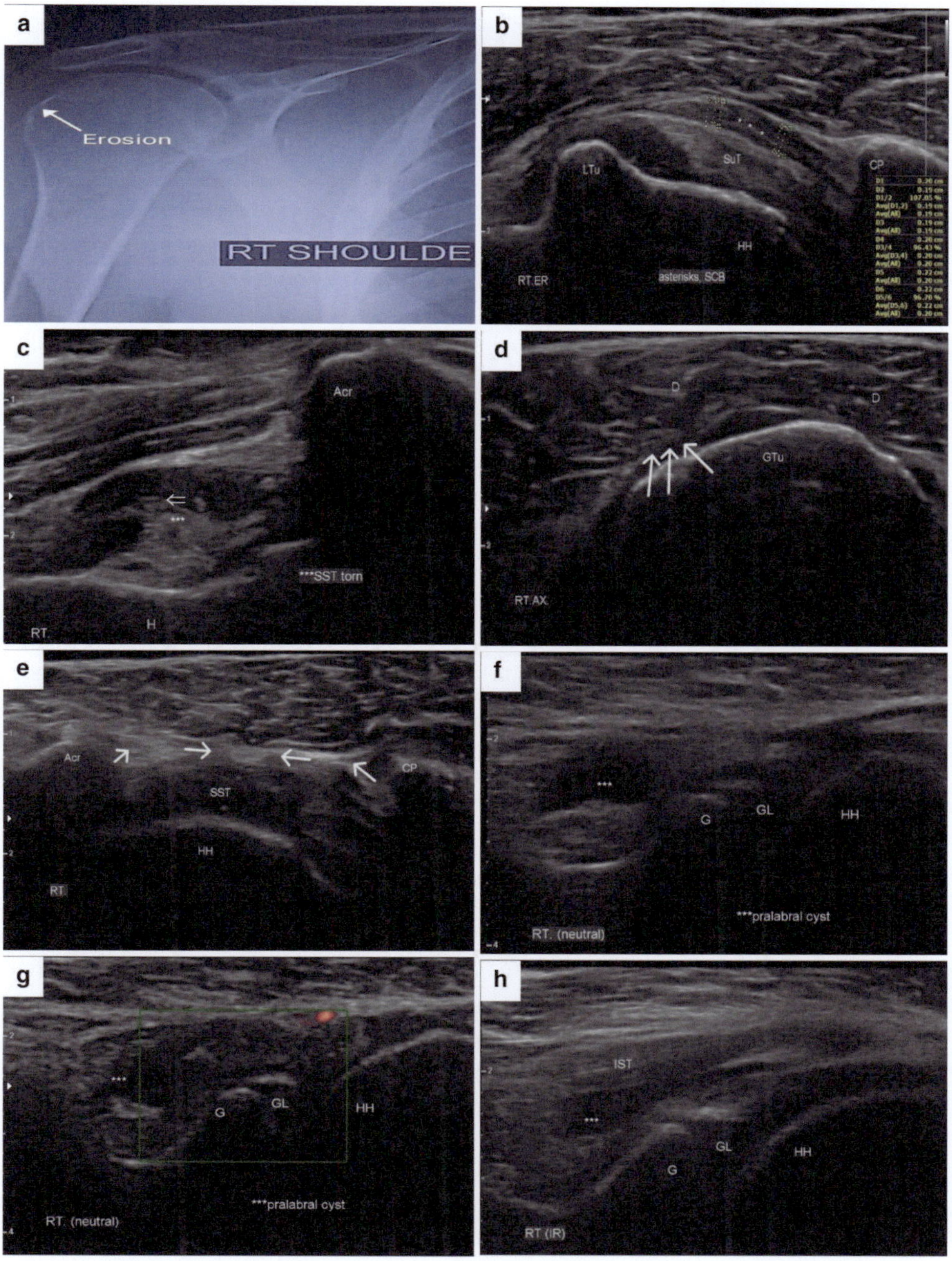

Fig. 7.50 Supraspinatus tendon tear with paralabral cyst. (**a**) X-ray shoulder revealed radioopacity and cortical erosion over the GTu (white arrow). (**b**) Axial scan of the anterior shoulder at the coracoid process level revealing SCB bursal thickening (asterisks). (**c**) Longitudinal scan on the lateral shoulder revealed a thick and hypoechoic SASD bursa (double arrows) and thick, hypoechoic-echogenic SST (asterisks). (**d**) Short axis scan of the GTu depicted SST (white arrows) absent with deltoid herniation. (**e**) Short axis scan at acromion and coracoid processes level demonstrated thick and hypoechoic SST under the CAL (white arrows). (**f–h**) Short axis scans of the posterior GH joint explored an anechoic, noncompressible cyst communicating with the joint cavity through the torn GL (asterisks). *AX* short axis, *GTu* greater tuberosity, *GH* glenohumeral, *G* glenoid, *GL* glenoid labrum, *H* humerus, *HH* humeral head, *IST* infraspinatus tendon, *LHBT* long head of the biceps tendon, *LAX* long axis, *LTu* lesser tuberosity, *SCB* subcoracoid bursa, *SST* supraspinatus tendon, *SOH* shaft of the humerus

print at the greater tuberosity (GTu) completely absent (Fig. 7.50d), alongside deltoid herniation. Additionally, a cortical defect was observed in the greater tuberosity. The subcoracoid bursa (Fig. 7.50b) was noted to be thickened without anechoic and compressible accumulation. Laterally, the subacromial subdeltoid bursa (SASD) appeared thick and hypoechogenic; nevertheless it did not bunch at the acromion during shoulder abduction. The SASD bursa did not extend over the hyperechoic transverse humeral ligament. The coracoacromial ligament remained fibrillar and not thickened (Fig. 7.50e). Posteriorly, the cartilage covering the humeral head appeared echogenic, although the thickness of the humeral head (HH) was maintained. The posterosuperior glenoid labrum was hypoechoic and contained an anechoic cleft within it. Furthermore, an anechoic compressible collection was detected medially, beneath the infraspinatus tendon and over the glenoid labrum, becoming more pronounced during external rotation (Fig. 7.50f–h).

Impressions Incomplete full-thickness supraspinatus tendon tears, subcoracoid bursal thickening, posterosuperior glenoid labrum tears, and paralabral cysts.

Case Summary 51 A 48-year-old male presented with a history of persistent right lateral knee pain accompanied by localized swelling at the joint line. The patient attributed the onset of symptoms to a recent incident related to an unaccustomed knee position while attempting fall prevention. He denied experiencing any other symptoms and showed no signs of joint effusion, audible crepitus during movement, or significant wasting of the thigh muscle. Tenderness was noted upon palpation of the lateral knee joint line. X-ray imaging revealed no evidence of osteophyte formation, suggesting that further investigation of the joint via ultrasound revealed the following information.

Ultrasound Findings The anterior joint recess did not exhibit any distension from a compressible collection. Later, the lateral collateral ligament appeared thick and hypoechoic (Fig. 7.51a–b). A smooth, immobile, noncompressible mass was observed posterolaterally on the lateral femoral condyle (Fig. 7.51c–d). The lateral meniscal body displayed an anechoic cleft within it (Fig. 7.51a–b). No anechoic, compressible, superficial Baker's cyst was identified posteriorly, nor was there any compressible, anechoic collection around the semimembranosus tendon. The posterior horn of the medial meniscus was intact.

Impression Knee lateral meniscal tear with calcified mass over the lateral femoral condyle.

Case Summary 52 A 50-year-old male patient presented with complaints of pain and swelling in his right elbow; this patient exhibited inflammatory characteristics and responded well to diclofenac sodium and steroid treatment but returned to follow-up with pain recurrence upon discontinuation of medication. He denied experiencing pain in other joints, as well as heel pain, neck pain, or low back pain. The patient tested negative for rheumatoid factor, and the erythrocyte sedimentation rate was elevated. Physical examination revealed a limited range of motion in the affected joint, with flexion and extension being particularly restricted. X-ray of the elbow revealed soft tissue swelling. Undifferentiated inflammatory arthritis was the provisional diagnosis. Ultrasound examination of the elbow was performed.

Ultrasound Findings Examination of the anterior radial and ulnar joint recesses indicated a notable thickening of the synovial membrane, which was marked by hypoechoic synovial hypertrophy and increased Doppler activity (Fig. 7.52a–b). This synovial hypertrophy was similarly noted in the medial and posterior recesses. In the posterior region, the synovial membrane appeared thick, hypoechoic, and hypertrophied (Fig. 7.52c), with elevated Doppler signals suggesting increased vascularity (Fig. 7.52d). The lateral aspect of the elbow showed that both the common extensor tendon and the radial collateral ligament remained intact

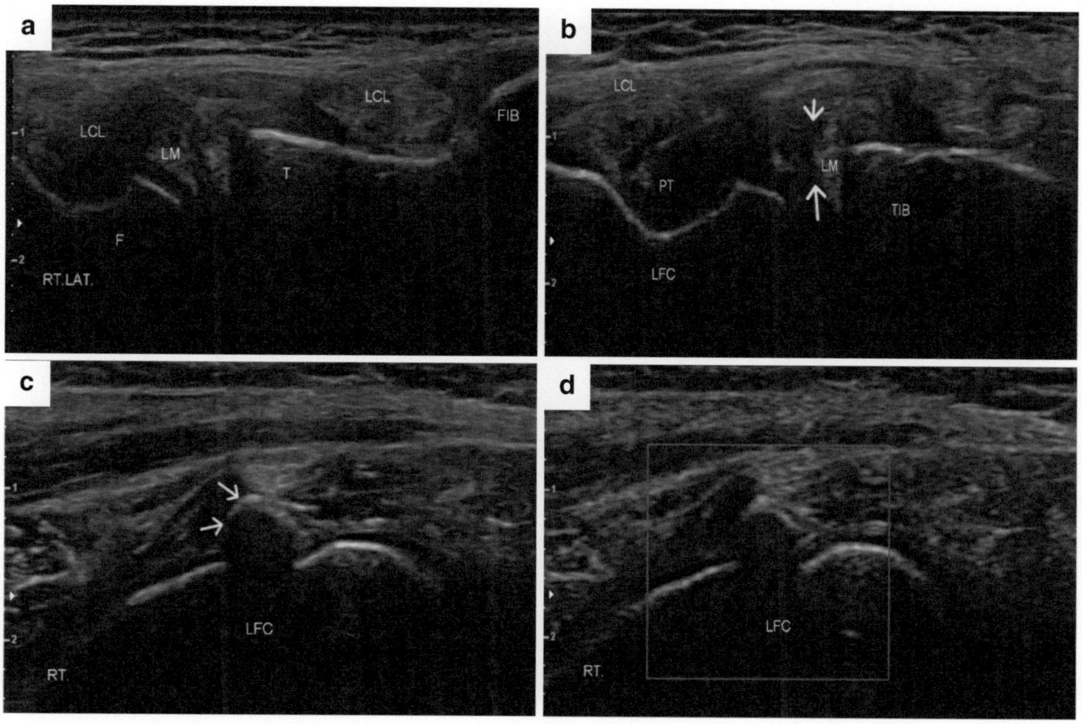

Fig. 7.51 Knee lateral meniscal tear. (**a, b**) Longitudinal scans of lateral knee revealed an anechoic cleft (white arrows) within the LM, meniscus was extruded laterally. (**c, d**) Short axis scans over the LFC condyle explored a hyperechoic mass with posterior acoustic shadowing (arrows). *LFC* lateral femoral condyle, *LM* lateral meniscus, *LCL* lateral collateral ligament

and fibrillar. Furthermore, the distal attachment of the long head of the biceps tendon was verified as intact in the anterior area. In the posterior region, both the triceps muscle and tendon were confirmed to be intact during both dynamic and static assessments.

Impression Elbow inflammatory synovitis.

Case Summary 53 A 35-year-old man was referred for an ultrasound evaluation of his right shoulder after experiencing a sudden emergence of symptoms while performing strenuous screw-fitting activities. At the moment of injury, he noticed a distinct popping sound emanating from his right shoulder. This incident was followed by the development of pain, restricted mobility, and swelling in the shoulder region. The patient highlighted considerable challenges in executing external rotation movements. Furthermore, an examination under ultrasound was performed.

Ultrasound Findings An echogenic lesion was detected in the area of the clavicular head of the right pectoralis major muscle, which presented an increased Doppler signal. Furthermore, a retracted segment of the torn clavicular portion of the pectoralis major muscle was noted, accompanied by the presence of hematoma (Fig. 7.53a–b).

Impression Pectoralis major muscle tear.

Case Summary 54 An adolescent male novice soccer player exhibited intermittent discomfort and pain in the lower outer region of his right leg (Fig. 7.54a), particularly when walking or performing weight-bearing daily physical activity. Further examination via ultrasound was performed.

Ultrasound Findings The peroneus longus muscle protruded through the interrupted fascial

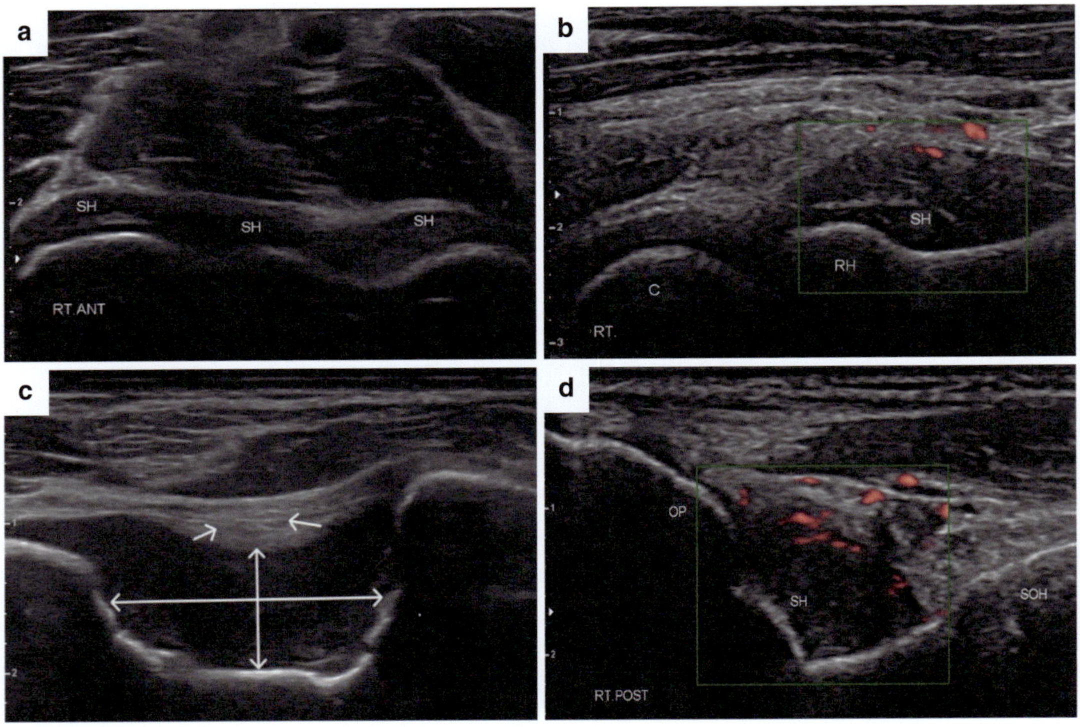

Fig. 7.52 Elbow inflammatory synovitis. (**a**, **b**) Transverse scans of the anterior partially flexed elbow revealed thick, hypoechoic synovium and echogenic cartilage. (**c**, **d**) Short axis scans of the flexed posterior elbow depicted noncompressible SH (**c**) (double arrows) in the posterior joint capsule (single arrows) with an increased Doppler signal (**d,** red dots). *C* capitellum, *OP* olecranon process, *RT* right, *RH* radial head, *SH* synovial hypertrophy

plane (Fig. 7.54b–d), with greater visibility on a short-axis image (Fig. 7.54d).

Impression Peroneus longus muscle herniation.

Case Summary 55 A 33-year-old male reported experiencing persistent and intense pain in his right shoulder, accompanied by symptoms indicative of impingement. During the physical examination, there was selective atrophy of the infraspinatus muscle area (Fig. 7.55a). Ultrasound examination of the posterior shoulder was performed.

Ultrasound Findings At the spino-glenoid notch, an anechoic, poorly compressible cystic mass with posterior acoustic enhancement was documented (Fig. 7.55b–c). There was no increased Doppler activity in the cyst wall.

Impression Paralabral cyst with infraspinatus muscle atrophy.

Case Summary 56 A man presented with a swollen and warm right ring finger (Fig. 7.56a) and experienced restricted mobility for several months. His condition improved with the use of pain relief medications. The patient was referred by a medical specialist to a physiatrist for a more comprehensive assessment via ultrasound.

Ultrasound Findings The subcutaneous fat appeared thick and hypoechoic (Fig. 7.6b–d). At the level of the proximal interphalangeal joint, bone erosion in the proximal and middle phalanges and joint space reduction were noted (Fig. 7.56c–d). The flexor digitorum superficialis and profundus tendons exhibited swelling, thickening, and hypoechoic echotexture, with loss of the fibrillar pattern (Fig. 7.56c–d). Furthermore,

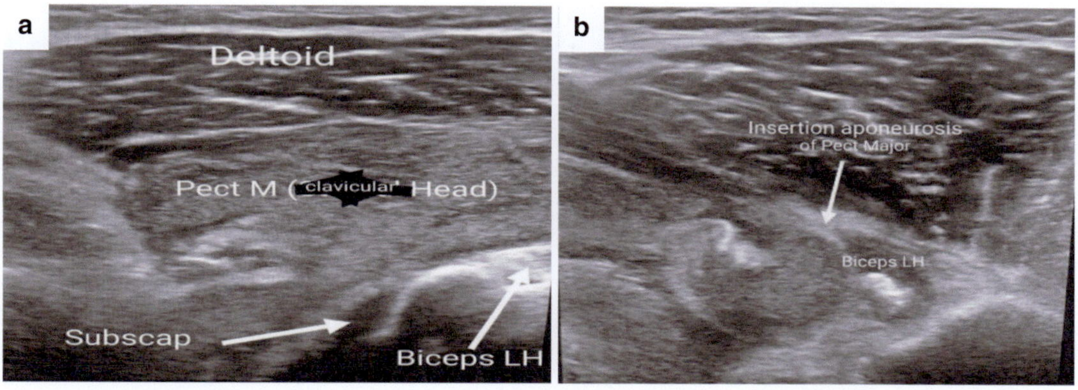

Fig. 7.53 Pectoralis major muscle tear. (**a**) Short axis scan of the anterior shoulder at the lesser tuberosity revealed torn, echogenic, and retracted clavicular part of the pectoralis major muscle in relation to the LHBT and subscapularis tendon (arrows). (**b**) Short axial scan of the anterior shoulder depicted aponeuretic insertion of retracted pectoralis major muscle (arrow) to the humerus in relation to LHBT. *LHBT/Biceps LH* long head of the biceps tendon, *Pect M* pectoralis major, *Subscap* subscapularis

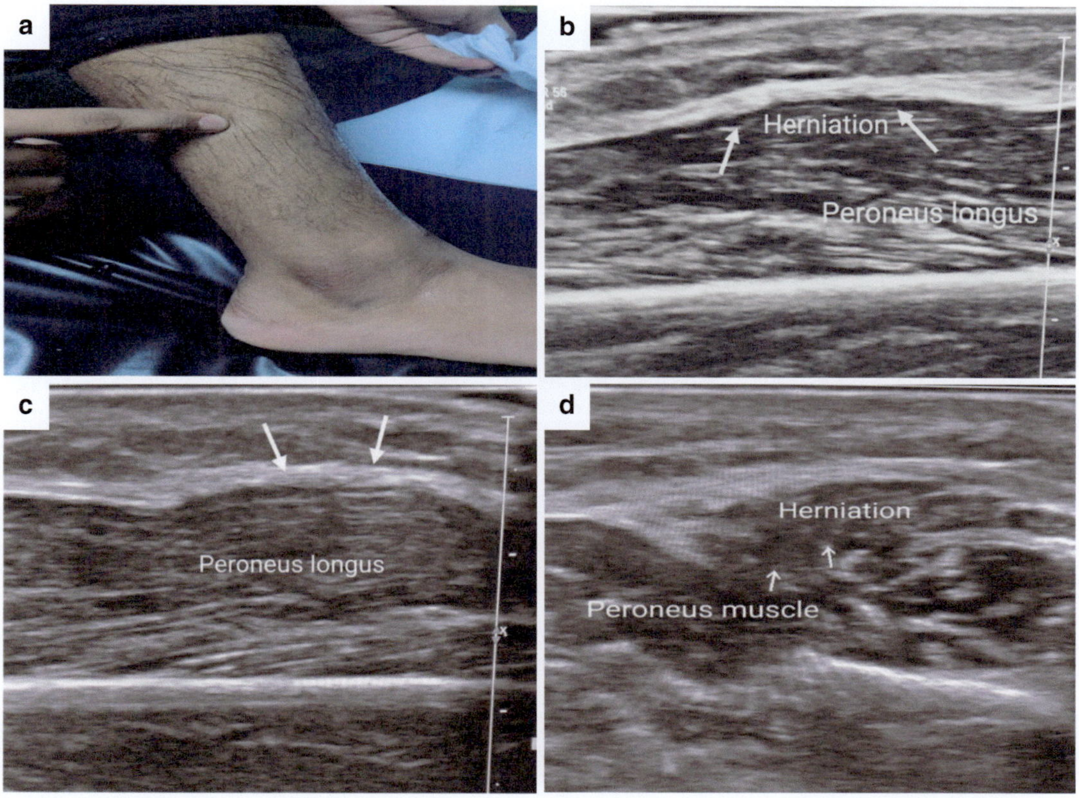

Fig. 7.54 Peroneus longus muscle herniation. (**a**) Index finger indicates focal area of pain at the lower one-third of the outer leg. (**b–d**) Longitudinal (**b**, **c**) and short axis (**d**) scans of the outer leg revealed hypoechoic and thick peroneus longus muscle herniated through the fibrous septum defect (arrows). *PL* peroneus longus

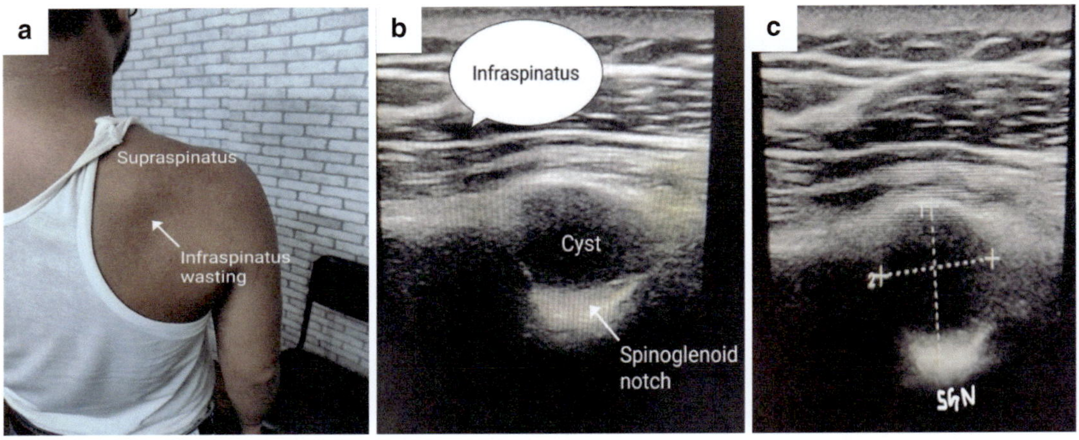

Fig. 7.55 Paralabral cyst with infraspinatus muscle atrophy. (**a**) The infraspinatus muscle area appeared wasted (white arrow). (**b**, **c**) Short axis scans of the posterior shoulder at the spino-glenoid notch (SGN) depicted the anechoic and noncompressible cyst. *SGN* spinoliglenoid notch

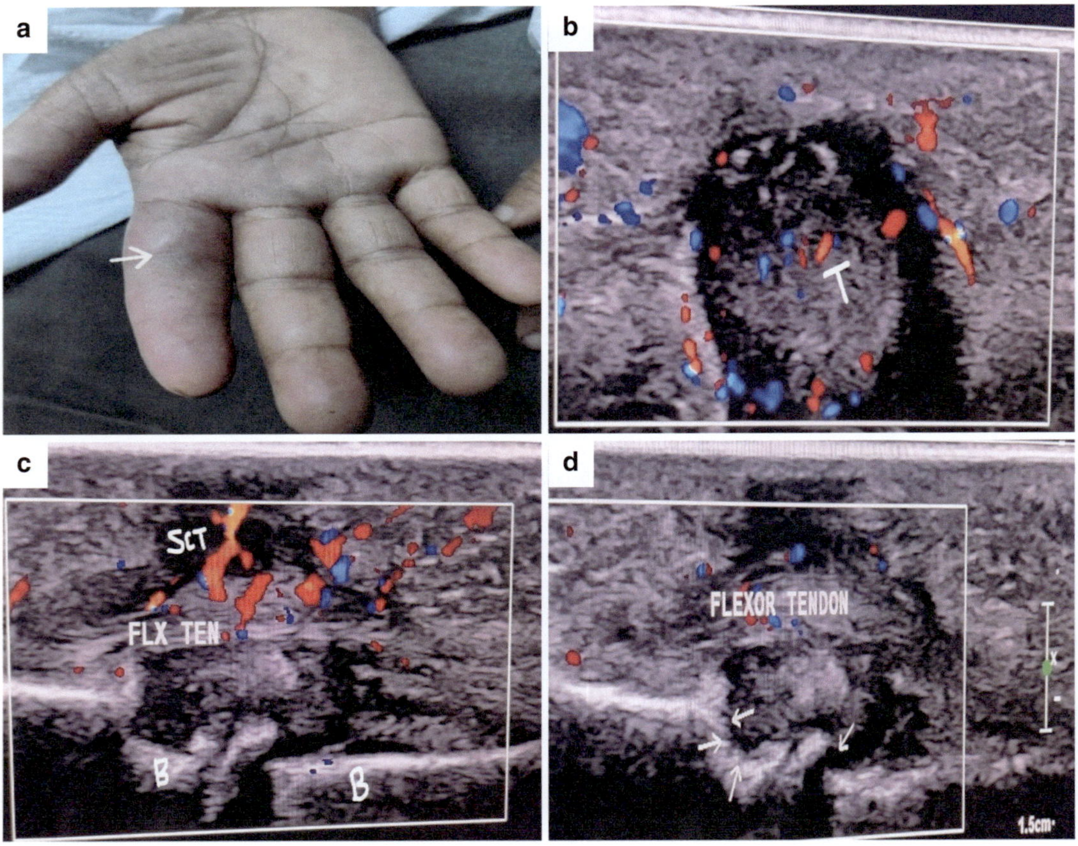

Fig. 7.56 Dactylitis. (**a**) Swollen volar aspect of the index finger (white arrow). (**b–d**) Short axis (**b, d**) and longitudinal (**c**) scans of the digit revealed a thick hypoechoic tenosynovial sheath around the hypoechoic-hyperechoic FLX TEN with increased Doppler activity (**b–d**). (**c–d**) Bone erosion (**d**, white arrows) with reduced interphalangeal joint space width. *B* bone, *FLX TEN* flexor tendon, *SCT* subcutaneous tissue, *T* tendon

an increase in Doppler activity was detected in the subcutaneous tissue and tendons (Fig. 7.56c–d).

Impression Psoriatic dactylitis.

Case Summary 57 A 29-year-old doctor described a sudden onset of swelling in his left calf, which was accompanied by increasing pain that eventually resulted in a sensation of tightness in the area (Fig. 7.57a). This condition affected the patient's normal walking speed during daily tasks. Although there was no direct trauma to the area, the incident might be associated with the unaccustomed body posture while lifting a weight. Upon physical examination, the findings included bruising on the left calf, a thinner appearance of the calf muscle, localized tenderness, and a noticeable difference in muscle tone compared with the right side. An ultrasound examination of the leg was performed.

Ultrasound Findings An anechoic and compressible mass was observed between the medial head of the gastrocnemius (MHG) and the soleus muscle (Fig. 7.57b–d). The MHG exhibited signs of tearing and roughness in the proximal region, although certain areas of the MHG appeared to be preserved (Fig. 7.57b–d).

Impression Medial head of gastrocnemius muscle tear.

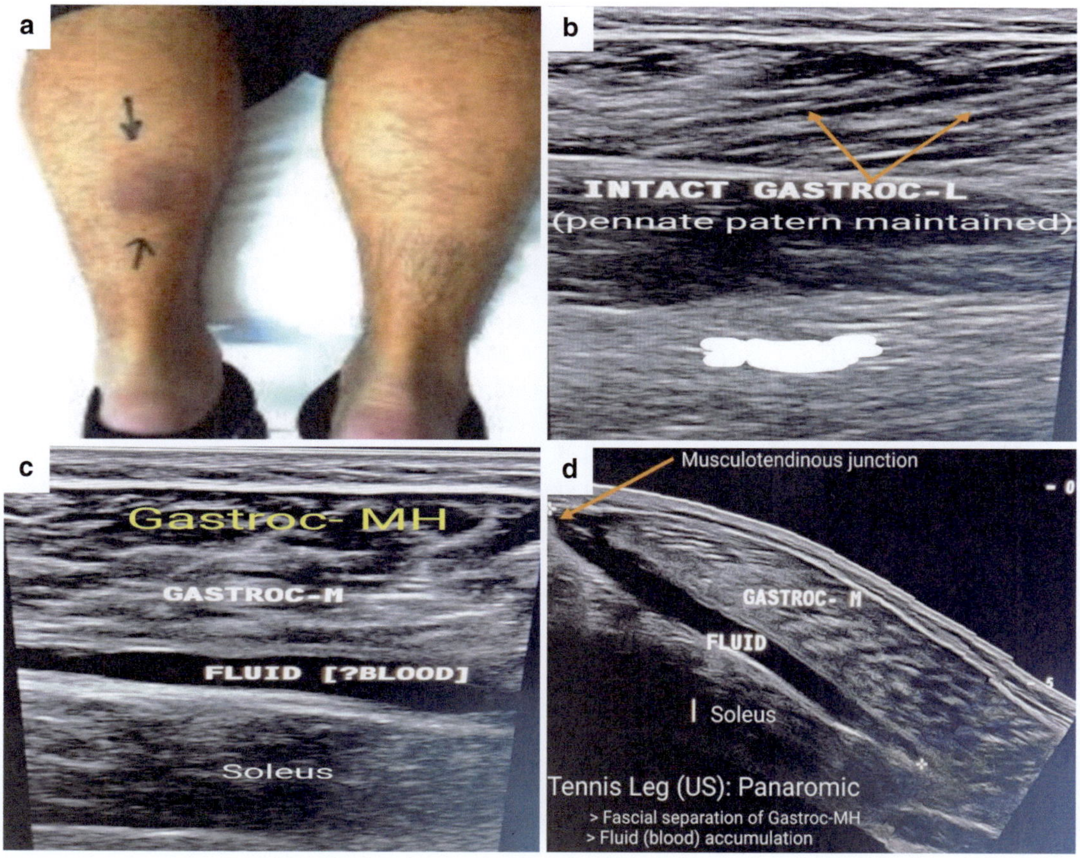

Fig. 7.57 Medial head of the gastrocnemius muscle tear. (**a**) Echymosis on the posterior leg (black arrows). (**b**) Longitudinal scan of the lateral leg revealed intact lateral head of the gastrocnemius muscle. (**c**) Longitudinal scan of the posterior leg depicted torn medial head of the gastrocnemius muscle with anechoic, compressible fluid (blood) collection above the soleus muscle. (**d**) Panoramic view explored blood accumulation between torn medial gastrocnemius and soleus. *MHG/Gastroc MH* medial head of the gastrocnemius

Case Summary 58 A 55-year-old patient complained of pain in the right shoulder joint and restricted mobility that had persisted for 3 months. He denied experiencing notable morning stiffness, headache, weight loss, or fever. There was no recent incident of falling, and he had no prior diagnoses of diabetes mellitus, hypertension, or ischemic heart disease. During the examination, the patient exhibited painful movements in the shoulder, a positive painful arc and Hawkin's maneuver, and a positive Apley's scratch test. Both shoulder abduction and external rotation were painful. Further evaluation under ultrasound was performed.

Ultrasound Findings The long head of the biceps tendon (LHBT) exhibited a fibrillar pattern, accompanied by peri-tendon compressible, anechoic effusion, and increased Doppler activity (Fig. 7.58a–c). A thick, hypoechoic synovial sheath surrounding the LHBT was noted (Fig. 7.58a–b). The subacromial-subdeltoid (SASD) bursa appeared thick and hypoechoic, with a thickness of 2.0 mm (Fig. 7.58d); nevertheless, the SASD bursa did not bunch while abducting the shoulder.

The bursal supraspinatus tendon (SST) appeared hypoechoic (Fig. 7.58e). Cortical irregularity with a partial thickness tear of the SST was revealed over the humeral head (Fig. 7.58e–f). A full-thickness tear of the SST was identified at the greater tuberosity footprint, characterized by a loss of cortical irregularity (Fig. 7.58g–h). Both abduction and external rotation were limiting, as revealed dynamically. The cartilage of the humeral head appeared echogenic; however, its contour was maintained, but cortical integrity was distorted (Fig. 7.58e–f). The triangular hyperechoic pattern of the posterosuperior glenoid labrum was absent, but no tears or extrusions were detected during dynamic scanning, and there was no visible glenohumeral joint effusion.

Impression A full-thickness supraspinatus tendon tear with a cortical defect and a long head of biceps tendon tenosynovitis.

Case Summary 59 A young male patient reported experiencing intense pain in the front and side areas of his chest after sustaining an impact during a football match the day before. He had trouble breathing deeply, and the discomfort intensified with physical movement, as well as during coughing and sneezing. An urgent ultrasound assessment revealed fractures in both the tenth and 11th ribs.

Ultrasound Findings Discontinuation of the 11th rib cortex was observed via both static and dynamic scans (Fig. 7.59a–b). The fracture was measured to be 1.44 cm away from the corresponding costochondral junction.

Impression Rib fracture.

Case Summary 60 A 35-year-old man reported practicing as a physiatrist, with the complaint of sudden and intense ankle pain and swelling that had progressed for a few days. He reported a previous history of occasional nonspecific joint discomfort. During the physical examination, Grade 2 tenderness was noted in the tibio-talar joint, and the patient exhibited a restricted range of motion. X-ray results of the foot revealed no notable abnormalities. He reported no additional joint issues, lacked a family history of chronic arthritis, and did not suffer from morning stiffness or any recent injuries to the joint. He had no diabetes mellitus or hypertension.

Ultrasound Findings The ultrasound assessment revealed an increase in the thickness of the synovial membrane in the talo-tibial joint, accompanied by a Doppler signal (Fig. 7.60a–b). Additionally, there was anechoic compressible fluid collection featuring a bright hyperechoic floating mass within the joint recess (Fig. 7.60a). Evidence of a double contour sign was also noted (Fig. 7.60a).

Impression Gouty arthritis.

Case Summary 61 A 23-year-old female patient had been suffering from swelling and discomfort in her left knee for the last 11 years, with

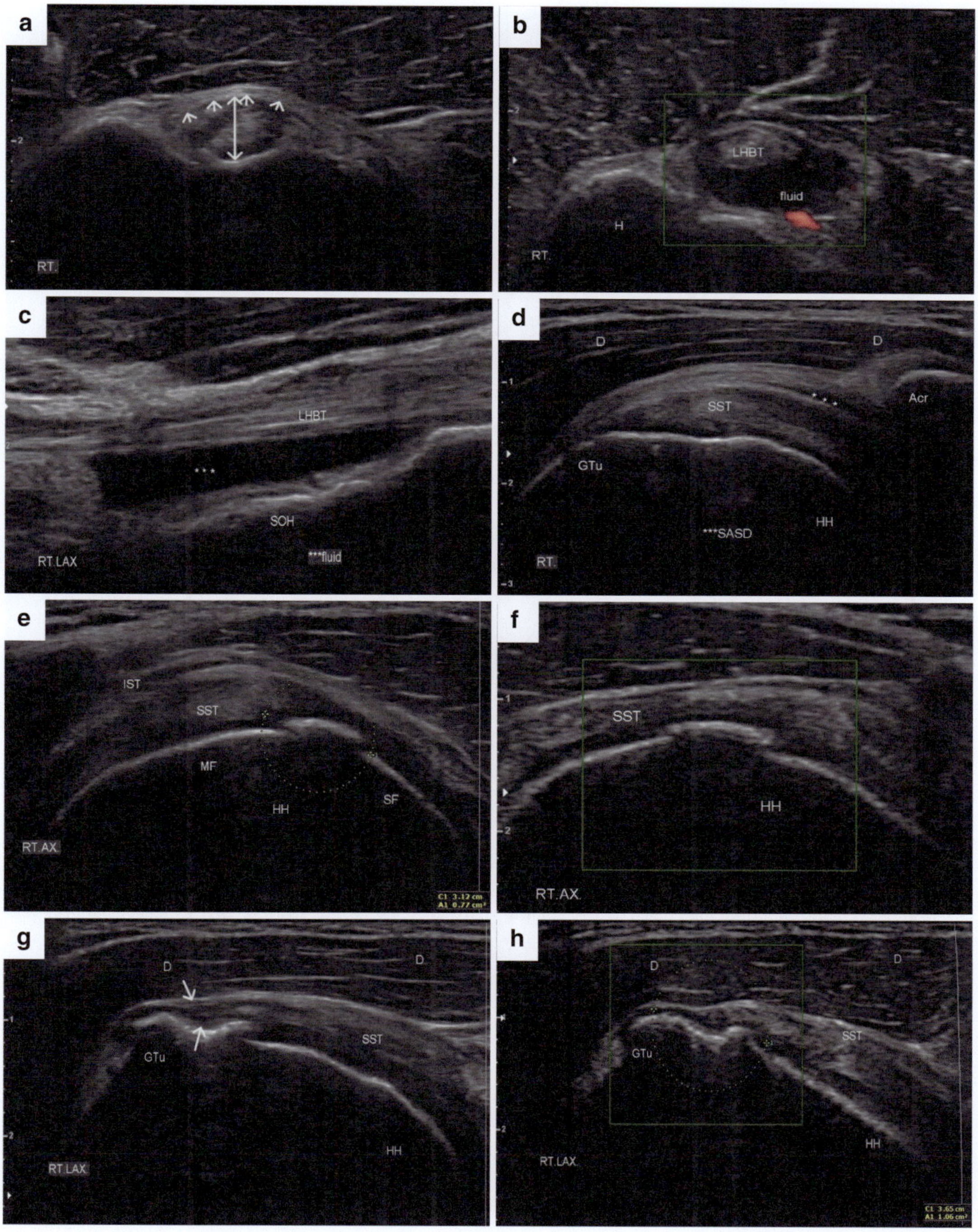

Fig. 7.58 Bicep's tenosynovitis with supraspinatus tendon tear. (**a**, **b**) Short axis scans of the anterior shoulder at the bicipital groove revealed the increased antero-posterior diameter of LHBT with thick and hyperechoic convex overlying THL (arrows). (**c**) Longitudinal scan of the anterior shoulder explored compressible, anechoic fluid accumulation behind the fibrillar LHBT (asterisks). (**d**) Longitudinal scan of the SST revealing an apparent hypoechoic SASD bursa. (**e**, **f**) Short axis scans depicted cortical defects (ellipse) over the HH with SST tear. (**g**, **h**) Longitudinal scans of the SST at the GTu insertion unveiled cortical irregularity (white arrows) and SST full-thickness tear. *AX* short axis, *GTu* greater tuberosity, *H* humerus, *HH* humeral head, *LHBT* long head of biceps tendon, *LAX* long axis, *LTu* lesser tuberosity, *SASD* subacromial subdeltoid, *SST* supraspinatus tendon, *SOH* shaft of humerus

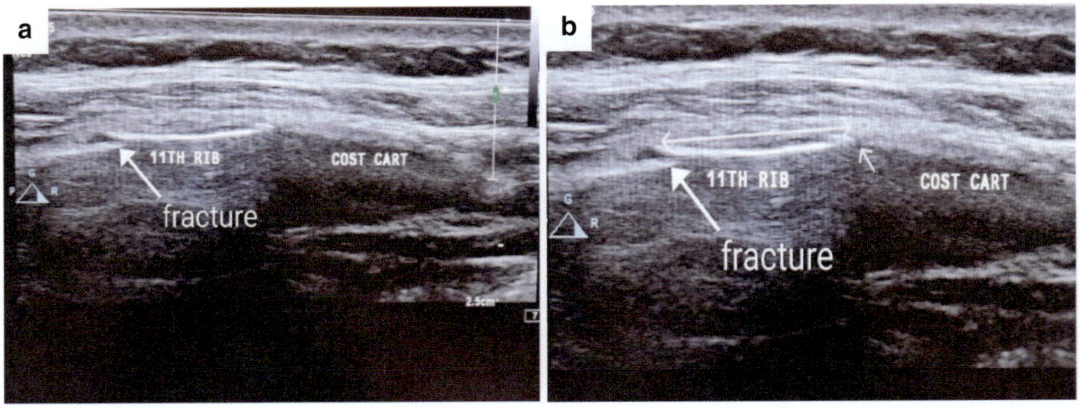

Fig. 7.59 11th rib fracture. (**a**) Longitudinal scan of the rib revealed cortical discontinuity (white arrow). (**b**) Longitudinal scan depicted rib fracture, located 1.44 cm away (double arrow) from the costochondral junction (small arrow). *COST CART* costal cartilage

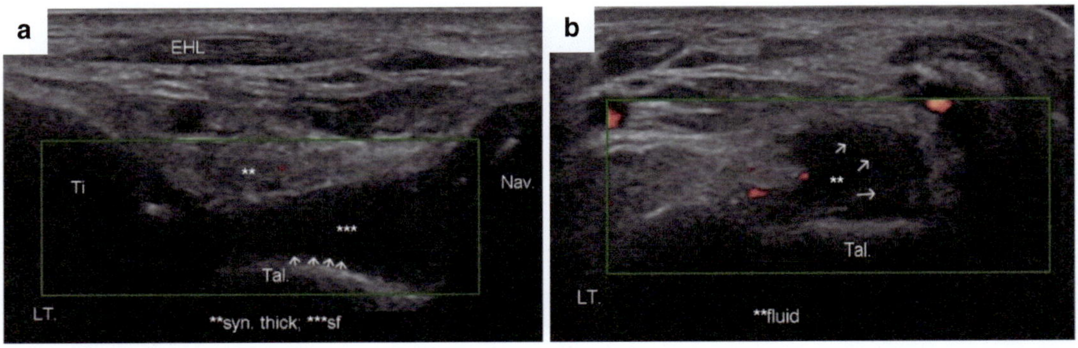

Fig. 7.60 Gouty arthritis. (**a**) Longitudinal scan of the anterior ankle revealed compressible and anechoic collection (asterisks) in the talocrural joint and a double contour sign (arrows) over the talar dome cartilage. (**b**) Short axis scan of the anterior ankle explored anechoic, compressible collection (asterisks) in the joint recess with synovial hypertrophy (white arrows). *EHL* extensor halluces longus, *Tal* talus, *Ti* tibia, *Nav* navicular

her symptoms gradually intensifying over that period. She did not exhibit any other symptoms and had not been previously diagnosed with rheumatoid arthritis. Laboratory evaluations revealed no notable serum inflammatory markers, except for a slight increase in the erythrocyte sedimentation rate on repeated occasions. An ultrasound examination was conducted to further assess her condition.

Ultrasound Findings The synovial membrane was observed to be thickened, exhibiting a heterogeneous appearance that was primarily hyperechoic and characterized by significant Doppler activity. This thickening of the synovial membrane resulted in compression of the prefemoral fat layer. Notably, there were no signs of erosion in the femoral or patellar regions, and the quadriceps tendon remained intact (Fig. 7.61).

Impression Pigmented villonodular synovitis. DD: Synovial sarcoma.

Case Summary 62 A 60-year-old male presented with pain localized to his left heel, which worsened while standing or walking but improved with rest. He reported no recent foot injuries or issues related to his footwear. During the physical examination, significant tenderness was noted at the inferior aspect of the heel,

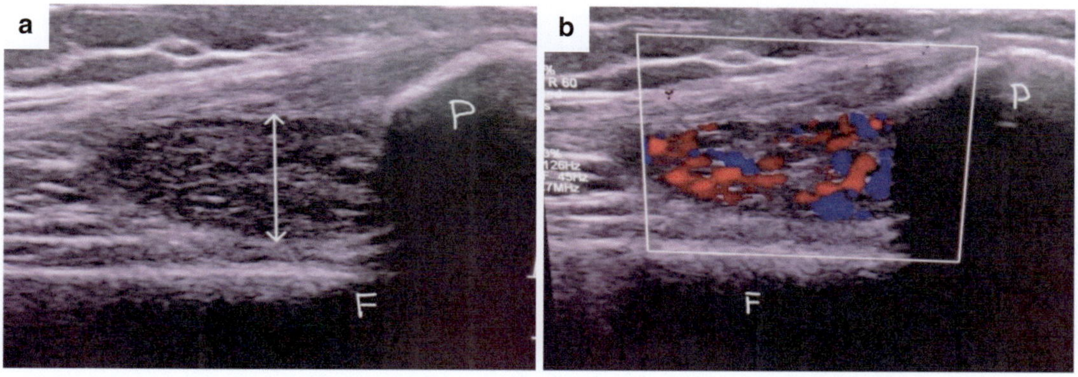

Fig. 7.61 Pigmented villonodular synovitis. (**a**, **b**) Longitudinal scan of the anterior joint recess revealed thick, hypoechoic, and noncompressible synovial membrane (double arrow) (**a**) with increased vascularity (**b**) (color spots). *F* femur, *P* patella

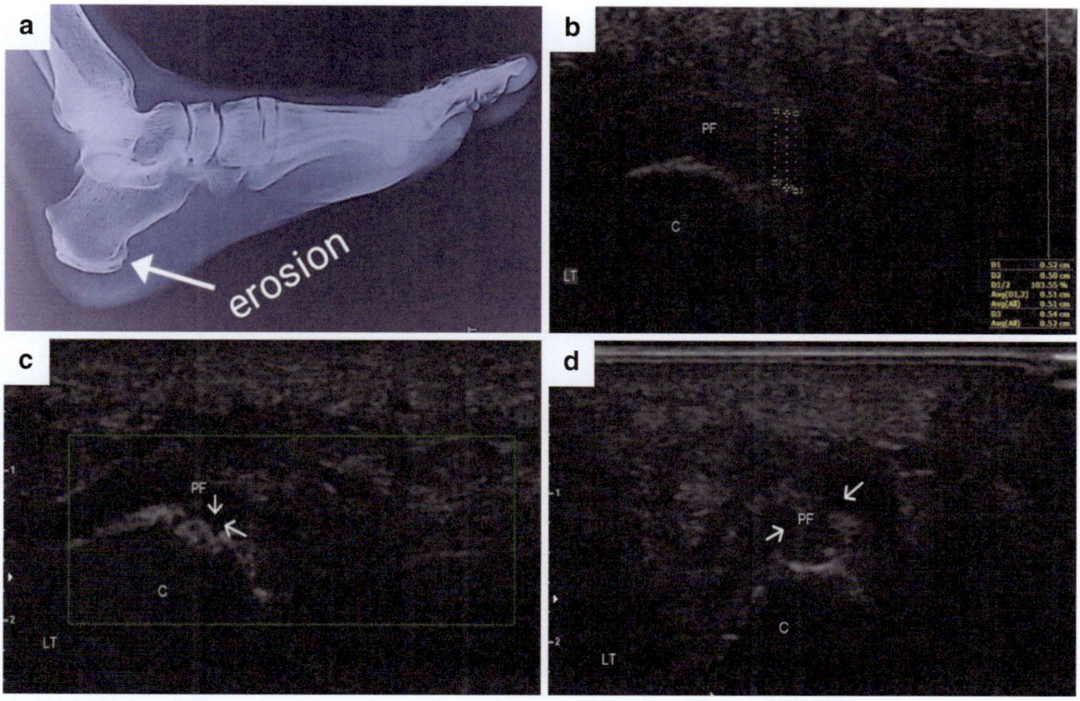

Fig. 7.62 Plantar fascia tear. (**a**) X-ray revealed cortical erosion at the inferior calcaneus. (**b**) Longitudinal scan of the inferior heel revealing the hypoechoic and thick PF. (**c**, **d**) Short axis scans of the inferior heel explored anechoic cleft within the hypoechoic plantar fascia on dynamic assessment (arrows) with cortical irregularity in the inferior calcaneus (arrows) (**c**). *C* calcaneus, *PF* plantar fascia, *RT* right

whereas evaluations for ankle and subtalar joint stability (negative anterior and posterior drawer tests) yielded normal findings. An X-ray revealed a punched-out cortical defect in the inferior calcaneus (Fig. 7.62a), along with adjacent soft tissue swelling. The erythrocyte sedimentation rate and C-reactive protein level were not increased. An ultrasound of the ankle joint was performed.

Ultrasound Findings The right inferior heel, where the plantar fascia (PF) is attached to the calcaneus, exhibited thickening and appeared hypoechoic, with a measured thickness of 5.2 mm (Fig. 7.62b). The anechoic cleft within the PF was demonstrated dynamically (Fig. 7.62c–d). The adjacent calcaneal cortex appeared irregular. There were no reports of increased Doppler activity in the area.

Impression Plantar fascia tear.

Case Summary 63 A young man sustained deep injury to his right elbow two months prior. He has now sought the expertise of an orthopedic surgeon due to weakness in his right hand. Physical examination revealed a wrist drop (Fig. 7.63a) and the inability to make the "OK" sign, known as the *Benediction sign.*

Ultrasound Findings Proximal to the radial tunnel, the radial nerve appeared thick and hypoechoic with loss of the fascicular pattern (Fig. 7.63b). The nerve was torn completely (Fig. 7.63c) just above the elbow crease before it divided into the posterior and anterior interosseous nerves (Fig. 7.63d).

Impression Wrist drop with radial nerve injury.

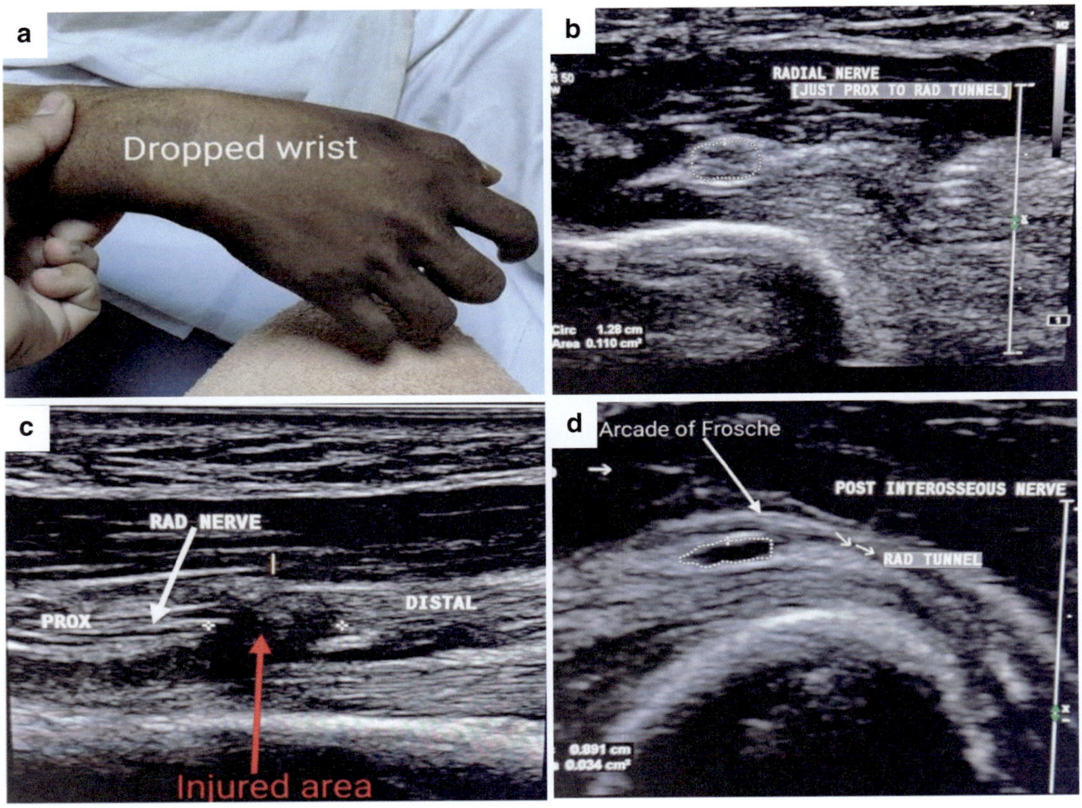

Fig. 7.63 Radial nerve injury with a wrist drop. (**a**) Wrist drop. (**b**, **c**) Short axis scans proximal to the radial tunnel revealed torn, thick, and hypoechoic radial nerve (**c**, red arrow). (**d**) Radial nerve with loss of fascicular pattern depicted at the Arcade of Frohse (large arrow), deep interosseous branch of radial nerve seen (small arrows) in the radial tunnel

Case Summary 64 A 50-year-old male with diabetes presented with intense pain and noticeable skin discoloration on his right thigh, which had developed over the past three to four days, leading to hospitalization. He is also experiencing a low-grade fever and a decrease in appetite. Ultrasound revealed typical findings of necrotizing soft tissue infection.

Ultrasound Findings The subcutaneous tissue exhibited swelling characterized by a cobblestone appearance of the underlying fat (Fig. 7.64a). Additionally, fluid accumulated within the fascia that extended from the inguinal ligament down to the tibia, tracing the course of the sartorius muscle. Within the hypoechoic sartorius muscle, a hyperechoic signal with a ring-down artifact was observed (Fig. 7.64b–d). Increased Doppler activity was also noted in the thick and hypoechoic sartorius muscle (Fig. 7.64d).

Impression Cellulitis with necrotizing fasciitis.

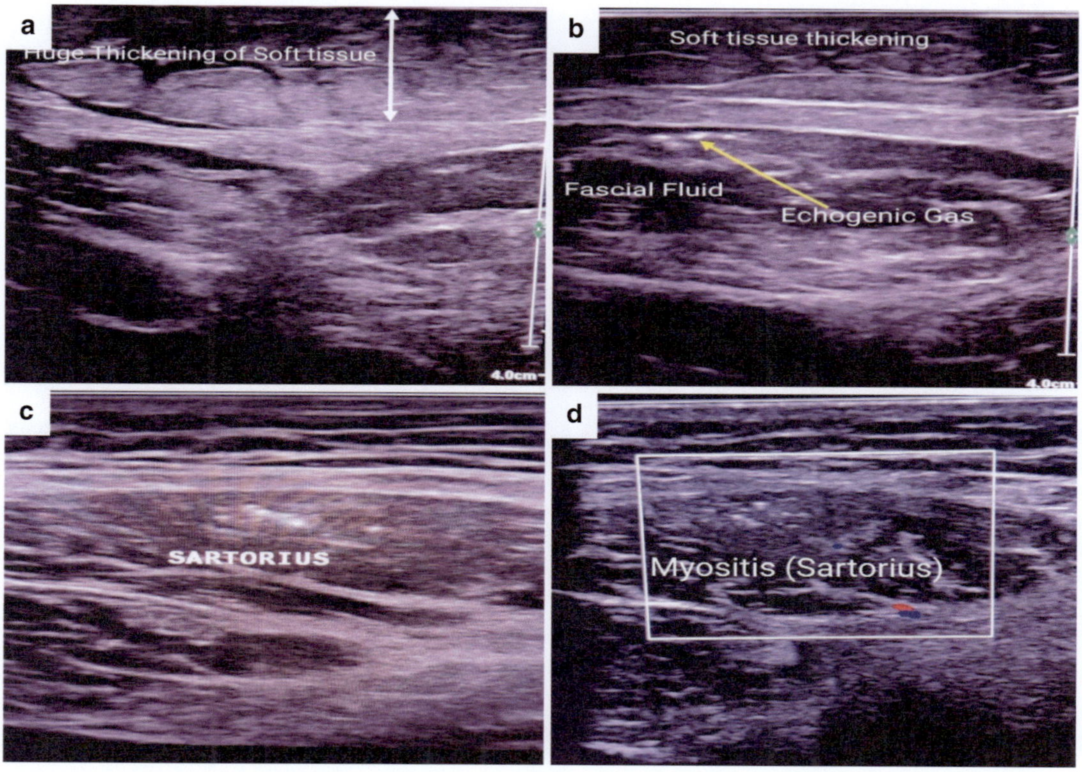

Fig. 7.64 Necrotizing fasciitis. (**a**) Longitudinal scan of the thigh revealed increased thickness of subcutaneous fatty tissue with anechoic fluid between fat lobules lead to cobblestone appearance. (**b–d**) Long axis scan depicted hypoechoic and increased thickness of the sartorius muscle (**b, d**) with hyperechoic gas (**b**, **d**) and ring-down artifacts (**b**, yellow arrow) within

Acknowledgments I would like to express my gratitude to Dr. Mohammad Moin Uddin, a consultant physiatrist at Apollo-Imperial Hospital in Chittagong, Bangladesh, for supplying the clinical data pertaining to cases 25, 41, 48, 54–59, 61, and 63–65. Additionally, I appreciate the contribution of Dr. Omer Mala Ahmed from Sulaimanya-Ranya Teaching Hospital in Iraq, who provided insights into the ulnar nerve epineural cyst case listed in number 47.

Conflict of Interest MAB is supported by a Faculty of Medicine and Health Executive Dean Stipend scholarship, University of Sydney, Australia, for his PhD course.

Suggest Reading

Journals Articles

Bruyn GA, Iagnocco A, Naredo E, Balint PV, Gutierrez M, Hammer HB, et al. OMERACT Ultrasound Working Group. OMERACT Definitions for Ultrasonographic Pathologies and Elementary Lesions of Rheumatic Disorders 15 Years On. J Rheumatol. 2019; 46:1388–1393. https://doi.org/10.3899/jrheum.181095.

Dalili D, Carne A, MacKay J, O'Connor P, Silver D, Robinson P, Mansour R, et al. Musculoskeletal ultrasound imaging standards in the UK: British Society of Skeletal Radiologists (BSSR) position statement, Br J Radiol 2021; 94: 20210198. https://doi.org/10.1259/bjr.20210198.

Costantino F, Carmona L, Boers M, Backhaus M, Balint PV, Bruyn GA, et al. EULAR recommendations for the reporting of ultrasound studies in rheumatic and musculoskeletal diseases (RMDs). Ann Rheum Dis. 2021; 80:840–847. https://doi.org/10.1136/annrheumdis-2020-219816.

Mandl P, D'Agostino MA, Navarro-Compán V, Geßl I, Sakellariou G, Abhishek A, et al. 2023 EULAR recommendations on imaging in diagnosis and management of crystal-induced arthropathies in clinical practice. Ann Rheum Dis. 2024;83:752–759. https://doi.org/10.1136/ard-2023-224771.

Hall MM, Allen, GM, Allison S, Craig J, DeAngelis, JP, Delzell, PB, et al. Recommended Musculoskeletal and Sports Ultrasound Terminology: A Delphi-Based Consensus Statement. J Ultrasound Med. 2022; 41: 2395–2412. https://doi.org/10.1002/jum.15947

Wakefield RJ, Balint PV, Szkudlarek M, Filippucci E, Backhaus M, D'Agostino MA, et al. Musculoskeletal ultrasound including definitions for ultrasonographic pathology. OMERACT 7 Special Interest Group. J Rheumatol 2005; 32: 2485–2487.

Oo WM, Linklater JM, Daniel M, Saarakkala S, Samuels J, Conaghan PG, et al. Clinimetrics of ultrasound pathologies in osteoarthritis: systematic literature review and meta-analysis. Osteoarthritis Cartilage. 2018; 26: 601–611. https://doi.org/10.1016/j.joca.2018.01.021.

Books

Kohler MJ. Musculoskeletal Ultrasound in Rheumatology Review. 2nd Edition. Switzerland. Springer Nature. 2021.

Yinh J, et al. Clinical Atlas of Musculoskeletal Ultrasound in Rheumatology. 1st edition. Springer Cham. 2024.

Web links

OMERACT Outcome Measures in Rheumatology. https://omeract.org/wp-content/uploads/2025/01/OMERACTHandbook-Chapter-3-Nov-1-2018.pdf.

AIUM Musculoskeletal ultrasoun: https://www.aium.org/practice-topics/musculoskeletal-ultrasound (learning and events).

Musculoskeltal Ultrasound Bachelor Class: https://123sonography.com/course/musculoskeletalusbachelorclass.

Social media

Musculoskeletal ultrasound club (https://www.facebook.com/groups/545078935502754/).

Part III

Multiple Choice Questions (MCQs)

Multiple Choice Questions (MCQs) and Answers

8

Md Abu Bakar Siddiq

Questions

1. Which year did OMERACT develop the first ultrasound definitions for rheumatic disease?
   (a) 1992
   (b) 1997
   (c) 2004
   (d) 2019
2. Which one is the OMERACT ultrasound elementary lesion?
   (a) Tenosynovitis.
   (b) Bone erosion.
   (c) Synovial effusion.
   (d) Synovitis.
3. A patient diagnosed with knee osteoarthritis reported the presence of a compressible, anechoic cystic mass located at the back of the knee, as observed through linear ultrasound imaging. *BC*, Baker's cyst; *LT*, left. Could you please specify the sonographic characteristics indicated by the arrows?

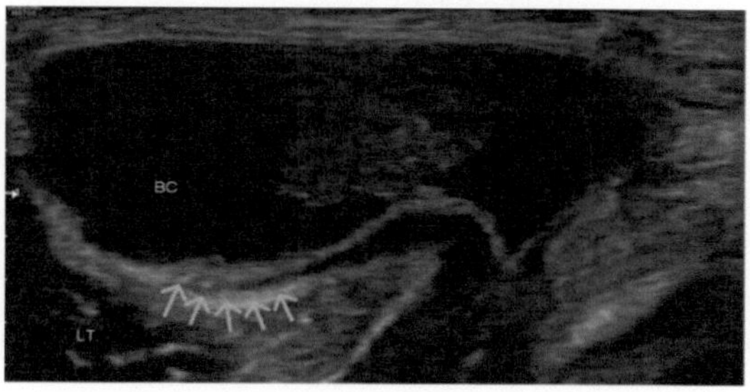

   (a) Posterior acoustic shadowing.
   (b) Posterior acoustic enhancement.
   (c) Reverberation artifacts.
   (d) Hyperechoic lesion in the posterior wall of Baker's cyst.
4. A patient presented with sensations of tingling along the distribution of the right median nerve (MN), accompanied by atrophy of the thenar eminence. The patient had a medical history of diabetes mellitus and hypertension. Tinel's and Phalen's signs yield positive results for MN compression. Clinically, carpal tunnel syndrome (CTS) was diagnosed. What ultrasound measurement of the MN indicates a severe CTS?

M. A. B. Siddiq (✉)
Department of Rheumatology, Royal North Shore Hospital, Northern Clinical School, Faculty of Medicine and Health, The University of Sydney, Sydney, NSW, Australia

Sydney Musculoskeletal Health, The University of Sydney, Sydney, NSW, Australia

Kolling Institute of Medical Research, St Leonards, NSW, Australia

School of Health Sports and Professional Practice (Rheumatology), University of South Wales, Pontypridd, United Kingdom

Department of Physical Medicine and Rehabilitation, Brahmanbaria Medical College, Brahmanbaria, Bangladesh
e-mail: msid8426@uni.sydney.edu.au

M. A. B. Siddiq (ed.), *Musculoskeletal Ultrasound in Rheumatic Diseases*,
https://doi.org/10.1007/978-981-96-5298-3_8

(a) Median nerve cross-sectional area > 15 mm.
(b) Median nerve cross-sectional area > 12 mm.
(c) Median nerve cross-sectional area > 10 mm.
(d) Median nerve cross-sectional area > 17 mm.

5. One patient presented with persistent pain and swelling in the right heel that had lasted for several months. Following a recent change in footwear, he experienced an exacerbation of heel pain during ambulation. Additionally, he experienced significant discomfort during the initial steps upon waking in the morning. Notably, the patient reported no other joint pain. An X-ray examination indicated the presence of a calcaneal spur, prompting further evaluation through ultrasound. Which sonographic characteristics are indicative of Haglund syndrome?
   (a) Retrocalcaneal bursitis, precalcaneal bursitis, and Achilles tendinopathy.
   (b) Retrocalcaneal bursitis, precalcaneal bursitis, and Achilles tendon rupture.
   (c) Achilles tendon rupture, calcaneal spur, and precalcaneal bursitis.
   (d) Retrocalcaneal bursitis, calcaneal spurs, and Achilles tendinopathy.
6. A patient presented with persistent pain and swelling in the right heel, which had been ongoing for several months, accompanied by morning stiffness. He reported that heel pain intensified during ambulation, particularly during the initial steps taken upon waking in the morning. Additionally, he reported a history of chronic spinal pain characterized by morning stiffness lasting approximately 1 hour, along with radiological evidence indicating the presence of syndesmophytes. Which ultrasound findings are consistent with enthesitis?
   (a) Calcaneal spur with increased Doppler activity.
   (b) Hypoechoic thick Achilles tendon with increased Doppler activity.
   (c) Calcaneal erosion with a thick hypoechoic Achilles tendon.
   (d) Hyperechoic thick Achilles tendon with increased Doppler activity.
7. Which one is not the absolute indication of shoulder ultrasound?
   (a) Rotator cuff tear.
   (b) Frozen shoulder syndrome in diabetes mellitus.
   (c) Glenohumeral effusion in rheumatoid arthritis.
   (d) Shoulder pain with a previous history of labral tear.
8. Low-level disinfections include all except?
   (a) Soap.
   (b) Dry heat.
   (c) Hand gloves.
   (d) Enzymatic cleaners.
9. A 30-year-old professional football player has been experiencing persistent pain in the right lateral elbow for several months. Upon examination, tenderness was noted over the lateral epicondyle, and Maudsley's maneuver yielded a positive result. X-ray analysis revealed no significant changes. In the ultrasound image, the arrow indicates which specific pathology?

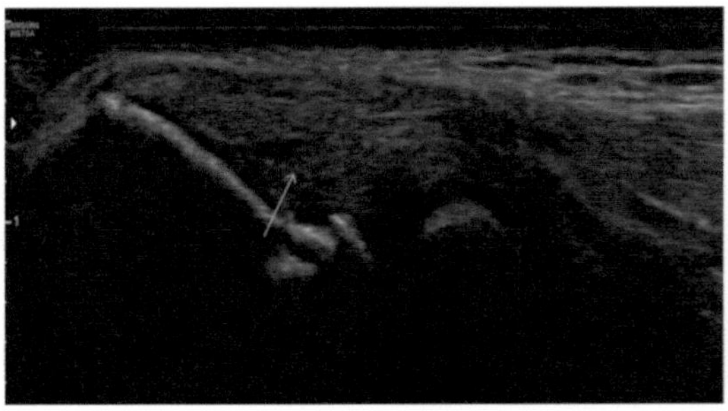

   (a) Hypoechoic and thickened common extensor tendon origin.
   (b) Hyperechoic and thickened common extensor tendon of the wrist.
   (c) Hyperechoic, thick, and fibrillar lateral collateral ligament.
   (d) Hypoechoic and thick lateral collateral ligament of the elbow.

10. A patient diagnosed with knee osteoarthritis presents with symptoms of pain and swelling in the knee. Clinical evaluation revealed a positive sign of joint effusion. Radiographic imaging revealed the presence of osteophytes along the joint line and subchondral sclerosis. Additionally, an ultrasound examination revealed pathological alterations in the anterior recess of the joint (white arrow). What is the underlying pathology?

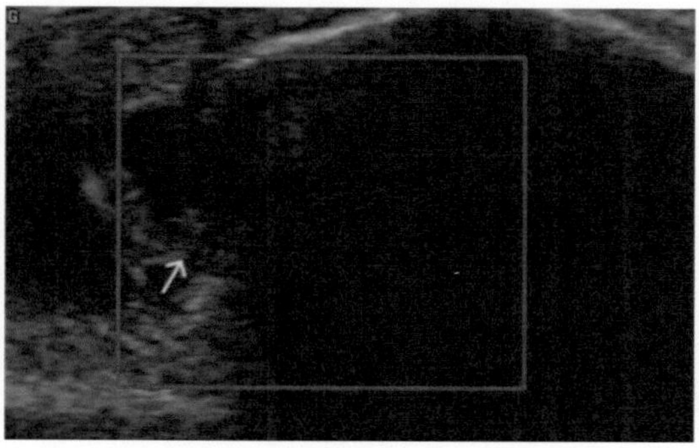

    (a) Loose body.
    (b) Synovial hypertrophy.
    (c) Synovial fluid.
    (d) Prefemoral fat.
11. A patient diagnosed with knee osteoarthritis underwent a linear ultrasound examination, during which the sonographer observed the presence of synovial hypertrophy. Which statement correctly defines synovial hypertrophy?
    (a) Thick and hypoechoic noncompressible synovial membrane with Doppler activity
    (b) Thick and hyperechoic compressible synovial membrane
    (c) Thick and hypoechoic compressible synovial membrane
    (d) Thick and hypoechoic noncompressible synovial membrane
12. Which lateral collateral ligament of the ankle component appears longest?
    (a) Anterior talofibular ligament
    (b) Posterior talofibular ligament
    (c) Calcaneofibular ligament
    (d) The lengths of the calcaneal and anterior talofibular ligaments are equal
13. Which statement is true for ultrasound artifacts?
    (a) Always misinterpret normal findings as pathologies
    (b) Artifacts may have diagnostic value
    (c) Artifacts occur with the grayscale mode only
    (d) An artifact only occurs when a sound reflects with a strong reflector bone
14. Sometimes, differentiating synovial effusion from synovial hypertrophy is difficult. What statement might assist in clarifying this distinction?
    (a) Compared with synovial hypertrophy, synovial effusion is more compressible and anechoic
    (b) Both synovial effusion and synovial hypertrophy are poorly compressible
    (c) Both synovial effusion and synovial hypertrophy are compressible and hyperechoic
    (d) Compared with synovial effusion, synovial hypertrophy is more compressible and displaceable
15. A 70-year-old woman with knee osteoarthritis reported to the physical medicine outpatient door department with sudden, severe, hot, and swollen right knee joints. Intense pain restricts the ability of the physician to examine the affected joint. An X-ray of the knee was performed, revealing the presence of marginal osteophytes, a reduction in joint space width, and changes in radio density associated with the medial meniscus. Which of the following options correctly defines the sonographic features of calcium pyrophosphate dihydrate deposition in the joint?
    (a) Sharp and smooth anechoic medial femoral articular cartilage with reduced thickness
    (b) Reduced articular cartilage thickness with hyperechoic deposits over the cartilage surface
    (c) Reduced articular cartilage thickness with hyperechoic deposits within the articular cartilage
    (d) Thickened synovial membrane with increased Doppler activity

16. A 30-year-old office employee reported experiencing pain in her right ulnar wrist, which primarily occurs during computer typing activities at work and has progressively worsened over the past 6 months. There was no history of recent trauma or any other joint pain or swelling. Upon clinical evaluation, tenderness was noted in the ulnar wrist region, particularly near the styloid process. What potential pathological findings might be observed via ultrasound?
    (a) Extensor carpi ulnaris tendinitis
    (b) Triangular fibrocartilage complex tear
    (c) Ulnar styloid process fracture
    (d) Pisiform bone avascular necrosis
17. A 30-year-old postpartum woman complained of right thumb base pain, which gradually progressed over the last 14 days, with more pain while her baby was lifted during breastfeeding. Upon clinical evaluation, there was notable localized swelling and tenderness at the base of the thumb, accompanied by a positive result on the Finkelstein test. Which anatomical structure could be involved in the pathology?
    (a) Adductor pollicis longus and extensor pollicis brevis tendons
    (b) Abductor pollicis longus and extensor pollicis brevis tendons
    (c) Abductor pollicis longus and extensor pollicis longus tendons
    (d) Extensor carpi radialis longus and abductor pollicis longus tendons
18. Which ultrasound feature has been introduced in the latest version of the OMERACT ultrasound?
    (a) Synovial effusion.
    (b) Tenosynovitis.
    (c) Bone erosion.
    (d) Synovitis grading.
19. To define increased vascularity in synovial tissue, which ultrasound feature is the most accurate?
    (a) Increased power Doppler activity.
    (b) Increased synovial thickness.
    (c) Increased synovial effusion.
    (d) Increased color Doppler activity.
20. One patient presented with complaints of right shoulder pain accompanied by restricted joint mobility persisting for the past 3 months. Notably, there was no joint line tenderness. The external rotation of the shoulder was painful and restricted, characterized by a snapping sensation during both internal and external rotation movements. The patient reported no issues with other joints. An ultrasound examination of the affected shoulder could identify specific pathological changes. An ultrasound of the respective shoulder could reveal which pathological change.
    (a) Subscapularis tendinitis
    (b) Subcoracoid bursal wall thick and hypoechoic
    (c) Subacromial-subdeltoid bursitis
    (d) Subacromial-subdeltoid bursal thickening
21. A 45-year-old male professional tennis player presented with a complaint of vague pain and weakness in the right posterior shoulder region. Upon examination, atrophy was noted in the infraspinatus area of the affected shoulder compared with the contralateral side, whereas the supraspinatus region appeared normal. The patient's medical history included shoulder dislocation that had been managed conservatively. He reported no difficulties with shoulder abduction, adduction, or rotation. Further examination via ultrasound could explore which pathology is involved.
    (a) Ganglion cyst at the supraspinatus foramen
    (b) Para-labral cyst at the spino-glenoid notch
    (c) Glenohumeral effusion
    (d) Infraspinatus tendon tear with fatty infiltration
22. When an area for nerve pathology at the carpal tunnel is scanned dynamically, which following statement helps in discriminating between nerves and tendons?
    (a) Tendons and nerves are both fibrillar and dynamically, they never move faster than tendons do

(b) The tendon is fascicular, the nerve is fibrillar, and later, it moves faster than the tendon
(c) The tendon is fibrillar, the nerve is fascicular, and the tendon moves slower than the nerve
(d) The tendon is fibrillar, the nerve is fascicular, and the tendon moves faster than the nerve

23. Which position is best for scanning the olecranon fossa?
(a) Elbow extension in the prone position
(b) Elbow flexion with the wrist extended
(c) Elbow flexion, shoulder extension, and wrist extension
(d) Elbow flexion, shoulder flexion, and forearm pronation

24. A 39-year-old agricultural worker presented with a complaint of right shoulder pain that had persisted for 5 days. Prior to this incident, he reported being in good health without any notable medical issues. In addition to shoulder pain, the patient experienced difficulty in both initiating and sustaining shoulder abduction. An X-ray examination was conducted, which yielded normal results. Further scanning via ultrasound revealed pathological changes that favored a complete tear of the rotator cuff. Select the correct response.
(a) On the longitudinal axis, there was an anechoic split in the supraspinatus tendon
(b) On the longitudinal axis, an anechoic split involving the whole width and depth of the supraspinatus tendon
(c) On the longitudinal axis, there was an anechoic split separating the supraspinatus tendon completely into two segments
(d) On the longitudinal axis, there was an anechoic split in the bursal supraspinatus tendon with subacromial bursal collection

25. Which statement is correct regarding ultrasound echogenicity?
(a) Skin and subcutaneous tissue is isoechoic
(b) Muscle is fibrillar and hyperechoic
(c) The nerve is fibrillar and hyperechoic
(d) Tendon fibrils and hyperechoic

26. A 40-year-old male patient arrived at the outpatient department of physical medicine and rheumatology and reported an abrupt onset of intense pain and swelling in his great toe. During the examination, the patient instinctively retracted the affected toe, making it challenging for the attending physician to conduct a thorough assessment. An X-ray examination indicated soft tissue swelling. Further ultrasound assessment revealed which following change indicating monosodium urate crystal deposition.
(a) Hyperechoic double contour sign in the synovial membrane
(b) Hyperechoic double contour sign over the cartilage surface
(c) Hyperechoic deposits within the articular cartilage
(d) Hyperechoic double contour sign within the articular cartilage

27. A 39-year-old female presented with a primary complaint of persistent pain in the left knee joint. She did not exhibit any additional joint pain, swelling, or deformities, and there was an absence of morning stiffness. The radiographic examination did not indicate any notable changes. Furthermore, serum biochemical analysis revealed no evidence of inflammatory biomarkers. An ultrasound examination revealed a thickened and branched synovial membrane, indicated by white arrows, along with increased Doppler activity. *Ax* axial scan, *SF* synovial fluid. What might be the potential pathology?

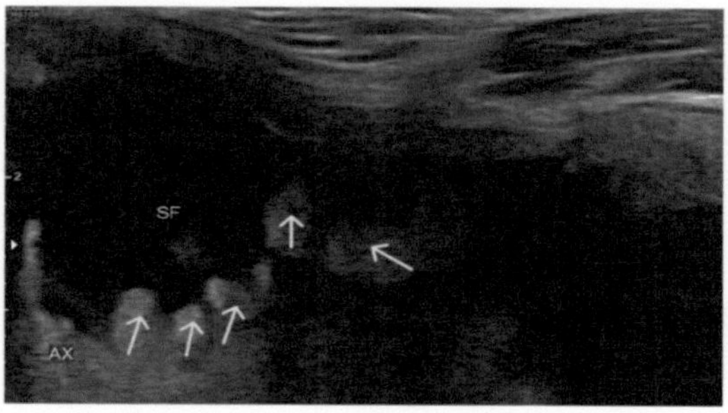

(a) Pigmented villonodular synovitis
(b) Hemangioma
(c) Synovial sarcoma
(d) Lipoma arborescence

28. A patient presented with discomfort characterized by pain and tingling sensations localized to the dorsal aspect of the wrist and the right thumb. Notably, swelling in the first extensor compartment of the wrist was observed. The combination of pain and tingling results in restricted motion of the thumb, significantly affecting the patient's ability to perform daily tasks. The patient did not report any neck pain, and a thorough examination of the nervous system yielded normal results. An ultrasound assessment of the first extensor compartment indicated the presence of thickened and hypoechoic tendons, accompanied by a loss of the normal fibrillar structure. Intralesional steroid injection alleviated the pain and swelling; however, the tingling sensation persisted. What could be the underlying cause of this condition?
    (a) Accessory muscle in the first compartment of the dorsal wrist
    (b) Coexistence of carpal tunnel syndrome
    (c) Coexistence of cervical radiculopathy
    (d) Wartenburg's syndrome
29. Which one is true for the OMERACT ultrasound feature for osteoarthritis diagnosis?
    (a) Measuring cartilage echogenicity and thickness changes.
    (b) Detection of increased synovitis.
    (c) Assessment of subchondral bone erosion.
    (d) Measuring secondary enthesitis.
30. Which one is the inflammatory elementary lesion of OMERACT ultrasound?
    (a) Synovitis.
    (b) Achilles tendinitis.
    (c) Pediatric synovitis.
    (d) Tenosynovitis.
31. Three months prior, a woman delivered a male infant and has since experienced discomfort characterized by pain and tingling sensations on the volar side of her hand, particularly affecting the three-and-a-half radial fingers, with symptoms worsening during breastfeeding. This clinical presentation raised the suspicion of carpal tunnel syndrome. Owing to the unavailability of nerve conduction study facilities at the medical center, an ultrasound examination of the volar wrist was performed. *FTs*, wrist flexor tendons; *LT*, left; *UV*, ulnar vessels. What observations can be made regarding the ultrasound features depicted in the provided image (dotted area)?

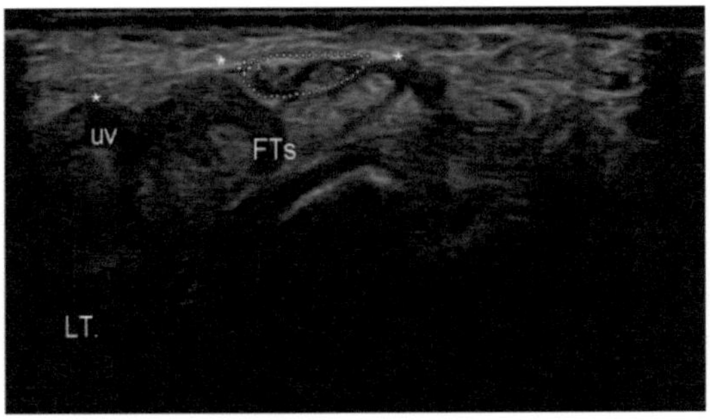

    (a) Median nerve trifurcation
    (b) Median nerve bifurcation with persistent median artery
    (c) Median nerve bifurcation with increased cross-sectional area
    (d) Ganglion cyst compressing the median nerve
32. A patient presented with complaints of pain localized to the lateral aspect of the knee, accompanied by tingling sensations in the same region that extended to the outer leg. Clinical examination revealed swelling of the knee joint, restricted range of motion, and tenderness along the medial joint line. To investigate potential intra-articular pathologies, particularly within the lateral compartment of the knee, ultrasound is recommended. The imaging results indicated the presence of an anechoic mass along the lateral joint line of the knee. What might this mass represent?
    (a) Compressible lateral meniscal cysts
    (b) Noncompressible anechoic meniscal cysts
    (c) Compressible meniscal cysts with increased Doppler activity
    (d) Noncompressible meniscal cysts with increased Doppler activity

33. A 67-year-old woman presented with complaints of pain in the right wrist that had persisted for several days. There was no recent history of trauma, falls, or any known inflammatory arthritis. However, the patient had been experiencing knee osteoarthritis for the past 5 years. An X-ray of the wrist was performed, which revealed a radioopacity located on the ulnar side of the wrist joint. An ultrasound was subsequently recommended, which identified a hyperechoic deposit in the meniscal analog in the same region. What potential pathology could be indicated by these findings?
    (a) Monosodium urate deposit
    (b) Calcium pyrophosphate dihydrate crystal deposits
    (c) Basic calcium deposits
    (d) Cortical erosion of the ulnar styloid process
34. Which principle is not encompassed by the ALARA (As Low As Reasonably Achievable) guidelines in ultrasound?
    (a) Ensuring that the appropriate examination presets are applied
    (b) Set the recommended limits of the mechanical index and thermal index
    (c) Minimizing the exposure time to sensitive structures to reduce side effects
    (d) Maximize the overall scanning time to gather more diagnostic information
35. High-level disinfections include all except?
    (a) Steam under pressure
    (b) Dry heat
    (c) Liquid chemical additives
    (d) Hand gloves and medical dressing
36. Which one is considered most advanced ultrasound imaging method for low-flow synovial vascularity?
    (a) Contrast-enhanced ultrasound Doppler activity
    (b) Shear wave elastography
    (c) Superb microvascular imaging
    (d) Power Doppler
37. A 33-year-old physician presented with a complaint of pain in the right heel. The discomfort is described as mild rather than severe, yet it has been particularly bothersome during the initial steps taken upon waking in the morning. There are no additional complaints of joint pain or swelling, nor is there any indication of low back pain accompanied by morning stiffness lasting over an hour. Upon clinical examination, tenderness was noted in the inferior aspect of the heel. An X-ray was performed, revealing no significant bony abnormalities. An ultrasound of the inferior heel was recommended for further evaluation. Which characteristic is indicative of plantar fasciitis?
    (a) Plantar fascia appears thick and hypoechoic
    (b) The plantar fascia appears thin, remains fibrillar, and hyperechoic
    (c) The plantar fascia appears thick, with anechoic cleft extending from the surface to the bone
    (d) Plantar fascia appears thick with increased Doppler signals
38. A 33-year-old physician presented with a complaint of pain in the right heel. An ultrasound examination of the inferior aspect of the heel demonstrated sonographic characteristics consistent with plantar fasciitis. What is the threshold value for ultrasound thickness that is utilized in the diagnosis of plantar fasciitis?
    (a) Plantar fascia thickness > 4 cm
    (b) Plantar fascia width > 4 mm
    (c) Plantar fascia thickness > 4 mm
    (d) Plantar fascia width > 4 cm
39. A patient presented with persistent pain in the anterior region of the knee and was referred for an ultrasound assessment. What is the most commonly utilized position for imaging the knee in this context?
    (a) Patients lying supine with knee flexion >50°
    (b) Patients lying supine with knee flexion <20°
    (c) Patients lying supine with their knees fully extended
    (d) Patients lying supine with knee flexion ranging from 20–30°
40. A 69-year-old man who presented with a gradual onset of pain in the right hip accom-

panied by brief morning stiffness and restricted range of motion in the joint was referred for an ultrasound examination of the affected area. Upon clinical evaluation, the hip exhibited a limited range of motion. What ultrasound characteristic indicate the presence of significant synovial effusion?
   (a) Anterior recess synovial effusion depth 3–5 mm
   (b) Anterior recess synovial effusion depth > 5 mm
   (c) Anterior recess synovial effusion depth > 15 mm
   (d) Anterior recess synovial effusion depth > 10 mm

41. A 23-year-old male from Bangladesh complained of low back pain accompanied by morning stiffness lasting over 1 h. Upon examination, there was a restriction in the range of motion of the hip, and both Patrick's and Gaenslen's tests yielded positive results. An ultrasound assessment of the hip joint revealed a thickened anterior joint recess, with an average thickness of 6.8 mm, and no compressible fluid collection was observed within the joint recess. What is the cutoff value for synovial hypertrophy in hip synovitis?
   (a) More than 5 mm
   (b) 2–4 cm
   (c) 2–4 mm
   (d) More than 5 cm
42. A 30-year-old professional hockey player presented with persistent dull pain on the right lateral aspect of the ankle, which followed a prior ankle sprain. Upon examination, swelling was noted in the anterolateral region of the ankle, accompanied by significant localized tenderness just anterior to the lateral malleolus. A clinical diagnosis of a lateral ankle sprain was made. Subsequent evaluation through ultrasound is warranted to identify the specific pathology associated with severe ankle sprain. What might the underlying pathology be?
   (a) Fibrillary anterior talofibular ligament with mild collection in the joint recess
   (b) Anterior talofibular ligament thick and hypoechoic with mild fluid in the joint recess
   (c) Both the anterior talofibular ligament and calcaneofibular ligament are torn
   (d) Only the calcaneofibular ligament is thick and hypoechoic
43. Which of the following statement favors posterior acoustic enhancement artifacts?
   (a) Happens when attenuation of the ultrasound signal passes through a cystic structure
   (b) Happened due to improper focal zone adjustment
   (c) Happens when the speed of sound waves at tissue interfaces varies
   (d) When sound passes through a calcified structure
44. In history, the first successful application of diagnostic musculoskeletal ultrasound has been in which condition?
   (a) Septic arthritis
   (b) Osteoarthritis
   (c) Rheumatoid hand
   (d) Baker's cyst
45. Which transducer manipulation technique has been correctly defined?
   (a) Compression—the transducer is moved across the body surface in any direction
   (b) The tilt transducer is moved along a fixed point in the long axis, changing the angle of insonation away from 90° to the skin surface while maintaining contact with the skin
   (c) The tilt transducer is moved along a fixed point in the short axis, changing the angle of insonation away from 90° to the skin surface while maintaining contact with the skin)
   (d) The sliding force on the transducer is applied toward the patient's body

46. Hyperechoic loose body (LB) seen in Baker's cyst (BC) with an area of darkness (white arrows). What could be the appropriate name for this ultrasound effect? *RT* right knee back.

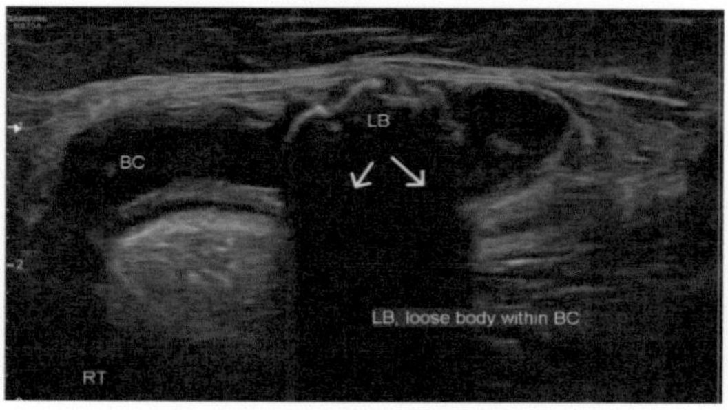

(a) Posterior acoustic enhancement
(b) Posterior acoustic shadowing
(c) Lateral acoustic shadowing
(d) Reverberation artifacts

47. A 65-year-old Bangladeshi presented with a painful and swollen great toe accompanied by hyperuricemia. An ultrasound examination of the toe was performed. *MTH*, metatarsal head; *PP*, proximal phalanx. Which ultrasound features support gout diagnosis?

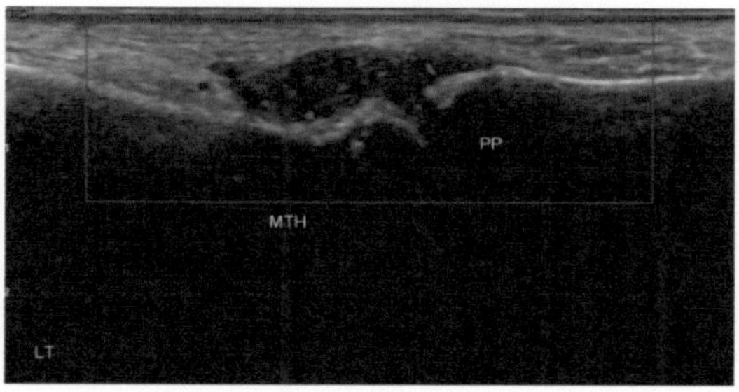

(a) Thickened, hypoechoic synovium
(b) Thickened, hypoechoic synovium with increased color Doppler activity
(c) Thickened, hypoechoic synovium with hyperechoic Doppler spots and power Doppler activity
(d) Hyperechoic synovium with cortical erosion

48. A 49-year-old male presented with complaints of pain and swelling in the posterior heel, which significantly affected his physical activity and overall performance. He reported no other joint pain or swelling. Radiographic imaging indicated the presence of a calcaneal spur. Subsequent ultrasound examination revealed specific features that supported Haglund's syndrome diagnosis. Which following statement correctly defines ultrasound Hugland syndrome? Single arrow, retrocalcaneal bursa; straight line, Achilles tendon; and double arrows, calcaneal spur.

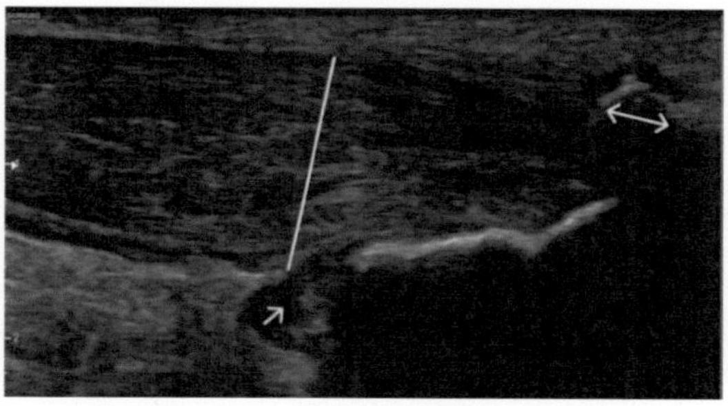

(a) Thickened, hypoechoic Achilles tendon, calcaneal spur, and retro-calcaneal collection
(b) Thickened, hyperechoic Achilles tendon, calcaneal spur, and retro-calcaneal collection
(c) Thickened, hypoechoic fibrillary Achilles tendon, calcaneal spur, and retro-calcaneal collection
(d) Thickened, hyperechoic Achilles tendon, calcaneal spur, and retro-calcaneal collection

49. Which of the following statement is correct about the body of the final ultrasound report except?
(a) Description of diagnostic features should be mentioned
(b) Mention of any contrast during ultrasound examination

(c) Correct mention of abnormal anatomic measurements if present
(d) Mention of ultrasound indication in the report

50. Which of the following statement correctly addresses advanced ultrasound imaging?
(a) Superb microvascular imaging has a lower resolution than power Doppler
(b) Contrast-enhanced ultrasound is useless for monitoring treatment efficacy
(c) Elastography effectively measures soft tissue elastic properties
(d) Elastography is useful for cortical erosion in rheumatoid arthritis patients

Answers: 1. c, 2. c, 3. b, 4. a, 5. d, 6. c, 7. b, 8. b, 9. d, 10. b, 11. a, 12. c, 13. b, 14. a, 15. c, 16. a, 17. b, 18. d, 19. a, 20. b, 21. b, 22. d, 23. c, 24. c, 25. d, 26. b, 27. d, 28. d, 29. a, 30. b, 31. c, 32. b, 33. b, 34. d, 35. d, 36. c, 37. a, 38. c, 39. d, 40. b, 41. a, 42. c, 43. a, 44. d, 45. c, 46. b, 47. c, 48. a, 49. d, 50. c.

MIX
Papier aus verantwortungsvollen Quellen
Paper from responsible sources
FSC® C105338
FSC
www.fsc.org

If you have any concerns about our products,
you can contact us on
ProductSafety@springernature.com

In case Publisher is established outside the EU,
the EU authorized representative is:
Springer Nature Customer Service Center GmbH
Europaplatz 3, 69115 Heidelberg, Germany

Printed by Libri Plureos GmbH
in Hamburg, Germany